Feelings of being
Phenomenology, psychiatry and the sense of reality

Matthew Ratcliffe
Reader in Philosophy,
Durham University, UK

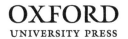
OXFORD
UNIVERSITY PRESS

OXFORD
UNIVERSITY PRESS

Great Clarendon Street, Oxford OX2 6DP

Oxford University Press is a department of the University of Oxford.
It furthers the University's objective of excellence in research, scholarship,
and education by publishing worldwide in

Oxford New York

Auckland Cape Town Dar es Salaam Hong Kong Karachi
Kuala Lumpur Madrid Melbourne Mexico City Nairobi
New Delhi Shanghai Taipei Toronto

With offices in

Argentina Austria Brazil Chile Czech Republic France Greece
Guatemala Hungary Italy Japan Poland Portugal Singapore
South Korea Switzerland Thailand Turkey Ukraine Vietnam

Oxford is a registered trade mark of Oxford University Press
in the UK and in certain other countries

Published in the United States
by Oxford University Press Inc., New York

© Oxford University Press, 2008

The moral rights of the author have been asserted
Database right Oxford University Press (maker)

First published 2008

British Library Cataloguing in Publication Data

Data available

Library of Congress Cataloging in Publication Data

Ratcliffe, Matthew, 1973-
 Feelings of being: phenomenology, psychiatry, and the sense of reality / Matthew Ratcliffe.
  p. ; cm. – (International perspectives in philosophy and psychiatry)
 Includes bibliographical references.
 ISBN 978-0-19-920646-9 (alk paper)
 1. Emotions. 2. Existential phenomenology. 3. Mental illness. I. Title. II. Series.
 [DNLM: 1. Emotions. 2. Existentialism. 3. Psychophysiology. BF 531 R233f 2008]
 BF511.R338 2008
 152.4–dc22   2008011166

Typeset by Cepha Imaging Pvt. Ltd., Bangalore, India
Printed in Great Britain
on acid-free paper by
Biddles Ltd., King's Lynn, Norfolk.

ISBN 978-0-19-920646-9

10 9 8 7 6 5 4 3 2 1

For Beth, with whom I feel at home in the world.

International Perspectives in Philosophy and Psychiatry

Series editors: Bill (K.W.M.) Fulford, Katherine Morris, John Z Sadler, Giovanni Stanghellini

Volumes in the series:

Forthcoming volumes in the series:

Acknowledgements

I am very grateful to a number of people for discussion and advice, including Steve Burwood, Giovanna Colombetti, Shaun Gallagher, Brian Garvey, Richard Gray, Paul Gilbert, Brady Heiner, Peter Hobson, Daniel Hutto, Martin Kusch, Kathleen Lennon, Richard Menary, Francis O'Sullivan, Darrell Rowbottom, Mark Rowlands, Maxine Sheets-Johnstone, Jan Slaby, Beata Stawarska, Achim Stephan, Tim Thornton, several colleagues and postgraduate students at Durham University and three anonymous referees. Special thanks to Bill Fulford for his encouragement and advice in relation to the initial proposal for this book, to Matthew Broome, Rachel Cooper, Peter Goldie, Simon James and Louis Sass for reading substantial chunks of an earlier version and offering very helpful suggestions, and to Amanda Taylor for reading the whole penultimate draft and making lots of insightful remarks. I would also like to thank my wife, Beth, for our many conversations about existential feeling, for bringing to my attention several descriptions of existential feeling in literature, for pointing out that everyday conversations don't refer to existential feelings quite as often as I think they do, and for reading and commenting on the entire manuscript.

Material from this book was presented to seminar audiences at the Universities of Cardiff, Durham, Lancaster and Surrey and at the National University of Ireland, Galway. I also presented related papers at conferences hosted by the Institute of Psychiatry in London and the Universities of Bonn, Cardiff, Hull, Osnabrück and Torun. I would like to thank all these audiences for their illuminating comments, criticisms and suggestions. I am particularly grateful to all those who attended the July 2007 meeting of the International Society for Phenomenological Studies at Asilomar in California, where, over five days, I received a great deal of insightful and encouraging feedback. I would also like to thank the British Academy for funding my attendance of this event.

Contents

Part II **Varieties of existential feeling in psychiatric illness**

Part III **Existential feeling and philosophical thought**

Introduction

The neglect of existential feeling

In recent years, there has been a resurgence of interdisciplinary interest in emotion. Amongst other issues, recent discussions have addressed the nature and role of emotion, the relationship between emotion and expression, the cultural variability of emotion, the narrative structure of emotion and how emotions differ from other kinds of mental state, such as moods and feelings.[1] A question central to current philosophical and scientific work on the topic is that of how emotions relate to bodily feelings. The latter, it is usually assumed, are experiences of bodily states and are, therefore, distinct from experiences of things outside of the body. In contrast, most emotions are intentional states that do not have the body as their primary object. Someone might be happy *about* an event, jealous *of* a person or afraid *of* a vicious, fast-approaching animal. In all these cases, the object of the emotion is not the body but something external to it. Thus, if bodily feeling is integral to emotion, it would seem that it is distinct from the world-directed aspect of emotion. Yet this is at odds with the nagging intuition that the feeling dimension of emotion is bound up with the world-directed intentionality of emotion. In the case of fear, for example, the *feeling* of fear permeates and shapes the experience of its object; it does not seem to be a bodily state that merely accompanies experience of an object external to the body.

In this book, I offer a phenomenological account of bodily feelings, which shows how they can be both *feelings of bodily states* and at the same time *ways of experiencing things outside of the body*. World-experience is not distinct from how one's body feels; the two are utterly inextricable. The experiential entanglement of body and world is more phenomenologically primitive than experience of either in isolation from the other. Even in cases where *either* the body *or* some other part of the world appears to be the sole content of an experience, that experience retains an underlying structure where body and world are inseparable—to experience one is to experience the other. This unity is obscured by a tendency in philosophy and other disciplines to interpret

---

[1] See the essays in Solomon ed. (2004) for a good survey of issues that are addressed by recent philosophical and interdisciplinary emotion research.

experience dualistically, as experience of bodily states on the one hand and experience of everything else on the other.

Most discussion of bodily feeling has focused specifically upon *emotional feelings*, the central question being that of how these feelings are associated with or integrated into emotions. In conjunction with this, there is a tendency to limit enquiry to fairly standard lists of emotions, which include anger, fear, joy, guilt, jealousy, envy, pride and so on. There is much debate concerning whether these various emotions together comprise a unitary or 'natural' kind of mental state and whether some are basic and others compound emotions.[2] However, although there are many different views regarding such issues, the lists of emotions that are offered up for discussion remain fairly consistent in their contents.

This book is specifically about feelings, rather than emotions. The emphasis on emotional feeling has, I think, led to the neglect of other kinds of feeling, which have so far resisted tidy classification and are not always constituents of or accompaniments to standard emotions. Amongst them are a distinctive phenomenological category of feelings that I call 'existential feelings'. These will be the focus of my discussion.

Existential feelings are central to the structure of all human experience. In addition, changes in existential feeling have an important part to play in many kinds of psychiatric illness. The nature and role of existential feeling in psychiatric illness and in everyday life has been obscured by an emphasis on certain familiar emotions and also by a tendency to misinterpret the structure of bodily feeling, stemming from the mistaken assumption that all feelings conform to a distinction between experience of 'internal' bodily states and experience of things 'external' to the body. Existential feelings are both 'feelings of the body' and 'ways of finding oneself in a world'. By a 'way of finding oneself in the world', I mean a sense of the reality of self and of world, which is inextricable from a changeable *feeling* of relatedness between body and world.

Hence existential feelings comprise a distinctive phenomenological category in virtue of two characteristics:

1 They are not directed at specific objects or situations but are background orientations through which experience as a whole is structured.

2 They are *feelings*, in the sense that they are bodily states of which we have at least some awareness.

Although they seldom feature in recent discussions of emotion, existential feelings are frequently alluded to in everyday discourse. People talk of situations

----

[2] See, for example, Griffiths (1997) for a discussion of basic emotions and for the view that 'emotion' is not a natural kind.

not feeling real and of things feeling surreal, strangely unfamiliar, uncanny, not quite right or too real. Associated with such talk are references to changed relations between self and world. The world can seem close or distant and our relationship with it can involve a general sense of belonging or estrangement. It will become apparent as the discussion progresses that the vocabulary used to describe these feelings is quite extensive. However, it is usually metaphorical or vague. There is no accepted taxonomy of existential feelings, their very nature makes them difficult to describe and they cannot be conveyed in terms of certain distinctions that have become entrenched both in academic and everyday life. I will suggest that some of the phenomena ordinarily referred to as 'emotions' and 'moods' fall into the category of 'existential feelings' but that most do not.

The role of existential feeling is perhaps most readily apparent when we consider those occasions where the sense of reality is diminished, fragmented or otherwise changed. We can do this by reflecting on some of our own experiences and on the descriptions offered by others. In psychiatry, there are frequent references to a range of such changes, associated with schizophrenia and other conditions. Reports by patients and clinicians often refer to a diminished or altered sense of reality, and to the self, the world and the relationship between them being somehow different. Such profound alterations in the structure of experience are usually associated with anomalous feelings. Indeed, these feelings often seem to be inseparable from distortions and diminutions of a sense of reality and of belonging to a world.

My primary aim here is to offer a phenomenological account of the structure of existential feeling in psychiatric illness and in everyday life, which shows how something can be a bodily feeling and also an existential orientation, a sense of the reality of the world and of one's being situated within it. In so doing, I will also distinguish some of the varieties of existential feeling.

One of the reasons why existential feelings are so difficult to describe is that the reality of the world and the sense of belonging to it are seldom explicitly reflected upon. We might debate over whether some entity is actually present or not, whether that particular entity or entities of its kind even exist, and whether we have sufficient warrant for believing in the existence of something. But no such metaphysical or epistemological discourse casts the sense of reality itself into doubt or even makes it explicit. We take reality and belonging for granted when we experience and think about things, even when engaged in most forms of philosophical enquiry.

Of course, plenty of philosophers have raised sceptical concerns regarding the existence of the external world and asked whether we have the kind of knowledge required to justify a belief in the world's existence. But, as I will show in Part III, such enquiries misconstrue the nature of the conviction that they claim to cast into doubt. The sense that 'the world exists' and that 'I am part of it' is not a matter of propositions that are assented to in the form of articulate beliefs. The conviction that the world exists is wholly different in character from the proposition that some entity within the world exists. It implicitly remains in place, even in those cases where a philosopher explicitly claims to doubt it.

Phenomenology and the sense of reality

The nature of our sense of reality and belonging is explored by various phenomenologists and it is to phenomenology that I turn in order to make the structure of existential feeling explicit. Edmund Husserl, the founder of phenomenology, is clear that the sense of reality is not comprised of a propositional attitude of the form 'I believe that p', where p is the proposition 'some entity called *the world* exists'. Rather, it is a pre-articulate conviction that is already in place before we explicitly assent to anything in the form of a propositional attitude. According to Husserl, the world's existence is something that we take for granted in our 'natural attitude'; it is presupposed throughout everyday life and by almost all intellectual enquiry too. Regardless of what we might doubt or assent to, we continue to take for granted a sense of being part of the world. This 'sense' is not itself held up as an object of doubt, even when people claim to sincerely doubt the existence of some entity called the world. As Merleau-Ponty (1964c, pp.163–4) emphasizes, the natural attitude is not something that we knowingly adopt; it is not a body of conceptual knowledge, a 'tissue of judicatory and propositional acts', but an 'opening' onto the world—an existential orientation that operates as a background to experience and thought, rather than an explicit content of experience or thought.

It is all very well to say such things but the question arises as to how the sense of reality, if we even accept that there is such a thing, can be explored philosophically. A central feature of Husserl's phenomenological method is a methodological shift that he calls the *epoché*. This is a suspension of the natural attitude and, by implication, a withholding of the assumption of the world's reality that is integral to the natural attitude. It does not involve doubting the reality of the world. When the phenomenologist withdraws from the natural attitude and thus from her ordinarily implicit commitment to the reality of the world, she leaves that commitment intact but 'brackets' it. From this disengaged perspective, she is able to study the structure of the natural attitude, including the sense of reality. This is something that she would not be able to do if she simply inhabited the natural attitude and, in so doing, implicitly accepted the reality of the world. Hence the phenomenologist is required to 'abstain' from her 'natural believing' in the reality of the world. In so doing, she acquires the ability to reflect upon the structure of everyday experience. The world of everyday social life (or 'life world') and also the scientifically described world both presuppose the natural attitude and, in bracketing that attitude, the phenomenologist is no longer committed to what is posited in either context. Instead she takes 'not just corporeal Nature but the whole concrete surrounding life-world' as 'from now on, only a phenomenon of being, instead of something that is' (Husserl, 1960, p.19).

This is not a *denial* of the world's reality. Husserlian phenomenology is neither a form of realism nor of idealism. It is not idealism because it preserves intact the sense that the world exists independently of our experiences of it and our thoughts about it. But it is not a form of realism either, as it does not accept the reality of things and begin from there. Instead it addresses, amongst other things, what the sense of reality consists of:

> That the being of the world 'transcends' consciousness [...] and that it necessarily remains transcendent, in no wise alters the fact that it is conscious life alone, wherein everything transcendent becomes constituted, as something inseparable from consciousness, and which specifically, as world-consciousness, bears within itself inseparably the sense: world—and indeed: 'this actually existing' world. (Husserl, 1960, p.62)

The sense of reality is something that is constituted by our experience but this does not entail that there is no reality other than consciousness, or that the 'real world' that we ordinarily take for granted does not exist. This is because the sense of reality that we have is a sense of a world that *does* transcend the experiences of individuals, a world that is not *contained* within one or more consciousnesses. But the phenomenologist, in suspending the natural attitude, has adopted a different perspective or orientation, from which the structure of background commitments that are integral to everyday experience and thought is described rather than assumed. Hence the structure of world-experience is not changed by the *epoché*. The sense of reality and belonging is preserved in its entirety:

> ... the world experienced in this reflectively grasped life goes on being for me (in a certain manner) 'experienced' as before, and with just the content it has at any particular time. It goes on appearing, as it appeared before; the only difference is that I, as reflecting philosophically, no longer keep in effect (no longer accept) the natural believing in existence involved in experiencing the world—though that believing too is still there and grasped by my noticing regard. (Husserl, 1960, pp.19–20)

The phenomenological enquirer has become disconnected from the way of experiencing that she ordinarily inhabits and is thus able to study its structure. So she does not offer a metaphysical or epistemological thesis but asks a different kind of question. Amongst other things, she asks what the sense of reality consists of, a sense that is presupposed by any question regarding what is and is not real or how we know what is and is not real.

Several authors have suggested that Husserl's conception of the natural attitude serves to cast light on the nature of changed experience in psychiatric illness and, more specifically, in schizophrenia. For example, Stanghellini (2001, 2004) refers to the natural attitude as a 'commonsense orientation' through which the world is experienced. He takes commonsense to be a practical, habitual, bodily appreciation of the world, rather than a body of conceptual knowledge.[3] Schizophrenia, he claims, is a 'crisis of commonsense', central to which is a loss of the sense of others as *people* (2001, p.201). He also addresses the relationship between a sense of reality and a feeling of being rooted in, or connected to, the social world, suggesting that the sense of reality is an '*experience of belonging*' (2004, p.69). Such claims complement the work of earlier authors working in the field of phenomenological psychiatry. Minkowski, for instance, claims that schizophrenia involves a loss of 'vital contact with reality', an absence of felt belonging (Minkowski and Targowla, 2001). Blankenburg (2001) appeals to the closely related notion of a loss of 'natural self-evidence', a breakdown of practical commonsense and a feeling of doubt regarding what was previously implicitly assumed.

An even closer parallel has been drawn between Husserlian phenomenology and schizophrenia, which emphasizes the similarity between schizophrenic experience and the *epoché*. Husserl's phenomenology demands a kind of detachment from one's own experiences, which are no longer *lived through* and instead become objects of reflection. There is a peculiar splitting of self, as one withdraws from one's experiencing whilst leaving that experiencing intact. Depraz (2003) and Stanghellini (2004, 2007) claim that schizophrenic people involuntarily perform the *epoché*, leaving their natural living and becoming detached onlookers upon their experiences:

> Phenomenologists believe that schizophrenic persons have the capacity to perform the reduction much better than ordinary people: they show an enhanced aptitude to the *epoché*. (Depraz, 2003, p, 189)

Such claims are misleading. Central to Husserl's method is the requirement that the sense of reality remains *intact*, that the structure of experience is preserved, thus allowing accurate phenomenological description of it. The phenomenologist withdraws from the everyday existential orientation in order to study its structure and, in so doing, she does not change its structure. Regardless of controversies surrounding how many variants of schizophrenia there are, and even whether there is such a thing as 'schizophrenia' (of which I will say more in Chapter 7), something that is clear is that many of those people diagnosed as schizophrenic undergo a significant *change* in existential orientation.

---

[3] See also Ratcliffe (2007, chapter 2) for a discussion of different senses of 'commonsense'.

When they do so, the original orientation or 'natural attitude' is no longer intact; the sense of reality is not preserved but profoundly altered.

Stanghellini (2007, p.132) acknowledges that, unlike the phenomenological *epoché*, the schizophrenic withdrawal becomes 'part of the natural attitude situated in ordinary life'.[4] But, given that it replaces the natural attitude, rather than leaving it intact, there is a significant difference between phenomenological and schizophrenic 'attitudes'.

I will however support the view that schizophrenia and other psychiatric illnesses involve changes to what Husserl calls the 'natural attitude'. Given such changes, a methodological shift that plays the role of the Husserlian *epoché* is required in order to interpret the relevant experiences. If an experience incorporates a change in the sense of reality, or even a loss of that sense, it cannot be adequately understood if it is interpreted against the backdrop of a presupposed sense of reality.

A word of caution is required at this point. It should not be assumed that there is a single sense of 'reality', which is integral to a constant, everyday, natural attitude that almost all of us unthinkingly inhabit. Reference to a host of subtly different existential feelings can be found throughout everyday life and such talk is certainly not restricted to a small number of highly unusual or obviously pathological experiences. For all of us, there are times when the world can feel *unfamiliar, unreal, unusually real, homely, distant* or *close*. It can be something that one feels apart from or at one with. One can feel like a participant in the world or like a detached, estranged observer, staring at objects that do not seem to be quite *there*. All experiences have, as a background, a changeable sense of one's relationship with the world. This background, I will suggest, is best understood in terms of feeling; ways of finding oneself in a world are, at the same time, feelings of the body. One of my central claims is that there is no single, constant 'natural attitude'; existential feelings vary in all sorts of subtle ways from person to person and from time to time. And the existential feelings of some people no doubt fluctuate more than those of others. Hence it would be a mistake to postulate only one everyday mode of existential feeling and then a few perturbations from it, which occur only in psychiatric illnesses, in exceptional situations or as a result of taking certain drugs.[5] I do acknowledge that

---

[4] Depraz (2003, p.192) similarly states that the schizophrenic *epoché* is an 'incarnation' of the Husserlian *epoché*, a way of living in the world rather than a theoretical perspective that is adopted.

[5] In this book, I focus on existential feelings in everyday life and in psychiatric illness. I do not discuss the wide range of feelings that can be induced by a variety of drugs. Nevertheless, I do acknowledge that there is a great deal to be said about the many effects that drugs can have on existential orientation, and also that existential changes in psychiatric illness are not always dissociable from the effects of medication.

existential changes involved in schizophrenia and other psychiatric illnesses are quite extreme, falling outside the range that most of us experience. Even so, the recognition that everyday life involves a plethora of different existential feelings, rather than one 'normal' existential orientation, serves to make certain pathological forms of experience more comprehensible and less removed from 'mundane' experience.

Given the range of existential feelings, talk of a single, constant 'sense of reality' is misplaced. As I will emphasize, the sense of reality is something that differs subtly in character from one existential predicament to another. To further complicate matters, existential feelings are sometimes referred to as changes in the sense of 'being' or 'existence', rather than 'reality'. These three terms are often used as synonyms, but not always. Someone might refer to losing the everyday sense of reality and at the same time being confronted with bare existence.

In the process of describing existential feelings, I will diagnose a range of commonplace philosophical maladies that serve to obscure them. As mentioned earlier, the nature of existential feelings (and indeed feelings more generally) has been obfuscated by the imposition of a clear-cut distinction between experience of body and experience of world. There are a host of other, closely related dualisms that also need to be discarded in order to appreciate the nature of our changeable sense of reality. A particularly troublesome one is that between cognition and affect but there are many others. Internal is contrasted with external, inside with outside, bodily with non-bodily, self with non-self, mind with world, mental with non-mental, subject with object, and the list goes on. None of these apply to the way in which we already find ourselves in the world before we conceptualize ourselves in such ways. Finding oneself in the world is unitary; feelings of the body are also ways of being in a world and the relatedness between self and world is more experientially primitive than the apprehension of either in isolation from the other. It is also important to emphasize that the everyday world is a world of other people, infused throughout with a sense of the personal. Others are not simply add-ons to an already established reality. To quote Wolfgang Blankenburg:

> Affectivity and the ability to judge, as we find it in *common sense*, refer back to an original unity of thinking, feeling and willing in human existence, which is primarily related to an intersubjective world. (2001, p.307)

Another inappropriate theoretical imposition that has obscured the nature of existential feeling is that of the 'propositional attitude'. It is frequently assumed by philosophers that all states of conviction can be conveyed in the form 'B believes that p', where p is any meaningful proposition you like, such as 'the car is red', 'nobody is in the room' or 'there is such a thing as schizophrenia'. But existential feelings do not conform to this assumption. The sense of reality, of belonging, of the world's existence, is not a matter of some proposition being accepted. Existential feelings comprise a more fundamental appreciation of reality than the various kinds of state that are referred to as 'beliefs' or 'propositional attitudes'. Furthermore, many pathological experiences that are frequently interpreted and explained in terms of changes in 'affect', coupled with pathologies of 'belief', are, I will argue, better interpreted as arising from altered 'feelings of being'.

This is not just a book about what phenomenology can contribute to psychiatry or, alternatively, about what psychiatry can contribute to phenomenology. The two are mutually illuminating. Certain misguided presuppositions have influenced recent philosophical enquiry into the nature of pathological experiences. Phenomenological accounts that dispense with these presuppositions therefore serve as a better interpretive framework through which to understand such experiences. Hence phenomenology can contribute to understanding in psychiatry. However, descriptions of pathological experience offered by psychiatrists and patients also aid phenomenological enquiry, in so far as they rest uncomfortably with phenomenological accounts of world-experience or draw attention to something that has been missed, and so prompt us to reconsider our phenomenological descriptions. So there is an ongoing hermeneutic between the two fields, where philosophical assumptions are questioned and refined through attention to work in psychiatry, and philosophical accounts of experience, in turn, contribute to an understanding of psychiatric illness. My aim here is to offer a phenomenological analysis of existential feeling and to show how this can be fruitfully applied to psychiatry and refined in the process. I do not set out to offer a comprehensive account of the varieties of existential feeling involved in psychiatric illness, although I do distinguish some of them.

Although I advocate a Husserlian methodological orientation of sorts, according to which we make the sense of reality a focus for enquiry rather than taking it for granted, I am very doubtful as to the prospect of a complete *epoché*. To bifurcate oneself in such a way that the stream of lived experience is perfectly preserved, whilst a reflective attitude is at the same time adopted towards it, strikes me as a phenomenologically impossible achievement. We can withdraw from aspects of experience and reflect upon them but we cannot bracket the entirety of experience in one go. Phenomenology does require adopting a kind of methodological orientation or stance, involving an appreciation of certain kinds of question that are seldom addressed by mainstream Anglophone metaphysics and epistemology. Amongst other things, we shift from asking what is real and how we know what is real to asking what the sense of reality (an aspect of our experience that such questions take for granted) consists of. However, a phenomenological stance does not provide us with access to the pure and unadulterated totality of possible experience. Phenomenological enquiry requires ongoing interpretation of experience, accompanied by progressive refinement and clarification of descriptions that are offered. This process can proceed gradually and collaboratively. One engages with and interprets the predicaments of others, as one reflects. And I regard the reports of clinicians and patients, in addition to the narratives and expressions offered by people more generally, as indispensable guides when it comes to exploring the phenomenology of existential feeling. My aim here is to pursue this kind of phenomenological enquiry, rather than to vindicate the thought of any particular phenomenologist, and I draw selectively on the works of several philosophers, principally Husserl, Heidegger and Merleau-Ponty. There are many significant differences between the methods of these thinkers and the phenomenological descriptions that they offer. Nevertheless, I hope it will become clear as the discussion proceeds that the lessons which I draw from them do complement each other and together contribute to a cohesive phenomenological account of existential feeling.

To further complicate the methodological issue, existential feelings are not just part of the subject matter of phenomenology; they also have an important *role* to play in phenomenological enquiry. Phenomenology requires suspending existential orientations—at least to some degree—in order to reflect upon their structure. But how can one suspend an inarticulate, practical, felt way of finding oneself in the world? Drawing on Heidegger and others, I will suggest that changes in existential feeling serve to reveal structures of experience that are ordinarily taken for granted. Without such changes, we might be oblivious to the sense of reality altogether; we might never 'see' it. But, when the structure of experience is disturbed in certain ways, what was in the background becomes conspicuous. I will propose in the final three chapters that existential feelings play a role in philosophy more generally—many significant differences between philosophies owe more to differences in existential orientation than they do to contrasting views regarding the cogency of explicit arguments.

Summary of the argument

Part I introduces the concept of existential feeling. The first chapter begins by reviewing some recent discussions of the relationship between emotions and bodily feelings, paying particular attention to those approaches that attempt to unite bodily feeling with the world-directed aspect of emotion. Although it is increasingly recognized that feelings can be about things other than the body, I suggest that none of these approaches offer a satisfactory phenomenological account of how this might be so. Then I consider the variety of feelings that people refer to in everyday life and observe that excessive emphasis on 'emotional feelings' has led to the neglect of other kinds of feeling, including existential feeling. In Chapter 2, existential feelings are introduced through a discussion of Heidegger's account of 'mood'. Heidegger claims that moods are not subjective states but existential orientations; they play a role in constituting the unitary structure of being-in-the-world and do not conform to distinctions between subject and object or inside and outside. I go on to point out some shortcomings of Heidegger's account and make a case for adopting the term 'existential feeling', rather than 'mood'. Following this, there are some preliminary reflections on existential feelings in psychiatric illness and everyday life. The chapter concludes by stressing the distinction between having a sense of reality and having a propositional attitude. Chapter 3 makes a case for the inextricability of body and world in existential feeling by drawing an analogy between existential and tactile feelings. In touch, perception of the body and perception of things outside of the body are indissociable aspects of a unitary perceptual experience. Existential feelings, I propose, not only have an analogous structure but also incorporate tactile feelings.

With this phenomenological account in place, Part II turns to the role of existential feelings in psychiatric illness, showing how the concept of existential feeling can be fruitfully applied to interpret pathological experiences and also how the study of such experiences can refine our appreciation of the nature and variety of these feelings. In Chapter 4, I further develop the view that many bodily feelings are not experiences of bodily states but ways of experiencing the relationship between body and world. Some such feelings, I argue, are not specifically focused experiences that have particular objects; they are existential backgrounds. This claim is supported by an appeal to several examples involving different kinds of existential feeling. The chapter concludes by showing how the phenomenological concept of an 'horizon', as employed by Husserl and Merleau-Ponty, can be used to convey how (a) existential orientations operate as backgrounds to experience and thought, and (b) these orientations can at the same time consist of feelings of bodily states. Chapter 5 turns to the Capgras delusion, which is generally characterized as the belief that one or more familiars have been replaced by impostors. I employ the delusion as a case study with which to demonstrate how something that is generally taken to involve affective anomalies and propositional attitudes is more plausibly interpreted in terms of changed existential feeling. Chapter 6 proceeds along similar lines, suggesting that explanations that appeal to altered feeling plus altered belief are guilty of double-counting.

The chapter begins by considering the Cotard delusion, the 'belief' that one is dead, nonexistent or disembodied. I argue that it is not a matter of diminished affect plus faulty reasoning, which together lead to the propositional attitude 'I am dead'. Instead, the utterances of patients express changed existential feeling. I go on to suggest that much the same lesson applies to the phenomenon of depersonalization. In Chapter 7, I address the topic of changed existential feeling in schizophrenia. Drawing on the work of Louis Sass and others, I argue that distinctions between positive and negative symptoms stem from the inappropriate imposition of a distinction between cognition and affect. Symptoms such as disorganized thought, delusions and thought insertion can all be understood, at least in part, in terms of changed existential feeling. The chapter concludes by addressing the difficult question of how many different kinds of existential feeling are involved in psychiatric illness. I draw some distinctions between the kinds of existential feeling that feature in autobiographical and clinical reports. In addition, I suggest that variants of existential feeling are highly unlikely to reliably track broad diagnostic categories, such as 'schizophrenia'.

Part III considers the role of existential feeling in philosophical enquiry, focusing throughout on the work of William James. Chapter 8 offers a rehabilitation of James's account of emotion. He is often charged with construing emotions as *feelings of bodily changes* and thus cutting them off from world-experience. However, by situating his work on emotion in the context of his other writings, I show that he does nothing of the sort. In fact, he acknowledges a range of feelings that do not feature in standard lists of emotions, and also recognizes their role in constituting a sense of reality. Variations in this sense of reality are, according to James, the sources of different philosophical stances or orientations. Chapter 9 takes, as its starting point, Sass's positive comparison between the 'hyper-reflexivitity' characteristic of schizophrenia and the philosopher's disposition towards detachment, abstraction and alienation from practice. Then I turn again to James, exploring and further developing his account of the relationship between feelings and philosophical thought. Following this, I consider what some more recent philosophers have to say about ground-floor philosophical commitments, focusing on Bas van Fraassen. I propose that existential feelings have an important part to play in the process of philosophical enquiry and that the ability to *shift* one's existential orientation is an important aspect of the rational, critical enterprise. Shifts in existential feelings can also play a more specific role in phenomenological enquiry, comparable to performance of a partial *epoché*. Hence they are integral to my own method. In Chapter 10, I round things off by addressing the question of what distinguishes pathological from non-pathological existential feelings.

I turn to so-called 'religious' experiences, which, I suggest, have changes in existential feeling at their core. My reason for looking specifically at these experiences is that there is considerable debate over whether they fall into the 'pathological' or the 'non-pathological' category. I argue that at least some of the existential feelings typical of 'religious' experiences can be distinguished from pathological existential feelings. In so doing, I offer a more general criterion for making the distinction. Central to all cases of what I call 'existential pathology' is either an impaired sense of others as people or an inability to connect with other people. The book concludes by commenting on the 'mechanistic' or 'naturalistic' worldview and proposing that, in its failure to acknowledge the way in which we find ourselves in the world, it amounts to an extreme but generally unacknowledged form of scepticism.[6]

---

[6] Throughout the book, I draw upon and develop points that I made in several previously published articles. Chapters 3, 5, 8 and 9 incorporate, in revised form, material from my articles 'Touch and Situatedness' (2008a), 'The Phenomenological Role of Affect in the Capgras Delusion' (2008b), 'William James on Emotion and Intentionality' (2005a) and 'Stance, Feeling and Phenomenology' (2008c), respectively. Other related articles include 'Heidegger's Attunement and the Neuropsychology of Emotion' (2002), 'Interpreting Delusions' (2004), 'The Feeling of Being' (2005b) and 'Existential Feeling and Psychopathology' (forthcoming).

Part I

The structure of existential feeling

Chapter 1

Emotions and bodily feelings

This chapter examines recent philosophical accounts of emotion and feeling, in order to make explicit some commonplace assumptions concerning the nature of bodily feeling. I begin by outlining two contrasting views, one being that emotions are bodily feelings and the other that they are judgements. The problem is that emotions seem to be both, and so the question arises as to how the feeling component can be united with the cognitive component. One solution is to maintain that emotions have at least two distinct ingredients, but this view does not accord with the relevant phenomenology; feelings seem to permeate the world-directed aspect of emotion. I therefore explore the possibility that feelings might be more than just experiences of bodily states, by focusing on three recent approaches that attempt to unite feeling with intentionality. I argue that all are incomplete in certain important respects. The chapter concludes by identifying existential feelings as an important phenomenological category and suggesting that an overhaul of some deep-rooted philosophical assumptions is required if we are to understand them. Central to this overhaul is the abandonment of the distinction between cognition and affect.

The dismissal of 'mere affect'

One of the main problems addressed by recent philosophical work on emotion is that of how emotions can be sophisticated cognitive states and, at the same time, have bodily feelings as a major component. This problem is exemplified by the contrasting views of William James, who claims that emotions are feelings of bodily changes, and Robert Solomon, who claims that they are judgements. I will start by discussing James's view and will then turn to Solomon.

Most accounts of emotion include some reference to James's well-known theory. It is often summarily dismissed, allegedly demonstrating in the process that emotions are not just bodily feelings. James (1884, 1890) famously challenges what he takes to be the conventional wisdom of his time by claiming that emotions are not mental states that follow perception and *cause* bodily changes. Instead, the relevant bodily changes are solicited by perception in a reflex-like manner and the feeling of these changes simply *is* the emotion:

> Our natural way of thinking about these standard [strong, occurrent] emotions is that the mental perception of some fact excites the mental affection called the emotion, and that this latter state of mind gives rise to the bodily expression. My thesis on the contrary is that *the bodily changes follow directly the* PERCEPTION *of the exciting fact, and that our feeling of the same changes as they occur* IS *the emotion.* (James, 1884, pp.189–90)

However, he does not restrict his account to these 'standard' emotions and claims that even subtle intellectual and aesthetic emotions, such as pleasure in a piece of music or satisfaction at having solved a problem, involve bodily feeling too. Without the feeling, there would be no emotion.

Recent criticisms of the theory take issue with its apparent implication that emotions are wholly distinct from cognition. These criticisms can be differentiated into philosophical objections and objections based upon scientific findings. I will address the scientifically based objections first.

James assumes that the relevant bodily feelings are sufficiently complex and diverse to distinguish the plethora of different emotions we feel. However, a well-known experiment by Schachter and Singer (1962) is often taken to show that, in different kinds of situation, experimental subjects undergoing the same physiological changes will interpret those changes in terms of very different emotions. This suggests that bodily feelings are not sufficiently differentiated to account for the full complexity of emotional experience and that an element of cognitive appraisal is also involved.

In addition to this, critics have addressed the implication that a subject who is unable to feel the relevant bodily changes will have no emotions. James himself recognizes this implication and proposes a hypothetical experimental test of his theory:

> A case of complete internal and external corporeal anaesthesia, without motor alteration or alteration of intelligence except emotional apathy, would afford, if not a crucial test, at least a strong presumption, in favour of the truth of the view we have set forth; whilst the persistence of strong emotional feeling in such a case would completely overthrow our case. (1884, p.203)

In the absence of such a case, it is often assumed that the retention of emotions in people with severe spinal cord lesions, which prevent neural communication between brain and body, also amounts to decisive evidence against James's theory.[1] For example, Greenfield (2000, p.98) claims that James's 'old, and now discarded' theory cannot accommodate this finding.

----

[1] So far as I know, there has never been a case of complete loss of bodily feeling without loss of motor capacities, awareness or thought. Cole (1995) discusses Ian Waterman, who

However, both of these alleged refutations are contentious to say the least. For example, de Sousa (1990, p.55) notes that 'the range of physiological changes taken into account in Schachter and Singer's experiment is much too narrow to count seriously against James's view'. He suggests that the relevant physiological changes may after all be complex and differentiated enough to facilitate the wide range of emotions that we experience. The claim that James's theory is falsified by the retention of emotions in subjects with spinal cord damage has been challenged by Damasio (2000, p.289), amongst others. Damasio makes three central points against the evidence from spinal cord lesions. To summarize:

1 Information concerning many of the relevant physiological changes could be transmitted to the brain via nerves such as the vagus, which enter the brain stem at a level too high to be impaired by spinal cord damage.

2 Hormonal changes will still be communicated to the brain via the blood-stream.

3 Some diminution of emotion is indeed found in many patients with spinal cords lesions.

Damasio's own theory of emotion is essentially an updated and elaborated Jamesian view, which maintains that 'the body is the main stage for emotions' (2000, p.287). However, there are at least three significant differences between the two. First of all, Damasio claims that many emotions involve 'virtual' representations of bodily changes by the brain, rather than the detection of actual bodily changes. This lends further support to the claim that retention of emotion in the case of spinal cord damage is compatible with the bodily nature of emotion, as virtual changes might be wholly unaffected. Second, Damasio offers a more specific account of the brain areas involved in causing and detecting the relevant bodily changes. He acknowledges that James was 'of necessity, somewhat vague about the brain aspect' of his theory and that many of James's speculations about brain physiology need to be reconsidered (Damasio, 2000, p.38). But he agrees broadly with James (1884, p.188), in rejecting the idea of a specific area dedicated to the emotions and in emphasizing the importance of physiological changes. The third difference is terminological. James takes emotions to be feelings of bodily changes, whereas Damasio takes them to be sets of bodily changes (including changes in the brain), which may or may not be felt. Hence James's 'emotions' become Damasio's 'feelings'.

As illustrated by the considerable amount of attention that Damasio's work has received, a Jamesian view of emotion is still taken very seriously by many

suffered de-afferentation and consequent loss of proprioception. But Waterman and others with similar conditions retain at least some feeling above the neck.

neurobiologists and other scientists. However, James is far less popular amongst philosophers working on emotion, many of whom have given him a very bad press. A resurgence of philosophical interest in emotion during the last forty years is closely associated with an increased appreciation of the cognitive dimensions of emotion. As Downing (2000, p.247) remarks, 'almost everyone writing on these issues would assent to one point: it has been this focus on cognitive evaluation which has opened up the overall discussion in the first place'. The term 'cognitive' is used in a number of different ways. But, by describing emotions as cognitive, philosophers tend to mean at least that they are intentional states of some kind. They either *are* or at least *involve* evaluations, appraisals or judgements, which are often taken to incorporate concepts and propositional attitudes (although it is also worth keeping in mind that terms such as 'appraisal', 'judgement' and 'evaluation' are used in a variety of ways too). In addition, it is increasingly emphasized that emotions are not just brief episodes of bodily arousal but longer term processes that are woven into our perception of, and thought about, the world. This 'cognitive turn' does not bode well for James. In identifying emotions with feelings of bodily changes, he appears to ignore altogether the cognitive aspects of emotion. As Downing goes on to say, 'James and Lange identified emotion simply and squarely with conscious body sensation, nothing more. A view which almost no one today, myself included, would want to defend' (2000, p.248).[2]

Such dismissals of James's position presuppose a distinction between cognition and 'mere feeling' or 'affect'. Any account identifying emotions exclusively with bodily feelings is charged with 'trivializing' them by rendering them non-cognitive. Emotions clearly play a central role in our mental lives and behaviour but they can only do this if they incorporate world-directed intentional states. If emotions are just feelings, then they are either intentional states that can have only the body or parts of it as their intentional objects or, alternatively, they are not intentional states at all. But it is clear that most emotions do have intentional objects other than the body. Emotions are not just *caused* by events in the world; they are also *about* such events. As a big shark approaches a swimmer at high speed, the swimmer is not 'afraid' in some objectless sense; she is afraid *of the shark*. Solomon (1993, p.91) and Gordon (1987, p.88) both go so far as to claim that James's view renders emotions epiphenomenal; cut off from the manner in which the triggering object is experientially presented, evaluated and acted upon. The bodily responses, including—James says—behaviours such as fleeing, occur before they are felt

---

[2] James's theory is often associated with the very similar view of C. G. Lange. Hence the James–Lange theory.

and so the feeling is not itself causally efficacious. In addition, the feeling is not *about* the object of the emotion. This latter concern is also raised by Brewer:

> [James's] identification of emotional experiences with feelings of bodily changes leaves their object entirely external to the nature of the experiences themselves, as if one first felt afraid all right, but then had to go on to look out for some likely candidate object of one's fear. [....] That one is afraid *of that particular object or event* is absolutely perspicuous, and intrinsic to the experience itself. So it looks as though we need to combine elements from both James own theory and the idea of emotions as presenting specific worldly objects in some way with which he contrasts it. (2002, p.27)

Thus bodily feelings, it is maintained, are not world-directed intentional states. An exclusive emphasis on feelings therefore fails to connect the emotion with its object, whereas even casual phenomenological reflection reveals to us that emotional experiences *do* have objects. Such criticisms tend to assume that feelings are unsophisticated, somehow trivial and quite unlike rich emotional engagements with things in the world. For example, Solomon (1993) insists that 'emotions are something far more sophisticated than mere feelings' (p.102); they 'are not merely "affects"' (p.108). Feelings, he says, 'no more constitute or define the emotion than an army of fleas constitutes a homeless dog' (p.97). He not only rejects the identification of emotion with feeling but denies even that feelings play an essential *part* in emotional experience, claiming instead that the relevant feelings merely *accompany* emotions.

Solomon on emotion and the meaning of life

According to Solomon, emotions are not feelings but judgements, which are indispensable to our ability to think and act. A wedge is drawn between emotions and feelings—emotions are of pivotal importance in our lives and so cannot be feelings. Throughout his book *The Passions*, Solomon distinguishes 'intelligent, cultivated, conceptually rich engagements with the world' from 'mere reactions or instincts', identifying emotions with the former (1993, ix).[3] Emotions are, he says, 'constitutive judgements', meaning that they are not judgements about pre-conceived objects but judgements that serve to make their objects what they are. By analogy, the announcement that a piece of wood placed upon a chess board will count as a King is not a judgement about a pre-existent chess piece; the judgement makes the piece what it is. However, emotions are unlike the pronouncement 'this is the King' insofar as they need not be articulate. Emotions, Solomon says, are not linguistic attitudes towards

---

[3] I refer here to the revised edition of *The Passions*. The book was originally published in 1976 and played a key role in reinvigorating philosophical discussion of the emotions.

the ingredients of an already experienced world. Instead, they are constitutive of *experience*. An object of fear is not first experienced and then feared. The fear is integral to the manner in which it is experienced, to the experiential shape it takes on. Things appear the way they do *through* our emotions.

Solomon's account of the role of emotion hinges on a distinction between the scientifically described world and the world as we experience it. The objective world of empirical science is bereft of value, purpose and practical significance but the everyday world is certainly not. We do not knowingly 'project' value and significance upon things that are first revealed to us in a neutral, detached, objective fashion. The world that we take for granted as a backdrop to all our activities, the world that motivates us and solicits us to act, is already configured in terms of our values and purposes. Solomon is not entirely clear on the relationship between these two 'worlds' but he seems to regard the scientifically described world as a selective abstraction from the everyday world. In describing the role of emotion, he emphasizes the world that we actually experience:

> My concern is with the world we *live* in, not the lifeless complex of facts and hypotheses that one finds so elegantly described, without a trace of passion, in the pages of our best science textbooks. (Solomon, 1993, p.19)

Emotions are, he claims, the 'meaning of life' (1993, ix). This is not to say that they give our lives a meaning or purpose relative to the intentions of some being that is external to the world. Instead, Solomon is claiming that emotions are exclusively responsible for constituting the meanings *in* life, the meaningfulness of a life. They accomplish this by configuring our experience in such a way that things appear as salient, valuable, significant, threatening, worth pursuing and so on. We experience our emotions first and foremost *as* the world that we inhabit, rather than as internal constituents of our psychology. And that world is not experienced as something set apart from our projects, from our sense of who we are and what we strive for. The world, as experienced, embodies what we take to be significant, what we care about, what we identify with and what drives us. It reflects the kinds of people we take ourselves to be or aspire to be. Emotions thus 'define us, our selves, and the world we live in' (1993, xv).

Solomon does not think that we are at the mercy of our emotions, which—in setting up the world for us—determine our preferences and motivations before rational deliberation and choice can even get started. Rather, drawing on Sartre, he claims that an emotion is a 'purposive strategy', the aim of which is to 'maximize our sense of personal dignity and self-esteem' (1993, xvii). We configure the world in such a way that it suits us. It might seem to us that the emotionally shaped world is a passive imposition upon us.

However, Solomon claims that our constitutive judgements are, in some sense, our choices. We do not choose our emotions explicitly on every occasion, in the way that we might choose to buy a car. But we do not choose our beliefs in this way either. And, just as we are responsible for managing our beliefs through rational deliberation, we are responsible for managing emotional configurations of the world. What one 'feels' emotionally is not what is inflicted upon one; it is 'what one chooses and accepts' (1993, p.23).

The claim that emotions are shaped by reasoning is plausible in some cases. For example, Solomon (1980) claims that there is a difference between feeling angry and actually being angry. I might be angry with a friend for failing to intervene in a difficult situation on my behalf. However, once I realize that her intervention could only have made things worse and that this is why she refrained from acting in the way I had hoped she would, my anger might fade or be displaced by a different emotion. Although the associated feeling remains, the anger itself is gone. Rational reappraisal of a situation serves to change the emotion, suggesting that emotions are not passive feelings that are thrust upon us but ways of judging a situation that we are responsible for. Of course, examples like this are contentious. In some situations, the anger might persist despite the knowledge that it is unwarranted. One might know full well that one's being in a bad temper with someone is symptomatic of too much alcohol or not enough sleep the night before, rather than anything the person has actually done, and yet persist in being unpleasant to him regardless. So the extent to which we regulate our emotions by means of rational deliberation is debatable.

Solomon would retort that the commonplace failure to rationally regulate emotion does not imply its impossibility, just as dogmatic adoption of unfounded beliefs does not imply the impossibility of rational re-appraisal. There is a difference between what we actually do and what rational beings ought to do. Even so, the question remains as to whether all our emotions are susceptible to rational intervention. And there may be some heterogeneity here, with different emotions being susceptible to rational intervention in different ways and to differing degrees.

Something that Solomon does not make sufficiently clear is the distinction between two different roles that emotions seem to play in his account. The claim that they either are rational judgements, or at least involve rational judgements, might seem intuitive when we turn to specific episodes of emotion and perhaps also longer term emotional dispositions towards certain objects, people or situation-types. However, Solomon's account of the role and significance of emotion indicates that not all emotions take this form. When you are happy or sad about a specific event, you are already *in a world* and take for granted certain patterns of significance, practical salience and value.

It is because you already do so that you feel happy or sad about some events and not others. You wouldn't feel sad about a football team losing a match unless you already had a particular set of cares and concerns relating to that team. Specific emotional 'judgements' only arise because certain things are already deemed significant. It is not occurrences of fear, pride or disappointment that constitute the meaningfulness of a life but the context that is already inhabited, out of which certain events emerge as significant and thus as potential objects of such emotions. As Solomon (1993) says, the emotions are 'the system of meanings and values within which our lives either develop and grow or starve and stagnate' (1993, xvii). They 'create our interests and our purposes' (p.15). Importantly, he adds they are also interpersonal; they are what 'commit and bind us to other people' (p.20) and are therefore responsible for a meaningful and always *interpersonal* world. Now, we might regulate some emotions through reasoning but it is not clear that the pre-given world can be regulated in such a way. We do not encounter the world as an object of experience and take responsibility for the manner in which it appears—we inhabit it, we find ourselves in it. And, in so far as we inhabit it, we take it for granted rather than assuming responsibility for it. To invoke Husserl's term, we *already* dwell in the 'natural attitude' when we experience an occurrent emotion.

Perhaps we can be responsible for the way we find ourselves in the world, in some way and to some extent. If emotions do constitute it, recognition of that fact might itself serve to emancipate us from the illusion of pure passivity, allowing us the possibility of somehow regulating the experiential backgrounds that shape our activities. All the same, doing so is not the same as regulating specifically directed emotions. The world is not an object of emotion towards which we adopt a particular emotional attitude. It might be argued that emotions that embrace the world as a whole are what we call 'moods'. Indeed, Solomon refers to moods as 'generalized emotions' (1993, p.15). I will have a lot more to say about moods in Chapter 2. However, for the time being, suffice it to say that, if moods are regarded as generalized emotions, then they too will fail to accommodate the way in which we find ourselves in the world. An emotion can be more or less general but, if a mood is just a generalized emotion, it will—like any other emotion—presuppose a context of significance. The world is not an *object* of emotion, however general that object might be.

It might be that moods and emotions feed back into, and reshape, the context out of which they emerge. Even so, an account is required of how that context differs in its phenomenological character from an emotion or mood that is had within it. When we are afraid of an entity, our fear may be described as a state of the self (being afraid), an attitude towards something (fearing it) or as a way in which the object of emotion appears (threatening). But I do not relate to the world in this way. It is where I already am before I have any such emotion, a context in which I might find myself afraid or find an object threatening. The significance Solomon ascribes to emotions in making a life meaningful seems to apply only to a certain subset, those that constitute the experiential world we inhabit. And a standard inventory of emotions and moods, such as fear, anger, rage, joy, happiness, jealousy, pride, sadness and envy, does not capture the distinctive way in which we belong to the world. One possibility is that they can do so when some or all of them are brought together. However, it is not at all clear how a collection of states that arise in the context of a pre-given world could together make up the phenomenological character of the world in which they arise.

Thus, in attempting to convey the sense of belonging to a world, Solomon ascribes a world-constituting role to emotions in general and obscures an important distinction between explicit attitudes and the taken-for-granted background in which these attitudes are embedded. Furthermore, it is not at all clear what the relevant 'judgements' consist of or whether the judgements that constitute emotional experiences of particular objects are similar in kind to those that constitute a sense of belonging to the world. And, without the incorporation of feeling, it is hard to see what makes any judgement distinctively 'emotional'. In fact, as will become clear in the next few chapters, to strip world-constituting judgements of feeling is to take away from them precisely what constitutes the world.

One way of bringing in feeling is to maintain that the term 'feeling' is sometimes employed in a way that is synonymous with 'judgement'. This is the strategy adopted by Nussbaum (2001, 2004), who offers a view that is similar in many respects to that of Solomon. She shares his disdain for bodily feelings and claims that they merely accompany emotions. According to Nussbaum, emotions are judgements concerning matters important to our well-being, which acknowledge our neediness and our dependence upon factors beyond our control. They are complex, cognitive states and to *feel* an emotion is not to have a bodily twinge but to form a judgement. The term 'feeling' is, she maintains, ambiguous. It does not always refer to perception of a bodily state. In some uses, it is interchangeable with terms like 'perception' and 'judgement', being 'a terminological variant for them' (2004, p.195). Nussbaum suggests that this applies to emotional feelings. Bodily feelings are incidental to emotion and the feelings that really matter could just as well be called judgements or beliefs (2001, p.60).[4]

---

[4] Several other contemporary philosophers have offered detailed accounts of how emotions contribute to experience of their objects. For example, Roberts (1988) proposes that they are 'concern-based construals'. Having an emotion is analogous to experiencing a gestalt switch;

Uniting cognition and affect

In contrast to Solomon and Nussbaum, many philosophers have offered conciliatory accounts of the relationship between emotion and bodily feeling. It is to some of these that I now turn in order to further explore the nature of bodily feelings.

When faced with the task of reconciling the bodily nature of emotions with their world-directedness, one strategy is to adopt a hybrid theory, according to which emotions have both cognitive and affective constituents. Lyons (1980) offers an account along these lines, accepting that feelings and judgements both contribute to emotion: 'the concept of emotion as occurrent state involves reference to an evaluation which causes abnormal physiological changes in the subject of the evaluation' (p.53). He suggests that, for a mental state to be an emotion, it must have both components but that it is the type of evaluation, rather than the associated feelings, which serves to distinguish one emotion from another. So the difference between fear and anger, for instance, is not a matter of there being different kinds of bodily twinge but of something appearing frightening in the former case and annoying in the latter.

In construing an emotion as a state incorporating *both* bodily feelings *and* cognitive states, Lyons takes it as given that cognition and affect are distinct. Most recent philosophical accounts similarly respect the distinction between bodily feelings and the cognitive aspects of emotion, with the intentional directedness of emotions towards objects, events and situations in the world falling into the latter category. Bodily feelings, it is assumed, either do not have intentionality at all or are intentional states directed exclusively at the body or parts of it. Ben-Ze'ev, for instance, opts for the former:

> ...unlike higher levels of awareness, such as those found in perception, memory, and thinking, the feeling dimension [of emotion] has no significant cognitive content. It expresses our own state, but is not in itself directed at this state or at any other object. Since this dimension is a mode of consciousness, one cannot be unconscious of it;

one perceives the object differently. (In his more recent work, Solomon [2003, p.185] indicates that he is leaning towards a preference for the term 'construal' over 'judgement'.) De Sousa (1980, 1990, 2004) similarly emphasizes the role of emotion in perceptual experience. Like Solomon, he claims that emotions configure experience into patterns of significance. *They manifest themselves as 'determinate patterns of salience among objects of attention, lines of inquiry and inferential strategies'* (1980, p.137), rather than being articulate, propositional judgements. Patterns of salience bind aspects of the world together into meaningful configurations. Neither de Sousa nor Roberts insist on the stark contrast between bodily feeling and emotional judgement that Solomon and Nussbaum advocate. However, they do not offer detailed accounts of the role played by bodily feeling in emotion either. Neither do they emphasize the 'existential' dimension of emotional experience to the extent that Solomon does.

there are no unfelt feelings. [...] Despite the importance of feelings in emotions, equating the two is incorrect since emotions have an intentional component in addition to the feeling component. (2004, pp.252–3)

Given this conception of feeling, he, like Lyons, adopts a hybrid account, according to which emotions are comprised of 'cognition, evaluation, motivation and feeling', all of which are intentional except feeling (2004, p.259). The reasoning behind such views seems to go something like this:

1 Emotional experience involves bodily feeling, as is apparent from phenomenological reflection.

2 Emotions are world-directed intentional states, as is also apparent from phenomenological reflection.

3 Bodily feelings are not world-directed intentional states.

4 Emotions are therefore a combination of bodily feelings and something else.

The problem with this is that we can only reach (4) if we accept that the relevant phenomenology distinguishes the feeling component from the world-directed component; and this doesn't seem to be so. Nussbaum (2004) offers a moving account of how she felt during the time leading up to and including her mother's death. She states that receiving news of her mother's serious illness 'felt like a nail suddenly driven into my stomach' (p.184) and that later, upon hearing of her mother's death, 'my body felt as if pierced by so many slivers of glass, fragmented, as if it had exploded and scattered in pieces around the room' (p.185). Such descriptions at least *seem* to refer to bodily feelings (although this is not the interpretation Nussbaum herself offers). However, what felt like a nail driven into the stomach was not a bodily state but the recognition of a state of affairs external to the body. The feeling seems indistinguishable from the manner in which that state of affairs is experienced. It is the objects of emotion that *hurt* us. The nail being driven in *is* the emotional apprehension of a situation; the intentionality and bodily nature of the emotion are entangled.

It is this inseparability that motivates Nussbaum's view of emotions as judgements rather than bodily feelings. If the emotion is a way in which the situation is appraised, then it cannot be a bodily feeling, given the assumption that bodily feelings do not reach out beyond the body. But this assumption is questionable. Must it be the case that bodily feelings are merely experiences of bodily states? Interestingly, Nussbaum suggests that:

...we are not left with a choice between regarding emotions as ghostly spiritual energies and taking them to be obtuse nonseeing bodily movements, such as a leap of the heart, or the boiling of the blood. Living bodies are capable of intelligence and intentionality. (2001, p.25)

What is set up as a choice between 'feeling' and 'judgement' could thus be interpreted quite differently. Rather than pitting judgements against feelings and assuming that the world-directed feelings involved in emotions cannot be 'bodily feelings', one might question the distinction between experience of internal bodily states and experience of the world, emphasizing that it is through our living, feeling bodies that we experience, think about and act upon worldly things. The cognition/affect distinction is perhaps symptomatic of too strict a division between how we experience our bodies and how we experience everything else. It could be that world-experience is inextricable from bodily feeling and therefore fails to conform to a range of dualisms that are imposed upon emotion. Should we really be carving off body from world, internal from external, feeling from intentionality? A departure from such approaches is recommended by Peter Goldie and Finn Spicer. They note that, if a clear distinction between mind and body (or some descendent of it that just as effectively separates our mental lives from our living bodies) is accepted from the outset, debates then become focused around the issue of how two aspects of emotional life that have been cut off from each other can be stuck back together again. Instead of setting things up in this way, they recommend that we put such assumptions aside and consider 'the emotions in their own right' (2002, p.4). A few philosophers have recently offered approaches that attempt to wed the feeling dimension of emotion to world-directed intentionality. In the next three sections, I will discuss three such approaches, one of which is adopted by Goldie and also by Michael Stocker, another by Solomon in his more recent work, and the other by Jesse Prinz.

Emotions as embodied appraisals

Prinz (2004) follows James and Damasio in claiming that emotions are 'gut reactions' rather than cognitive states. In the process, he provides a detailed account of how something can be a bodily feeling and at the same time be about something outside of the body. He observes that the term 'cognitive' is seldom adequately defined and offers a definition according to which a state is cognitive if it (a) involves mental representations and (b) either originates from or is maintained by organismic control, which, he proposes, is something accomplished by 'executive systems' in the prefrontal cortex (2004, p.46). Prinz claims that most emotions are passive states, rather than states that we actively control; they are more like percepts that we are presented with than concepts that we manipulate. He attempts to reconcile this view of emotions as non-cognitive with the view that they are appraisals by maintaining that they are 'embodied appraisals'; bodily feelings that represent organism–environment relations:

> Appraisal theories claim that emotions necessarily comprise representations of organism–environment relations with respect to well-being. An embodied appraisal theory

says that such representations can be inextricably bound up with states that are involved in the detection of bodily changes. (2004, p.52)

How can perceptions of bodily states represent or be *about* organism–environment relations? Prinz adopts a teleosemantic theory of mental representation in order to explain how bodily feelings can be about something other than the body.[5] According to his account, X represents Y if it carries information about Y and is susceptible to error. Susceptibility to error is understood in terms of 'proper function'. The heart has the proper function of pumping the blood and it errs when it fails to do so. It has this function in virtue of the fact that organs of its kind have been evolutionarily adapted to pump the blood. Teleosemantic theories apply the same conception of function to mental states. According to Prinz, 'a mental state represents whatever it has the function of detecting' (2004, p.186) and its function is to detect something 'if it has been set in place by learning or evolution to detect that thing' (2004, p.54). Emotions such as sadness, he suggests, are indeed perceptions of bodily states but they also represent other things, in virtue of the fact that they are reliably associated with those things as a consequence of historical selection and/or learning. They 'track' their objects by 'monitoring changes in the body' (2004, p.86). This account allows that a representation can be a lot simpler than what it represents. So a simple, non-conceptual feeling can represent a complicated state of affairs. Prinz claims that the proper objects of emotion are not concrete entities, events or situations, but 'formal objects'; meaning more abstract relations such as loss, achievement or threat. Sadness, for example, reliably detects and therefore represents loss. He applies the same account to moods, which detect 'how one is faring overall' (2004, p.188).

A problem with this account is that it completely dissociates the intentionality of emotion from the relevant phenomenology. In addition to this, the criteria that something has to fulfil in order to be an intentional or 'representational' state are so minimal that all sorts of unlikely candidates turn out to be intentional in character. For example, it seems that pupil dilation is 'about' decreased light intensity, as it reliably detects decreased light intensity and has an appropriate history. The same goes for thermostats and smoke alarms, which reliably detect temperature and smoke, respectively. Any account that applies equally to human cognition and to smoke alarms will not cast light on the nature of emotional experience or experience more generally, given that

---

[5] The 'teleosemantic' approach to mental representation appeals to the notion of 'proper function' or 'biological purpose' in order to specify what a mental state is about, the aim being to provide a naturalistic account of intentionality (meaning an account that does not appeal to anything outside of the scientifically described world). It originates in the work of Millikan (1984) and Papineau (1987).

state X can meet all the requirements for representing Y without having any phenomenology. The account does not have the conceptual resources with which to address the phenomenology of feeling because it has nothing at all to say about experience. In fact, a feeling—emotional or otherwise—could be an experience of one thing but be 'about' something else. A feeling of hunger, for example, would surely 'represent' a relation between self and world, that of needing food. But this would not threaten in any way the claim that hunger is experienced exclusively as an internal, bodily state. If one wanted to show that the *experience* of hunger was not exhausted by the experience of a bodily state, this would be a very different matter.

There is nothing to stop people from using the term 'intentionality' to refer to an evolved, learned or designed correspondence between detectors and what they detect. But this is quite different from a phenomenological conception, and the two should not be confused. In what follows, I will concern myself only with intentionality construed phenomenologically (which is how the term 'intentionality' was originally used, before some philosophers started using it to mean something different). I will argue that all intentional states are structured by an experiential background and that this background always incorporates feeling. 'Intentionality', characterized as a relation between two objects in the world (one of which represents the other) and without any reference to the structure of experience, is either a misleading abstraction from the richness of experience or something else entirely.

In addition to dissociating the intentionality of feelings from their phenomenology, Prinz continues to assume the usual distinction between bodily feelings and world-experience. He claims that, in some occurrences of emotion, a cognitive judgement precedes the embodied appraisal and that, in such cases, only the latter is to be identified with the emotion. For example, 'when romantic jealousy occurs, there is first a judgement to the effect that one's lover has been unfaithful and then an embodied appraisal' (2004, pp.98–9).[6] But Prinz also acknowledges that emotion and judgement are not always separable in this way. He distinguishes 'state emotions', such as being in a state of panic, from 'attitudinal emotions', which are 'ways of construing objects or states of affairs emotionally', and concedes that, whilst the former consist

---

[6] This claim is contentious and the relevant phenomenology is, I think, considerably more complicated. The judgement that a lover has been unfaithful could originate in a feeling of suspicion. Indeed, feeling and judgement might well merge into one. It is not at all clear that they can be cleanly disentangled or that one but not the other should be treated as the emotion. Furthermore, the judgement that a lover has been unfaithful could be gradually formed over a prolonged period, its formation involving a range of feelings. Othello did not simply judge that Desdemona had been unfaithful and then feel jealous.

solely of embodied appraisals, the latter do not.[7] When you are angry about something, your thoughts about it are sometimes *part* of your anger (2004, pp.180–1). Thus it would seem that only an emotion that is felt as a bodily state, an emotion with an exclusively *bodily* phenomenology, has an embodied appraisal as its sole ingredient. At most, what Prinz shows is that some states with a bodily phenomenology are also about (in a non-phenomenological sense of 'about') something else too. This does not challenge the assumption that the relevant phenomenology is wholly internal. However, the intentionality of emotion that has troubled other philosophers is precisely the intentionality of *attitudinal* emotions. In these cases, the feeling does not just *track* something other than a bodily state; it also seems to contribute to the *experience* of what it tracks.[8]

Emotions as bodily judgements

An account that does address the phenomenology of feeling is offered by Solomon in some of his most recent work. The later Solomon concedes that the view he offered in *The Passions* is guilty of neglecting the body. He acknowledges that feelings are not, as he once maintained, a 'secondary concern' and that they do need to be accommodated by a theory of emotion (2003, p.189). Solomon suggests that this task requires abandoning the 'fuzzy and ultimately content-free notion of "affect"' and reconceptualizing feelings as ways of engaging with the world (2004a, p.85). He does not resign himself to the view that emotions are 'judgements plus affects' but makes a case for the incorporation of what are usually referred to as 'affects' into the category 'judgement'. Appealing to Heidegger (whose work I will discuss in Chapter 2), Solomon observes that most of our dealings with the world are practical, engaged, habitual and unthinking, rather than reflective and theoretical. Given this, he invokes the category of kinaesthetic judgements or '*judgements of the body*' (2003, p.191). An example of such a judgement would be reaching out to catch a ball and adjusting one's hand in a way that reflects the ball's speed,

---

[7] I am doubtful of the distinction between attitudinal and state emotions. I suspect that in at least some cases it is illusory, a linguistic artefact. For example, I can be angry with you and in a state of anger but I am not undergoing two different emotions; they are different descriptions of the same thing.

[8] Another philosopher who claims that an affect can be an appraisal is Greenspan (2004, p.132): 'Affect evaluates! Emotional affect or feeling is itself evaluative—and the result can be summed up in a proposition. I think we can have it both ways, that is, about emotions as feelings or judgements'. Unlike Prinz, she does not carve off the intentionality of affect from the experience of affect, but neither does she offer a detailed account of how it is that affect succeeds in evaluating.

size and shape. The adjustment of the hand *is* a judgement regarding the properties of the approaching object. Hence the judgement is not something that one consciously makes; it is embodied in the activity. Solomon argues that the so-called 'affective' dimension of emotion can be reinterpreted in terms of judgement, if it is modelled on these practical, habitual judgements:

> I now agree that feelings have been 'left out' of the cognitive account, but I also believe that 'cognition' or 'judgement' properly construed captures the missing ingredient. The analogy with kinesthetic judgements suggests the possibility of bringing feelings of the body into the analysis of emotion in a straightforward way. (2003, pp.189–90)

Solomon continues to maintain that emotional judgements are 'constitutive of experience' (2003, p.95), manifesting themselves as the meaningful, significant, everyday world that we take for granted in our activities. However, given the comparison with kinaesthetic judgements, his early emphasis on the extent to which we choose our emotions now appears unsustainable. Solomon claims that emotions are like perceptual judgements, in that they are 'pre-reflective and inarticulate' (2003, p.97). But we do not choose our perceptual judgements. He concedes this, to some extent at least, and renounces his strong claim to the effect that we are always responsible for all of our emotions. Emotional judgement is, he now claims, 'a complex, multidimensional phenomenon, some aspects of which are clearly within our control and some of which are not' (2003, p.210). So we can admit that some habitual judgements are not under our control in any informative sense, whilst maintaining that others, perhaps the majority, are. Solomon also recognizes that the line between what we are and are not responsible for is blurred; not every-thing can be categorized either as 'deliberate action' or 'straightforward passivity' (2004b, p.15).

In acknowledging the heterogeneity of emotional judgements, Solomon waters down the category 'judgement' to such an extent that the claim 'emotions are judgements' does not appear to tell us very much anymore. He claims that non-human animals make judgements too, such as 'whether something is worth eating, worth chasing, or worth courting', acknowledging in the process that they are not responsible for their emotions (2003, p.187). But, if cases such as a fish being disposed to eat something and a cat being disposed to chase a mouse are to be admitted as judgements, then 'judgement' is broad enough to accommodate just about any behavioural disposition, however simple or automated.

Furthermore, it is unclear whether or not the category 'judgement' now incorporates *all* of those phenomena previously termed 'feelings' or 'affects'. If it does, then Solomon's account has dispensed with the distinction between cognition and affect only by widening 'judgement' to such an extent that it encompasses pretty much everything that an organism thinks, feels, does and undergoes. However, it is not clear that the analogy with kinaesthetic judgements is quite so accommodating. The judgement that a ball is approaching from a certain angle and at a certain speed, which is partly embodied in one's activities as one tries to catch it, is different in phenomenological character from a feeling of discomfort in one's abdomen. In the former case, the bodily judgement is integral to the structure of goal-directed activity. In the latter, the feeling is not so directly connected to interaction with worldly situations. So some feelings might be re-interpreted as non-conceptual, kinaesthetic judgements that cannot be dissociated from activity, but others are not amenable to such an analysis. The kinds of visceral feelings that are associated with emotion fall into the latter category. Do these remain 'mere feelings', fleas on the homeless dog of emotion, or are they somehow phenomenologically rich engagements with the world?

Of course, visceral feelings do influence our engagements with the world. Running to catch a ball is not so appetizing a prospect when you have a terrible pain across your abdomen. Feelings like this shape world-experience too; the world surely looks somehow different when one feels nauseous. But the question of how such feelings (emotional and non-emotional alike) structure our experience and influence our activity is not answered by an account that emphasizes kinaesthetic judgements. Some feelings are just too passive, too cut-off from specific practical activities to be regarded as kinaesthetic judgements. Hence the category 'judgement' is either too general to illuminate, insofar as it includes itches, indigestion, headaches, ball-catching and complex rational appraisals, or it continues to exclude some of the feelings that feature in emotion.

As mentioned earlier in this chapter, there is also a need to distinguish a sense of belonging to the world from those judgements that we make *within* a world. In Chapter 4, I will appeal to Husserl's account of kinaesthetic feelings in order to draw the distinction. In the process, I will endorse—to some extent—the approach taken by Solomon. However, Husserl's phenomenological account of these feelings differs from Solomon's. Central to my own account will be the role that Husserl ascribes to bodily feelings in setting up a space of *possibilities* that is presupposed by all instances of judgement.

Bodily feelings and feelings towards

It could be that some of the feelings involved in emotional experience are experiences of bodily states and that others are not. This view is endorsed by Goldie (2000, 2002, 2004), Stocker and Hegeman (1996) and Stocker (2004).[9]

---

[9] The relevant chapters of Stocker and Hegeman (1996) have Stocker as their sole author. Hence I refer to the view as his rather than theirs.

Goldie acknowledges that feeling and world-directedness are not always experientially distinct components of emotion and that 'emotional feelings are inextricably intertwined with the world-directed aspect of emotion' (2004, p.97). He suggests that emotional feelings fall into two categories. There are 'bodily feelings', which are intentional states directed exclusively at the body. These can 'borrow' world-directed intentionality from other intentional states that they arise in conjunction with. And there are also 'feelings towards', which are intentional states that do not have the body as their object. They cannot be analysed into a feeling component *and* a world-directed component, as the 'feeling towards' is inextricable from world-directed intentionality:

> Feeling towards is unreflective emotional engagement with the world beyond the body; it is not a consciousness of oneself, either of one's bodily condition or of oneself *as* experiencing an emotion. (Goldie, 2002, p.241)

Goldie recognizes that the intentionality and phenomenology of emotion are inseparable. Feelings have a phenomenology and the intentionality of emotion incorporates feeling. Therefore, the intentionality of emotion cannot be treated independently of a phenomenology that 'infuses both attitude and content' (Goldie, 2002, p.242).

A similar point is made by Stocker, who is critical of cognitive approaches that downplay feelings:

> Intellectualization involves dividing emotions, and other affectively laden elements, into two parts, one with affect and the other just with proposition-like content. It then involves repressing, dissociating from, or otherwise ignoring those affective elements, while keeping accessible what is 'of the intellect', the nonaffective component, such as thoughts as propositional content and the neutral, nonaffective holding of that content. (2004, p.144)

Stocker stresses that emotions are essentially *felt*. To accommodate the feeling dimension of emotion, he adopts a similar strategy to that of Goldie, distinguishing *bodily feelings* from *psychic feelings* and emphasizing the latter as constituents of emotion (Stocker and Hegeman, 1996, pp.18–19). He does not offer an account of what bodily feelings actually are but instead assumes that what is merely bodily cannot play a significant role in emotional experience.

Although these authors are right to recognize that some feelings are inextricable from experience of the world, I think they are mistaken in claiming that there are two different kinds of feeling involved. Goldie acknowledges that, in some cases, bodily feelings and feelings towards are seemingly inseparable: 'the bodily feeling is thoroughly infused with the intentionality of the emotion; and, in turn, the feeling towards is infused with a bodily characterization' (2000, p.57). Stocker similarly observes that 'various feelings seem at once both bodily and psychic' (Stocker and Hegeman, 1996, p.19).

However, because it is assumed from the outset that bodily feelings do not have world-directed intentionality, the distinction between experience of the body and experience of the world is preserved, with bodily feelings on one side and psychic feelings on the other.

If we aspire to respect the phenomenology of emotion, what is required is an account of how something can be both a bodily feeling *and* a feeling towards something else. After all, the motivation for invoking feelings towards or psychic feelings is phenomenological. And, as both Goldie and Stocker recognize, the phenomenology which motivates the view that at least some feelings are not just feelings of the body also fails to respect a clear distinction between feelings that are and feelings that are not of the body. Furthermore, if feelings towards or psychic feelings are not feelings of the body, it is not at all clear what they do consist of or what gives them their *felt* character.

My approach in what follows will be to argue that distinctions between world-directed and bodily feelings involve double-counting; bodily feelings just are feelings towards. Some are principally feelings towards the body or parts of it and others are feelings towards things outside the body. However, the phenomenology of feeling does not respect clear-cut distinctions between body and world. Most, if not all, feelings are not of *the world in isolation from the body* or of *the body in isolation from the world*. It sometimes looks as though this is the direction Goldie wants to take too: 'the phenomenology of emotion is such that we experience bodily feelings and feelings towards almost as one' (Goldie, 2002, p.247).[10]

Feeling is not 'mere affect'

So far, I have discussed three recent accounts that challenge the distinction between intentionality and affect, and suggested that they are all importantly incomplete. Prinz unites intentionality and feeling by ignoring experience altogether. Solomon widens the category 'judgement' to such an extent that it is unclear what a judgement is or how the judgements that some call 'feelings' differ from other kinds of judgement. Goldie and Stocker acknowledge the world-directedness of emotional feeling but continue to impose a distinction between bodily and non-bodily feelings. This distinction, I have suggested, does not respect a phenomenology that they themselves acknowledge. What is

----

[10] That bodily feelings and feelings towards are inextricable is suggested by Drummond (2004, p.115), although he does not go into the matter at length: 'I must emphasize that we must be careful not to distinguish these different kinds of feelings too sharply; they are intertwined with one another in complex and various ways. Indeed, they are the same feelings considered in two different relations, once in relation to the body and once in relation to the object'.

needed is an account of how something can be both a bodily feeling and a feeling towards. The remainder of Part I will be concerned with formulating a phenomenological account along just such lines. Bodily feelings, I will argue, are neither states that are altogether bereft of intentionality nor states that can have only the body or a part of it as their object. Instead, they are part of the structure of intentionality. To briefly explain, a feeling need not be, first and foremost, an experience of some part of the body where it is felt to occur. The feeling can be a way in which something other than the body is experienced, rather than itself being the object of experience. Things are experienced *through* bodily feelings and the body itself may or may not be the most salient *object* of feeling. Even when it is not the object of experience, it still *feels* in a way that is phenomenologically accessible.

In addition, it is not simply the case that bodily feelings can have *either* the body *or* something else as their object. A strict contrast between bodily and non-bodily objects of experience needs to be abandoned in order to understanding certain feelings. Solomon's work gestures towards a distinction between judgements that we make within a world and others that constitute a presupposed sense of belonging to the world. As discussed in the Introduction, a similar distinction is made by Husserl in his account of the natural attitude. In what follows, I will argue that this sense of belonging is constituted by feeling and that the relevant feelings are not experiences of *just the body* or of *just the world*. Rather the two aspects of experience are phenomenologically inextricable. My primary task will be to offer a phenomenological account of those feelings that constitute how we find ourselves in the world, what Solomon refers to as the 'meaning of life'. However, in the process I will also argue that feelings more generally are not simply of the body or of the world, but involve a relationship between the two in which one, the other or neither might occupy the experiential foreground.

The nature and role of feelings has been eclipsed by the commonplace assumption that all bodily feelings are experiences of bodily states and also by an over-emphasis on the issue of how they are integrated into *emotional* experience. Many of the feelings referred to in everyday conversation, in literature and also in the context of psychiatry are not to be found on standard lists of emotions, alongside fear, anger, happiness, disgust, sadness, grief, guilt, jealousy, joy, envy and so on. As noted by Campbell (1997, pp.4–6), 'conceptually well-behaved' emotions are only a 'subset of feelings'. Regardless of whether emotions *are* feelings or whether they *incorporate* feelings, the fact remains that most of the feelings that people refer to do not crop up in discussions of 'emotions':

> It is only sometimes that we express our emotions, express 'how we are feeling' by referring to a classic emotion, such as anger, jealousy, or love. Often our feelings are too nuanced, complex, or inchoate to be easily categorized. (Campbell, 1997, p.3)

In addition, many references to feeling suggest that the experiences in question are neither of bodily states nor of specific objects in the world. Consider the following list:

The feeling of being: 'complete', 'flawed and diminished', 'unworthy', 'humble', 'separate and in limitation', 'at home', 'a fraud', 'slightly lost', 'overwhelmed', 'abandoned', 'stared at', 'torn', 'disconnected from the world', 'invulnerable', 'unloved', 'watched', 'empty', 'in control', 'powerful', 'completely helpless', 'part of the real world again', 'trapped and weighed down', 'part of a larger machine', 'at one with life', 'at one with nature', 'there', 'real'.[11]

At least some of these seem to be ways of experiencing the self, the world and also the self–world relation, the three aspects being inextricable. They are existential orientations, ways of finding oneself in a world that operate as a background to all experience, thought and activity. We could perhaps widen the category of 'emotion' so as to encompass these feelings. Stocker takes this approach, in claiming that some emotions take the form of subtle, all-encompassing ways of experiencing, rather than being episodic relations to particular objects. They are, he says, 'diffuse, pervasive, and long lasting, forming our background, as well as the tone, the color, the affective taste, the feeling of activities, relations, and experiences' (2004, p.137). However, such feelings are not always categorized as emotions. For example, Stern proposes that there is a distinctive category of affective phenomena to be distinguished here, which has not been adequately explored. He refers to these affective phenomena as 'relational affects' and takes them to include relations such as the feelings of 'being loved, esteemed, thought wonderful, special, or hated, and the feelings of being secure, safe, attached, alone, isolated, or separated' (1993, p.207).

Both approaches have their problems. Widening the category 'emotion' so as to include existential orientations obscures the important difference between states that are intentionally directed at particular objects, events or situations in the world, and others that constitute backgrounds to all our experiences, thoughts and activities. The category of relational affects similarly fails to differentiate between object- or person-specific feelings of relatedness and an all-embracing background feeling of belonging. The world as a whole can sometimes appear unfamiliar, unreal, distant or close. It can be something that one feels apart from or at one with. One can feel in control of one's overall situation or overwhelmed by it. One can feel like a participant in the world or like a detached, estranged observer staring at objects that do not feel quite 'there'. Such relationships structure all experience. Whenever one has a specifically focused experience of oneself, another person or an inanimate object

---

[11] All of these examples were obtained by typing 'the feeling of being' into the Internet search engine Google on 12 February 2005 and selecting from the first 50 hits.

being a certain way, the experience has, as a background, a more general sense of one's relationship with the world. This relationship does not simply consist in an experience of being an entity that occupies a spatial and temporal location, alongside a host of other entities. Ways of finding oneself in a world are spaces of possibility, which determine the various ways in which things can be experienced. For example, if one's sense of the world is tainted by a 'feeling of unreality', this will affect how all objects of perception appear; they are distant, removed, not quite 'there'.

These ways of finding oneself in a world are usually described as 'feelings', rather than 'emotions', 'moods' or 'thoughts'. Of course, some of the 'feelings' I listed earlier might well have other ingredients and some may be directed towards situations *within* the world, rather than being all-encompassing existential backgrounds. For example, the feeling of being a fraud could involve an appraisal of one's status, abilities and conduct in a specific context. In addition to a 'bodily feeling', there might be elaborate, intertwined narratives concerning one's relationships with others, plus an evaluation of one's abilities. Many other 'feelings' are clearly not just 'ways of finding oneself in the world'. Take, for example, 'the feeling of being a true American', which involves interpretations of nationality and nationhood, or 'the feeling of being rejected by God', which is a specifically theistic interpretation or expression of one's predicament. The term 'feeling' is also employed to describe what it is like to be in quite specific situations. Think of 'the feeling of being on Brighton beach on a hot summer day'.[12] So Nussbaum (2001, 2004) is right to point out that 'feeling' has diverse uses. Even so, I suggest that certain uses of the term 'feeling' do pick out a distinctive phenomenological category. Feelings belong to this category in virtue of two shared characteristics. First of all, they are not directed at specific objects or situations but are background orientations through which experience as a whole is structured. Second, they are *bodily feelings*. As these feelings constitute the basic structure of 'being there', a 'hold on things' that functions as a presupposed context for all intellectual and practical activity, I refer to them as *existential feelings*.

Much of the language used to convey existential feelings is metaphorical, and the metaphors employed generally allude to relationships between the body and the world. For example, the world can feel 'overbearing', 'overwhelming' or 'suffocating'. One can feel 'trapped' in a situation, 'invulnerable' or 'part of something greater', and the world as a whole can be 'distant' or 'close'. I will argue that this kind of language is no accident. The feelings that

---

[12] Again, these three examples are taken from the first 50 hits that appeared when I used Google to search for 'the feeling of being'.

such talk expresses are indeed *bodily* but they are, at the same time, ways of relating to the world.

As stated in the Introduction, this is a book about existential feelings in psychiatric illness and everyday life, rather than about emotions. But I should at least say something about the relationship between the two. There are numerous competing conceptions of emotion. According to Damasio and several others who offer neurobiological accounts, emotions are physiological states that need not be felt. When they are felt, the '*feelings are the mental representation of the physiologic changes that occur during an emotion*' (Damasio, 2004, pp.52–3). If some such account of emotion is accepted, then existential feelings are clearly different from emotions, as existential feelings are—in some sense at least—felt. They are not like Damasio's 'feelings' either, as the latter have only the body as their object.

However, in this chapter I have emphasized recent accounts offered by philosophers, as my concern is with the phenomenology of feeling rather than with non-conscious bio-regulatory processes. Most philosophers regard emotions as complicated mental states of which we have at least some awareness, thus implying that certain neurobiological accounts over-simplify things considerably. As Solomon (2004*b*, p.19) stresses, 'an emotion is *not* what happens in the first 120 milliseconds of arousal'. Emotions can take the form of brief episodes, more enduring states or processes, and most, if not all, emotions are intentional in character. If a richer conception of emotion is adopted, some kind of hybrid account might well turn out to be the right way to go, according to which all emotions involve feelings but at least some of them have other ingredients too. According to Goldie, an emotion can be:

> … a relatively complex state, involving past and present episodes of thoughts, feelings, and bodily changes, dynamically related in a narrative of part of a person's life, together with dispositions to experience further emotional episodes, and to act out of the emotion and to express that emotion. (2000, p.144)

I do not wish to deny this, although I do claim that the inclusion of additional ingredients should not be motivated by the assumption that bodily feelings can only be *of* the body or parts of it, given that these feelings are not just experiences of bodily states. I also allow that the emotions, whichever conception one adopts, might turn out to be quite a heterogeneous group, as suggested by Griffiths (1997) amongst others.

How do emotions, conceived of in this way, differ from existential feelings? Existential feelings, I claim, are not hybrid states. They are non-conceptual *feelings* of the body, which constitute a background sense of belonging to the world and a sense of reality. They are not evaluations of any specific object, they are certainly not propositional attitudes and they are not 'mere affects'.

They can be sporadic or sustained and can even amount to entrenched dispositions or temperaments, but they are never absent; all experience is structured by some variant of existential feeling. When one experiences an emotion, one already finds oneself in the world. And the way in which one finds oneself in the world disposes one to certain kinds of emotional experience. However, I grant that there is two-way interaction here; emotional episodes, amongst other things, can serve to reshape backgrounds of existential feeling.

The part played by existential feelings in our experience is thus different from that played by most of those states that philosophers refer to as emotions. Whereas emotions are usually directed towards specific objects, events or situations, existential feelings are not *about* anything specific. More importantly, although emotions might structure the ways in which objects are experienced, they are not responsible for our sense of the *being* of those objects. An escaped lion sitting in one's garden might appear as a *frightening lion* but the emotion directed towards it does not exhaust the sense of its existence, of *there being a lion there*. Existential feeling, in contrast, is not just a matter of relatedness; it is a background that comprises the sense of 'being' or 'reality' that attaches to world-experience. For example, people speak of feeling detached from things and, at the same time, of things not seeming quite 'real'. Specifically directed emotions presuppose this background and so, whatever such emotions turn out to consist of, existential feelings are more fundamental to world-experience.

Existential feelings are most amenable to phenomenological reflection when they shift. When this happens, what was an unreflective experiential background becomes conspicuous in its absence. So, in order to make explicit the nature, role and variety of existential feelings, I will focus on some ways in which the structure of world-experience can change. In so doing, I will further emphasize the need to set aside contrasts between internal and external, cognition and affect, and subject and object. Chapter 2 will turn to Heidegger's work, both to reflect upon changing existential feeling and to assist in the escape from body-world dualism.

Chapter 2

Existential feelings

In the last chapter, I proposed that bodily feelings are not just feelings of internal bodily states; they can also contribute to experiences of things outside of the body. In addition, I suggested that certain *feelings* are not experiences of specific entities or of entities in general. Instead, they are ways of finding ourselves in the world, existential backgrounds that shape all our experiences. In this chapter and the next, I will further develop and defend these claims. The aim of the current chapter is to describe the experiential role of existential feeling. Then, in Chapter 3, I will offer a phenomenological account of how something can be both a bodily feeling and an experience of something other than the body.

I have already noted that when philosophers reflect upon experience, they usually impose distinctions between body and world, subject and object or internal and external. These distinctions stem, in part, from a tendency to construe experience as the standoffish, spectatorial contemplation of objects by a curiously detached subject, who is set apart from the world that she somehow experiences. As I will show in this chapter, such thinking fails to recognize the way in which we already *find ourselves in a world* when we encounter something in that way. However detached we might become in relation to a particular object of experience, that experience still presupposes a background orientation, a variable sense of belonging and of reality. I describe the role of this background by drawing on some themes in Heidegger's work. First of all, I sketch the way in which Heidegger challenges commonplace conceptions of experience. Then I show how this paves the way for his characterization of *mood* as something that we find ourselves *in*, which does not conform to a distinction between experience of 'internal' states and of an 'external' world. Following this, two weaknesses in his account are considered and, in the process, the rationale for adopting the term 'existential feeling' instead of 'mood' is made clear. The remainder of the chapter embarks upon a preliminary exploration of the phenomenology of existential feeling, by looking at how it features in autobiographical accounts of schizophrenia and depression, and in literary descriptions of experience. In the process, I discuss the tendency in philosophy of mind and philosophical psychology to over-emphasize *propositional attitudes*. I argue that, like the tendency to conceive of experience as a detached, spectatorial affair, this serves to obscure the phenomenology of existential feeling.

Heidegger on practical understanding

Heidegger is highly critical of the persistent neglect and misinterpretation of affective states in philosophy. He notes how, according to the 'traditional view':

> …affects and feelings come under the theme of psychical phenomena, functioning as a third class of these, usually along with ideation [*Vorstellen*] and volition. They sink to the level of accompanying phenomena. (1962, p.178)[1]

In other words, they are construed as superficial subjective colourations that taint our cognition of the objective world and are therefore of marginal interest when it comes to understanding how we experience, think about and practically engage with the world. Heidegger's own account is a complete reversal of this position. He insists that affective states and, more specifically, moods are not mere icing on the cognitive cake. They are not 'subjective' or 'psychic' phenomena but amount to a background sense of being situated in a world. Although this background is something that we seldom reflect upon, it shapes all our experiences, thoughts and activities. Whatever we experience, we already have a sense of being *there*, of being part of the world. This is not something that can be understood if we think of experience exclusively in terms of a subject gazing upon an object; that kind of thinking is something Heidegger seeks to escape from. Thus, in order to appreciate his account of the experiential role of mood, it is important to understand something of how it fits into his broader project.

Heidegger's primary concern in *Being and Time* is the question of the meaning of Being. The 'Being of beings' is, he says, not 'a being' (1962, p.26). Rather, it is a meaning-giving background that is presupposed by the intelligibility of all the worldly beings that we experience. We can assert of any being that it 'is' or that it 'is not' but all such judgements presuppose a sense of what it is to 'be'. Even if we recognize that something is not, in so doing we presuppose an understanding of what it would mean for that thing to be. Now it might seem that our sense of what it is for something to be is exhausted by the recognition that it occupies a particular spatiotemporal location. Likewise, experience of

---

[1] I shall be referring to Macquarrie and Robinson's 1962 translation of Heidegger's *Being and Time*. Quotations have been amended, with the term 'being' in place of 'entity' and 'attunement' in place of 'state of mind' for *Befindlichkeit*. 'Being' [*Sein*] is capitalized so as to distinguish it from 'being' [*Seiende*]. I will also draw on Heidegger's *Basic Problems of Phenomenology* (Heidegger, 1982) and his essay 'What is Metaphysics?' (Heidegger, 1978a).

oneself as part of the world might be thought to consist in the recognition of oneself as a certain kind of entity occupying a specific place in a spatiotemporal framework, alongside lots of other entities. However, Heidegger claims that such views privilege the epistemic standpoint of a voyeuristic observer, who gazes upon things and registers what is 'out there'. He maintains that this emphasis on detached contemplation has served to obscure the nature of our understanding of Being. The history of philosophy consists, he claims, in a progressive misinterpretation of what that understanding consists of. The misinterpretation and eventual forgetting of Being is possible because our understanding of Being is implicit; it is something that all thoughts and experiences presuppose but is not itself an object of experience and thought, at least not ordinarily.

Heidegger seeks to emancipate himself from this history of misinterpretation and make the sense of Being explicit. The first question to ask is 'where do we start?', given that the usual starting point is inappropriate. Heidegger begins by turning to ourselves. We are the beings that have an implicit understanding of Being. Hence phenomenological enquiry should focus on us in order to investigate what that understanding consists of. Heidegger christens the focus of his investigation '*Dasein*' (meaning roughly 'being-there' or 'being-here'), in order to distance himself from traditional philosophical conceptions of the self as a detached 'subject' that relates to entities in an objective, external world by reaching out to them with its intentional states. He contends that, in construing world-experience in terms of subjects hooking up with objects, philosophers have obscured the way in which we most fundamentally relate to the world and have consequently obscured the nature of our understanding of Being:

> …in this characterization of intentionality as an extant relation between two things extant, a psychical subject and a physical object, the nature as well as the mode of being of intentionality is completely missed. (1982, p.60)

His conception of us as *Dasein*, unlike traditional conceptions of the subject, does not carve us off from the world but emphasizes the fact that we are situated in the world. We find ourselves in it, rather than gazing upon it from some mysterious external standpoint.

The next step is to address how beings are actually experienced by *Dasein*. The usual place to start is with beings as encountered through a detached, somewhat theoretical stance; beings that are encountered as 'present-at-hand' [*Vorhanden*]. However, Heidegger considers the possibility that beings as encountered in some other way might provide a better clue to the structure of our understanding of Being, a more appropriate starting point for his phenomenological enquiry. He notes that much of the time we do not come across beings in a standoffish way, as present-at-hand objects. Instead, we encounter them as 'ready-to-hand' [*Zuhanden*]. That is, as things to be used in a context of ongoing activity.[2]

These two ways of relating to beings are quite different in their phenomenological character. I might stare at an entity in a detached fashion, contemplating its shape, its position and its various features. If we model all experience on this kind of encounter, then subject becomes detached from object, viewer from viewed. But, as I am writing this paragraph, consider my relations with the various objects around me. I do not look upon the computer keyboard in such a way; I use it. And I do not first perceive the keys as discrete entities, then assign a functional role to them and finally act upon them. Rather, I encounter the keyboard as something useable, as something that has immediate practical significance in the context of my project. Indeed, the term 'encounter' is perhaps misleading. I do not 'encounter' the keyboard at all, in the sense of coming across it as an entity that is distinct from what I am doing. I do not contemplate it as an 'object' whilst I type; it is a participant in my activities. The keyboard is understood practically, in the context of certain dealings, and this is quite different from an explicit, theoretical understanding of it as something presented to my gaze.[3] Furthermore, it is not understood as an isolated entity but as something that is bound up with numerous other tools that are seamlessly integrated into my current project, including the chair I am sitting on, the glass of water I unthinkingly sip from and the mouse that I skilfully move without reflecting upon my actions. My office as a whole takes the form of a functionally interrelated web of equipment, where everything has its place in relation to everything else—the telephone, the pile of articles, the note with reminders of several dozen things I need to do on Monday, the shoes on the floor, the light switch, the table, the kettle, the cups, the sugar bowl and the coffee jar. All of these are tacitly understood in terms of their practical significance and, in many cases, their established functions. I do not pit myself against them as I use them. When I skilfully use a tool such as a pen, my experience does not make a clear distinction between me and it. The pen and my hand merge seamlessly in a context of practical activity. Understanding beings as ready-to-hand thus differs from present-at-hand contemplation in two important respects. First of all, ready-to-hand beings are not related to each only in so far as they occupy positions in a common space–time; they knit together as a cohesive functional whole. Second, as we skilfully employ tools and become unreflectively absorbed in our activities, we do not cleanly distinguish ourselves from them.

....

[2] See *Being and Time*, Part 1, Division 1, III: 'The Worldhood of the World'.

[3] See also Merleau-Ponty (1962, p.144) for a description of the phenomenology of typing.

Of course, the difference between unthinking practical activity and a reflective contemplation of objects that wholly removes itself from their practical significance is a matter of degrees. As I turn to look at my glass of water, I do see an object; the glass does not wholly 'disappear' into my activities. However, it is not completely purged of its functionality either. It still appears as something to be used in a particular way, and is positioned functionally in relation to a host of other items. As will become clear towards the end of this chapter, experiencing something as wholly stripped of its practical significance and extricated from any relationship to potential activities is highly unusual.

In emphasizing readiness-to-hand [*Zuhandenheit*], Heidegger does not want to claim that presence-at-hand reduces to readiness-to-hand or rests on top of it in a relation of asymmetric dependence. He explicitly states that the practical attitude does not have 'priority' over the theoretical attitude (1962, p.238). His aim is to draw attention to the way in which philosophical thinking has been restricted by its exclusive emphasis on presence-at-hand [*Vorhandenheit*], which is in fact only one of the ways in which we encounter beings. However, he does maintain that an emphasis on readiness-to-hand is more phenomenologically illuminating when it comes to revealing the understanding of Being that is implicit in our experiences of things. In order to characterize that understanding, we must first characterize what is understood. What we understand is not just some specific being but the 'world' in which such beings are encountered. Regardless of whether we contemplate something or use it, our experience is never of that thing in isolation from everything else. All experiences incorporate the sense that we are *in* the world; we encounter things within that presupposed context.

If we consider only presence-at-hand, the experience of belonging to a world might be characterized as that of being an entity with a particular location relative to other entities. But Heidegger suggests that our sense of being part of the world is not like this at all. The world is not experienced in an object-like way. Instead, it is a realm of practical, purposive relations that we *inhabit*. Any encounter with an object, present-at-hand or ready-to-hand, is embedded in this pre-understood context of purposive relations. To illustrate this, Heidegger reflects upon what we experience when our relations with tools break down. The keyboard that disappears into my activities becomes conspicuous or 'un-ready-to-hand' when it fails to function. As I type and nothing appears on the screen, the keyboard is extricated from my activities and appears as something that stands in the way of my project. Equipment can become conspicuous in various ways—when it is damaged, missing, inappropriate or otherwise disruptive. And this, Heidegger says, is a first step on the way to contemplation of it as present-at-hand. It becomes partially removed from a network of functionality, disconnected from a project. As we look upon it, the possibility arises of its further extrication from our dealings, of its appearance as pure presence-at-hand, with all its practical significance lost. Understanding something as present-at-hand thus requires a kind of withdrawal from the ready-to-hand, a loss of immediate practical significance. In this transition from readiness to presence, something else happens too:

> When an assignment to some particular 'towards-this' has been thus circumspectively aroused, we catch sight of the 'towards-this' itself, and along with it everything connected with the work—the whole 'work-shop'—as that wherein concern always dwells. The context of equipment is lit up, not as something never seen before, but as a totality constantly sighted beforehand in circumspection. With this totality, however, the world announces itself. (1962, p.105)

When something breaks down, the associated experiential change is not restricted to the item in question. As a project is disrupted, so is unthinking practical immersion in it. We momentarily stop taking for granted a web of practical purposes and instead become fleetingly aware of it; the whole context of our equipmental dealings is lit up. Hence it is when practical dealings get disrupted that our background understanding of the world comes briefly into focus. This world is not an object and it is not the totality of objects. It is a teleological background structure, a realm of practical significance that one finds oneself bound up with before one looks upon or uses anything. The experience of being *there* is not a matter of being plonked into a spatial location but of being practically situated in an interconnected web of purposes, an appreciation of which is inseparable from practical activity. We are not *in* the world like peas sitting passively in a pod. Our activities and our sense of being part of the world are inextricable; the world shows up as a space of practical, purposive possibilities that we are entwined with.

Having characterized how we find ourselves in the world, Heidegger is now able to enquire into the structure of our understanding of Being. The world is an enabling context for any encounter with beings, whether practical or theoretical. To describe the understanding that makes this context possible is to offer a description of our understanding of Being. The kind of 'possibility' in question is not a matter of causal facilitation but of a tacit understanding that renders the world *intelligible*.

Heidegger's discussion proceeds in two stages. He first characterizes our understanding of Being as 'care' [*Sorge*]. The world is a web of purposive relations: the 'in-order-to', the 'towards-which', the 'towards-this' and the 'for-the-sake-of' (1962, p.415). So the structure of care consists of whatever it is that makes such relations possible. Care is a condition of possibility for apprehending the world as a significant whole, as an arena of possible projects, goals and purposes. Heidegger offers a lengthy discussion of the constituents of care and then goes on to consider what might be presupposed by the possibility of care itself, maintaining that our understanding of Being is ultimately comprised of temporality. As my aim here is to explore the phenomenological contribution made by affective states, I will leave most of this aside and address only one aspect of care: mood [*Stimmung*].

Heidegger on mood

The possibilities of purposively engaging with anything, of striving towards a goal, of valuing something, of registering something as practically salient and of pursuing a project all presuppose a sense of things 'mattering' to us (Heidegger, 1962, p.176). We don't assign values to preconceived present-at-hand objects but inhabit a context of significance through which things are encountered as mattering. According to Heidegger, it is moods that allow things to matter. He states that one of three inextricable ingredients of care is *Befindlichkeit* (e.g. 1962, p.172), the other two being understanding [*Verstehen*] and discourse [*Rede*]. '*Befindlichkeit*' is not an easy term to translate. Dreyfus (1991, p.168) notes that no English term seems to capture its sense and settles for 'affectedness'. Harr (1992, p.159) similarly describes it as 'primordial affectivity' or 'affectedness'. Macquarrie and Robinson, in their translation of *Being and Time*, rather misleadingly refer to it throughout as 'state of mind'. Although this might seem to approximate the meaning of the German term, it is inappropriate when applied to Heidegger's view. In challenging the subject–object distinction and emphasizing practical engagement with equipment over detached cognition of objects, Heidegger rejects distinctions such as that between an internal 'mind' and an external 'world'. Such distinctions fail to convey the ordinarily taken-for-granted structure of experience, which involves unitary, purposive belonging, rather than minds making contact with an external world. Even when an experience does incorporate a contrast between oneself and something else, that experience continues to presuppose a unitary structure of belonging and it is *Befindlichkeit* that makes this structure possible. In what follows, I will adopt Stambaugh's translation of it as 'attunement' (from her 1996 translation of Heidegger's *Being and Time*), a term that does not presuppose anything of the subject–object or internal–external model of experience and thought that Heidegger is trying to leave behind.

By 'attunement', Heidegger seeks to convey the way in which moods constitute a sense of belonging to the world. They do so by revealing the world as a realm of practical purposes, values and goals. The world that we take for granted in our activities is a background of significance, a space of potential purposive activities that frames all our experiences. So a mood does not 'colour' some already experienced world. It is what opens up a world in the first place; it is through moods that we find ourselves in a world. For Heidegger, mood is *primordial*, meaning that it is presupposed by the intelligibility of all our experiences, thoughts and activities. Moods are not subjective or psychic phenomena. We do not experience them as mental states inside of us, to be contrasted with a non-mental outside. When we distinguish inside from outside we do so against the backdrop of a pre-given world that is opened up by mood: 'a mood assails us. It come neither from 'outside' nor from 'inside', but arises out of Being-in-the-world, as a way of such Being' (1962, p.176).

Hence moods do not feature in our phenomenology as states of 'subjects'. A subject does not *have* a mood but is *in* a mood. Regardless of whether we encounter something as present-at-hand or ready-to-hand, we already find ourselves in the world where that encounter takes place. It is mood that constitutes this presupposed sense of belonging to the world, the context in which encounters with things are experientially possible: '*The mood has already disclosed, in every case, Being-in-the-world as a whole, and makes it possible first of all to direct oneself towards something*' (1962, p.176). Intentionality is not therefore a matter of an otherworldly subject reaching out so as to mysteriously hook up with an entity or collection of entities called 'the world'. This is a misleading abstraction, which leaves out the fact that, before one directs oneself towards anything, one is already *there*. A mood is not an intentional state directed at either the self or something other than the self and it is not a more encompassing intentional state directed at lots of things. It is a condition of possibility for any specifically directed intentional state.[4]

As moods are constitutive of our understanding of Being, we cannot escape them altogether. The only way to escape a mood is by way of another mood. Even when we are not aware of being in a particular mood, the apparent lack of mood is itself a mode of attunement, a way of finding oneself in the world: 'The pallid, evenly balanced lack of mood [*Ungestimmtheit*], which is often persistent and which is not to be mistaken for a bad mood, is far from nothing at all' (1962, p.173).

....

[4] Strasser (1977, chapter 7) offers a similar phenomenological description of *Stimmung* (translated here as 'disposition', rather than 'mood'). For Strasser, as for Heidegger, 'mood' or 'disposition' is not a specifically directed intentional state but something that is presupposed by all such states; it is 'the medium and ground of all experiential life', 'the elementary foundation of experience' (p.182). Strasser also stresses that it is neither subjective nor objective but a unified sense of being in the world that is phenomenologically prior to any distinction between subject and object: 'Do I [ ] lay hold of myself in disposition as a kind of conscious island? One would be very hard pressed indeed to maintain that. Rather, in actual being disposed, no I, no object, no boundary between I and object really appear. [...] I and world are embedded in an undivided experience of totality' (p.188).

What about emotions? Heidegger is not very clear on the relationship between moods and emotions. However, his view seems to be that moods are presupposed by occurrent emotions. Take an instance of fear. This is something that happens in the world rather than something that constitutes Being-in-the-world as a whole. It is a relationship between a person and the object of her fear, which incorporates a way of experiencing self, the object of fear and the relationship between them; the self is 'afraid', the object is 'frightening' and she is 'frightened of it'. But, before one feels afraid, one already has a sense of belonging to the world, of being in a situation *in* which one is afraid. Despite this, Heidegger refers to fear as a 'mood'. But I do not think he is claiming that the *occurrence of fear* is the mood. Instead, he is suggesting that the relevant mood is itself the *possibility of fear*. In other words, one is attuned to the world in such a way that experiences of object-directed fear are possible. Fear, he says, is 'a slumbering possibility of Being-in-the-world', which 'has already disclosed the world, in that out of it something like the fearsome may come close' (1962, p.180). As he goes on to explain, only a being capable of being threatened, a being whose own being matters to it, can be afraid. Hence occurrent emotions presuppose a background of values, purposes and projects that makes it possible for things to matter to us and for us to experience relations such as being under threat.

Heidegger goes on to distinguish different kinds of fear. Commonplace fear is of something familiar. There is also 'dread' [*Grauen*], a fear of the unfamiliar. If we combine the suddenness of the threat with dread, we get 'terror' [*Entsetzen*]. He adds that other kinds of fear include 'timidity, shyness, misgiving, becoming startled' (1962, p.182). In so doing, he seems to run three different things together—specific intentional states, the presupposed moods that make these possible and, in the case of timidity and shyness, character or personality traits. We need not insist on a firm phenomenological distinction between short-lived moods and a more enduring character. At least some of those attributes that are referred to as 'character' and 'personality' traits might well consist of longer term moods or enduring dispositions towards certain kinds of mood. (This is the line that I will take in Chapter 9, when I discuss philosophical 'temperaments'.) But the distinction between intentional states and the moods that they presuppose is more important. Heidegger maintains that moods are not just generalized emotions, where emotions are understood as intentional states directed at particular objects. Hence he makes an important distinction that is not made so clearly by Solomon. As discussed in Chapter 1, Solomon does treat moods as generalized emotions:

> The difference between an emotion and a mood is the difference in what they are *about*. Emotions are about particulars, or particulars generalized; moods are

about nothing in particular, or sometimes they are about our world as a whole. (Solomon, 1993, p.112)

However, the difference between emotions and Heideggerian moods is not just a difference in the generality of their objects. They play very different phenomeno-logical roles: moods set up the world in which we can have specific, object-directed emotions. This phenomenological distinction serves, I think, to clarify what Solomon seeks to convey with the claim that emotions are what make life meaningful. An emotion is, he claims, 'a structure of my world' (1993, p.100), rather than a specific occurrence. Every emotion 'presupposes the entire body of previous emotional judgments to supply its context and its his-tory' (1993, p.137). But, in regarding moods as emotions that are directed at the world as a whole, he fails to characterize the distinctive way in which certain 'emotional' states constitute a sense of belonging that is presupposed by any object-directed state, regardless of how many objects that state might encompass.

It is important to note that the aspect of experience that Heidegger draws attention to is not something that could be brought to light by relying exclu-sively on the metaphysical and epistemological resources of empirical science. In order to enquire into what our sense of the Being of beings consists of, one cannot content oneself with determining what *is* and what *is not* the case. An enquiry into our *sense of what it is for something to be* requires a very differ-ent kind of questioning. We cannot pursue it if we simply presuppose, as empirical scientific enquiry does, an understanding of what it is for some-thing to be. Furthermore, the empirical sciences make certain epistemological assumptions that are not conducive to phenomenological enquiry. Heidegger proposes that the theoretical, detached perspective, which science takes to be epistemically privileged, is in fact just one way of encountering beings; it by no means discloses *how the world is* in a way that is more fundamental than practical attitudes. Hence both philosophy and the empirical sciences have obscured the nature of our understanding of Being by putting one form of understanding (detached cognition) on a pedestal and mistakenly construing it as a privileged vantage point upon the world.

Heidegger claims that all our theoretical and practical activities unavoidably presuppose the world that is disclosed through mood:

> Any cognitive determining has its existential-ontological Constitution in the [attune-ment] of Being-in-the-world; but pointing this out is not to be confused with attempting to surrender science ontically to 'feeling'. (1962, p.177)

He is not suggesting that affective states *replace* theoretical contemplation and rational deliberation. Rather, he is saying that mood is *prior* to them. When science enquires as to what *is*, the world disclosed through mood is something that it already takes for granted but fails to acknowledge. Science does not start off from nowhere. It is embedded in a pre-understood everyday world that is opened up by mood:

> The basic structures of any such area [a science] have already been worked out after a fashion in our pre-scientific ways of experiencing and interpreting that domain of Being in which the area of subject-matter is itself confined. (1962, p.29)

So the sciences, according to Heidegger, cannot legitimately lay claim to an all-encompassing perspective on moods and emotions.

Given that a theoretical, scientific approach is, according to Heidegger, an inadequate means of understanding the phenomenological role of mood, we might wonder how that understanding is to be obtained. In brief, Heidegger's answer is that a particular mood itself serves to reveal to us the way in which moods attune us to the world. There is, he suggests, a fairly consistent, every-day mode of attunement to the world, which most of us are immersed in most of the time.[5] In this state, we are oblivious to the role of mood. We take the familiar world for granted and the mood that makes it possible remains hidden. But occasional perturbations in everyday attunement diminish the sense of practical familiarity, significance and belonging. Sometimes, the world seems *unheimlich* [uncanny]; somehow strange and unfamiliar. (The term '*unheimlich*' is usually translated as 'uncanny' and I will adopt this convention here. However, it should be kept in mind that the German term better conveys the relevant sense of 'not feeling at home in a situation'.) The practical familiarity through which we encounter things is eroded and our 'hold' on the world is weakened. The culmination of this erosion is a mood that Heidegger calls anxiety [*Angst*]. His discussion seems to suggest that anxiety manifests itself as a brief *episode*, rather than an enduring state. It differs from

---

5 According to Heidegger, this everyday way of finding oneself in the world is itself partly responsible for the pervasive misinterpretation of our predicament. In everyday life, the world that is disclosed to us is a public world, configured in terms of practical norms that people unthinkingly abide by. There is a tendency to interpret our activities in terms of these norms, drifting along and doing 'what one does', letting situations guide us. In so doing, we forget that our Being is not exhausted by the possibilities that this world lays out for us. Heidegger suggests that there is a sense of security gained through 'falling' into the publicly interpreted world; it involves a 'tempting, tranquillizing' alienation (1962, p.223). Everyday obliviousness to the constitution of Being-in-the-world and the nature of *Dasein* amounts to what he calls 'inauthenticity', an inadvertent abdication of responsibility for one's projects and activities, where responsibility for 'what is to be done' is transferred to the public norms that configure situations. In Chapter 9, I will argue that something like this does indeed happen. Most ways of being in the world involve obliviousness to the structure of being in the world.

emotional episodes, such as fear, as it does not have a specific intentional object: 'that in the face of which one has anxiety is not an entity within-the-world' (1962, p.231).[6] Anxiety is a complete loss of everyday practical familiarity, an absence of any sense of connectedness to things:

> Here the totality of involvements of the ready-to-hand or present-at-hand discovered within-the-world, is, as such, of no consequence; it collapses into itself; the world has the character of completely lacking significance. (1962, p.231)

The mood that ordinarily binds us to the world breaks down and Heidegger refers to the sense of utter unfamiliarity that arises through this as the 'nothing'. This 'nothing', he explains, is not itself a being. It is a disintegration of everyday belonging; the apprehension of a total absence of significance. One is no longer *there* anymore and all that remains is the feeling of having 'no hold' on anything (Heidegger, 1978a, p.101).

In addition to being an object of Heidegger's enquiry, anxiety plays an important methodological role. It is itself the means whereby the structure of everyday attunement is made accessible to phenomenological reflection (1962, pp.226–7). In everyday life, it is easy to take the world for granted but, when the mood that constitutes a sense of belonging breaks down, what one was previously oblivious to becomes conspicuous in its absence. Of course, it might be objected that occurrences of anxiety are not like that at all. But Heidegger insists that 'real' anxiety is rare and different from various experiences that we might ordinarily refer to by using the term (1962, p.234).

Existential feeling as a phenomenological category

My account of the nature and role of existential feeling will draw on Heidegger's conception of mood. Of central importance are his claims that experience incorporates a background sense of belonging to the world and that this background is changeable in structure, as illustrated by what he calls 'anxiety'. However, Heidegger's account suffers from some serious weaknesses. First of all, he restricts his discussion to only a few variants of mood, focusing on the contrast between everyday mood and anxiety. He also mentions 'elation' (1962, p.173) and, as discussed above, some varieties of fear. A later work also includes a lengthy description of kinds of boredom (Heidegger, 1983, Part I).

---

[6] In Ratcliffe (2002), I suggested that anxiety be treated as an 'emotion' rather than a 'mood', given that it is a brief occurrence rather than a longer term state. I now think that this was a mistake. Calling Heideggerian anxiety an emotion fails to make clear the distinction between within-world emotions and existential orientations that are presupposed by all such emotions.

Heidegger does acknowledge that there is more to be said about the varieties of attunement:

> The different modes of [attunement] and the ways in which they are interconnected in their foundations cannot be Interpreted within the problematic of the present investigation. The phenomena have long been well-known ontically under the terms 'affects' and 'feelings' and have always been under consideration in philosophy. (1962, p.178)

Although at least some of Heidegger's 'moods' have no doubt been discussed by others using the terms 'affect' and 'feeling', it is important to distinguish affective states understood as within-world attitudes from those affective states that constitute the world we inhabit. Although there have been plenty of attempts to distinguish and classify within-world emotions, feelings and affects, nobody has offered a comparably detailed phenomenological account of the various different ways in which we can find ourselves in the world. In addition, some of the predicaments that Heidegger does discuss require more fine-grained differentiation. Consider anxiety, for instance. It is arguable that Heideggerian 'anxiety' encompasses a range of subtly different experiences. For example, Glas (2003) describes a number of what he calls 'fundamental', 'basic' or 'existential anxieties', all of which he regards as ways of being in the world, rather than focused conscious states. One form of anxiety he describes is a feeling of disconnectedness from the world:

> What prevails is a tormenting feeling of distance, the awareness of an unbridgeable gap. This feeling can amount to the awareness that one lives in a vacuum and is about to suffocate, or that one lives in an unreal world in which things [are not] what they seem to be and in which attempts to connect fail as if there were a glassy wall between the person and the surrounding world. (2003, p.238)

This looks fairly close to Heidegger's account of 'anxiety revealing the nothing', but Glas distinguishes it from several other kinds of existential anxiety, including anxiety concerning meaningless, anxiety in the face of death and anxiety before existence itself, any one of which might be plausibly identified with Heidegger's anxiety.

Much the same applies to a less pronounced sense of the 'uncanny', which is also an existential predicament that comes in several different forms, rather than something that varies only in its intensity. Freud's (2003) discussion suggests (perhaps unintentionally) that the term 'uncanny' is used to refer to several different kinds of experience. The uncanny, he says, belongs to the 'realm of the frightening' (2003, p.123). However, he goes on to claim that it can involve a feeling of 'helplessness', which is 'the same sense of the uncanny'. Then he refers to a sense of the 'fateful' and the 'inescapable' (2003, p.144). Now an unfamiliar world might appear through a general atmosphere of fear but this need not amount to a feeling of helplessness. And helplessness need not be accompanied by a sense of fate or inevitability. If the uncanny is to be understood in a permissive way, it is not clear that the relevant experience need include fear at all. An all-enveloping sense of weirdness or mysteriousness differs from a frightening estrangement or unsettledness. It may even be possible to *enjoy* certain feelings of not being at home in a situation, of things not seeming quite right. Newfound detachment might include indifference to a situation that one was previously caught up in and oppressed by. Indeed one might revel in being able to wander around feeling utterly dislodged from everything and thus emancipated from the pressures of commitments that once seemed so pressing and inescapable. Of course, 'the uncanny' could simply be defined in such a way as to restrict it to the frightening. But the question would then remain of how a range of closely related variants of experiential defamiliarization, from which it had not previously been adequately distinguished, are to be characterized.

Freud's discussion of the uncanny emphasizes the role of 'repression'. The uncanny is not, as might at first seem, an experience of things as 'unfamiliar'; its 'common nucleus' is a sense of something *familiar* that has been repressed. So the unfamiliarity that characterizes it is not to be *contrasted* with familiarity, given that a feeling of familiarity continues to lurk at the heart of the experience. The kind of unfamiliarity involved is thus a variant of the familiar; 'this uncanny element is actually nothing new or strange, but something that was long familiar to the psyche and was estranged from it only through being repressed' (2003, p.148).

In offering a phenomenological account of the nature and role of existential feeling, I will not be appealing to Freudian repression. Even so, I think that Freud's explanation of the uncanny manages to pick up on an important feature of certain experiences that are described in terms of *feelings of unfamiliarity*. We might come across something and declare it to be unfamiliar, meaning that we do not recognize it and believe we have not previously encountered it. However, the unfamiliarity at play in the uncanny is not an *absence of the feeling of familiarity* but a *feeling of unfamiliarity*. In experiencing something as unfamiliar in this way, there is an awareness of its not being quite right—we feel that something is *missing*. For Freud, it is this sense of absence that is to be explained in terms of the familiar being repressed. But, even if we reject this explanation, the point remains that the unfamiliar is not just an absence of the familiar (something I return to in Chapter 5). This also applies to Heideggerian anxiety. When the uncanny culminates in anxiety, there is a positive apprehension of 'the nothing'. The feeling of something being missing from the experience is itself a conspicuous feature of the experience.

Heidegger does not always make clear this difference between a loss of something from experience and a feeling of loss.

Another weakness in Heidegger's account of mood is that it does not address the role played by the body in experience, even though the emphasis on practical activity and purposive orientation surely implies a central role for the body. As noted, Heidegger remarks that his 'moods' have been referred to by others as 'feelings'. But he does not tell us whether moods are in any sense 'feelings' and, at one point, he contrasts moods as 'existential modes' with 'degrees of "feeling-tones"' (1962, p.181). So a puzzle remains as to whether and how these 'moods', once they have been salvaged from a history of misinterpretation, relate to the feeling body. Without some further characterization of what moods are, we are left with the conclusion that a mood is simply *whatever it is that plays the relevant phenomenological role*. Heidegger does acknowledge his neglect of the body: 'this "bodily nature" hides a whole problematic of its own, though we shall not treat it here' (1962, p.143). In his later *Zollikon Seminars*, he recalls this remark and goes on to discuss the phenomenology of the body (2001, pp.80–92).[7] However, he does not explicitly relate the body to mood, and it remains unclear how he understands the relationship between mood and our bodily phenomenology.

One reason for adopting the term 'existential feeling' rather than 'mood' is that—as Chapters 3 and 4 will show—certain bodily feelings do indeed play the role of what Heidegger calls 'mood'. Something can be both a bodily feeling and a sense of belonging to the world. Another reason is that, in using the term 'mood' (or the German term *Stimmung*, which has slightly different connotations) there is the risk of restricting one's enquiry to an overly limited range of feelings. Something I will emphasize throughout is that there is a considerable variety of existential feelings. They can be (a) short-lived, (b) sustained over a period of time or (c) retained over the course of a life as habitual temperaments; but the English term 'mood' only seems suited to (b). In addition, most of the phenomena that I call existential feelings are indeed referred to by people as 'feelings', rather than as 'emotions' or 'moods'. A focus on the latter two terms therefore serves to distract attention from many of the existential predicaments that people attempt to express. The term 'emotion' might invoke the usual list of states, such as 'anger', 'fear', 'happiness', 'sadness', 'shame', 'guilt', 'regret' and so forth. And 'mood' might make one think of 'misery', 'elation', 'boredom' or just of 'good' and 'bad' moods. However,

---

[7] There are further references to the body in the 'Conversations with Medard Boss, 1961–1972', which are published with the seminars (Heidegger, 2001, pp.157, 170, 200–1, 231–4).

'belonging', 'familiarity', 'completeness', 'estrangement', 'distance', 'separation' and 'homeliness' are usually referred to as feelings. One can speak of the 'feeling of being' or the 'feeling of reality', whereas the 'emotion' or 'mood' of being or reality sounds peculiar at best.

Some states that are referred to as 'moods' and 'emotions' do fall into the category 'existential feeling' but others do not. The 'emotion' of intense grief might take the form of an all-enveloping alteration of relatedness to things, but fear of a particular entity does not. The moods discussed by Heidegger are existential feelings. However, the term 'mood' is used quite loosely and can also refer to experiences that have specific objects. One can be in a bad or grumpy mood *with* somebody or *about* something in particular. Such moods do not seem to be all-encompassing existential orientations. They are states that one experiences or attitudes that one adopts when one is already *in* a world. The experiential backgrounds that constitute a sense of belonging to the world and a sense of reality play a quite distinctive phenomenological role. The terms 'mood' and 'emotion' do not adequately distinguish them and so there is the need to recognize a distinctive category of feeling phenomena— 'existential feelings'.

An alternative term that could be used to refer to existential feelings and feelings more generally is 'affect'. For instance, Sass (2004*b*) does so in discussing changed existential orientation in psychiatric illness.[8] One problem with 'affect' is that different people mean different things by it. For example, Hobson (2002) takes it to be a feature of interpersonal relatedness. Solomon (1993), in contrast, is dismissive of 'mere' affect, which he construes as an awareness of internal bodily states. Others use it in a physiological rather than phenomenological sense. For example, in a discussion of monothematic delusions, Davies *et al.* note that patients, although aware that their experience is in some way different, need not be aware of their reduced affective response, which is a matter of 'unconscious affective processing' (2001, p.140). Hence it is important to distinguish *experienced feeling* from *physiological affect*. 'Existential feeling' is a phenomenological category, and there is unlikely to be a reliable correlation between the level of physiological affect and the phenomenology of feeling. By analogy, consider waking up with a numb hand, having slept upon one's arm. It is not that the hand, in the absence of feeling, simply disappears from experience. Physiologically speaking, 'feeling' is diminished or absent from the hand but the numbness is not just an absence of feeling. There is a *feeling of numbness*; one experiences the absence. The lack

---

[8] Stanghellini (2004, pp.39–40) describes the same kinds of changes in terms of Heideggerian 'mood'.

of sensation in the hand makes it an especially salient object of experience, rather than something that recedes altogether from experience. Similarly, a pronounced existential feeling could arise through a lack of physiological affect, rather than an excess.

Some use 'affect' as a very general term to cover all those states that we might think of as emotional; it is 'used to designate a wide range of states which attract emotional vocabulary' (Gerrans, 1999, p.595). In psychiatric diagnosis, it is often used to refer to a patient's *observable* emotional responsiveness to stimuli. This is how Bleuler (1950) employs it when describing the affective changes seen in schizophrenia ('schizophrenia' being a term that he introduced in the same work). It is still used in much the same way in DSM IV-TR, where it is stated that, in schizophrenia:

> Affective flattening is especially common and is characterized by the person's face appearing immobile and unresponsive, with poor eye contact and reduced body language. (2004, p.301)

A clinician could observe such 'affective' changes in a patient without engaging in any way with the patient's phenomenology. Treating affective changes as objective symptoms to be observed from a dispassionate perspective is a far cry from enquiring into the phenomenological role of affect, the way in which it contributes to a patient's existential orientation.

So why use 'affect' rather than 'feeling', when the former is employed in a variety of different ways, which are sometimes vague? Sass raises the following concern about 'feeling':

> The term 'feelings' has a more subjective focus: unlike emotion, it refers not so much to an attitude toward the world as to a state of or within the self, one that does not elicit any action tendency or sense of urgency. (2004*b*, p.133)

However, I suggest that the supposed 'subjective focus' of 'feeling' is a symptom of its philosophical neglect and misinterpretation, rather than of connotations that attach to the term throughout everyday discourse. We do refer to ways of finding ourselves in the world as 'feelings'.

The nonsense charge

I have claimed that all experience presupposes a background of 'existential feeling', a changeable sense of reality and belonging. However, my case in support of this consists mainly of phenomenological assertions, drawn for the most part from Heidegger. In the absence of additional support, these assertions could simply be dismissed, and my claims about existential feelings along with them. In fact, a critic could go further than this and argue that talk of feelings of 'existence', 'unreality' and the like does not even mean anything.

This charge was famously levelled against Heidegger by Carnap (1959). According to Carnap, Heidegger's references to 'the nothing' depart from established word meanings to such an extent that the result is nonsense. He focuses on Heidegger's discussion of anxiety and the nothing. Heidegger claims that the 'nothing' revealed in anxiety is more fundamental to our phenomenology than the 'not'. When we say that something is 'not' the case, we negate a proposition. The 'nothing', however, is something that we actually experience—it is 'there'. Our appreciation of 'negation', of something's not being the case, is derived from this.

In contrast, Carnap maintains that everyday use of the word 'nothing' is parasitic on logical negation. If we assert 'there's nothing there', we mean something along the lines of 'it is not the case that entities of some type or types occupy a particular place'. Heidegger's use of 'the nothing' therefore strays from everyday use. However, it is clear that he is not using the word 'nothing' in a completely different but equally meaningful way, as his discussion continues to draw on familiar connotations of the word. Carnap's conclusion is that Heidegger's talk of the nothing means nothing. This view is given further weight by several obscure claims that Heidegger makes regarding the nothing and the limits of logic. For example, he states that 'the idea of "logic" itself disintegrates in the turbulence of a more original questioning' (1978a, p.105). If logic does not apply when we reach this 'primordial' level of experience, and if word meaning is no longer respected, what we get is meaninglessness.

Carnap proposes that assertions such as Heidegger's retain the illusion of meaning because the reader still associates the words with their familiar uses, giving the text a *feeling of meaning*. This feeling is all there is to it. He thus accuses the likes of Heidegger of kindling feelings in the reader, of the kind that a musician or artist might hope to evoke, by using the inappropriate medium of pseudo-philosophical prose:

> Perhaps music is the purest means of expression of the basic attitude because it is entirely free from any reference to objects. The harmonious feeling or attitude, which the metaphysician tries to express in a monistic system, is more clearly expressed in the music of Mozart. [...] Metaphysicians are musicians without musical ability. (Carnap, 1959, p.80)

Carnap's critique is grounded in his own account of linguistic meaning. For Carnap, a sentence is meaningful if (a) it is an observation sentence that can be verified by certain states of affairs in the world or (b) it is deductively implied by one or more observation sentences. This sort of meaning verificationism has fallen out of favour for several reasons, including its assumption of a clear distinction between observation and theory, its failure to accommodate apparently meaningful sentences that cannot be verified and the fact that it does not itself conform to the criteria for meaningfulness it offers. Despite this, the mud has still stuck to Heidegger. Indeed, Carnap's influential critique is partly responsible for the near absence of positive references to Heidegger in twentieth-century Anglophone philosophy.[9]

It is possible to agree with the various charges levelled at Heidegger by Carnap without at the same time endorsing Carnap's own account of meaning. Many philosophers place considerable emphasis on the methodological requirement that we abide by the norms of propositional logic. It seems to them both obscure and far-fetched to claim that there is a realm of experience presupposed by logic, which can be disturbed in such a fashion that the intelligibility of logic itself crumbles. In addition, it is frequently assumed that objective, empirical science is the best tool we have for revealing the way the world is. There is no place for anything like 'the nothing' in a scientific view of the world.

The root of the problem is that Heidegger's philosophical starting point is radically different from the starting points of many who do not take him seriously. Meaning, for Heidegger, is *not* to be contrasted with 'mere feeling'. The source of all meaning, the framework of intelligibility within which logic resides, is something pre-articulate and felt. In order to even contemplate this possibility, it must first be admitted that there is indeed something like the 'question of Being'. However, as illustrated by Carnap's doctrine of meaning, some philosophical approaches deny that there is any such question.

If meaning is already assumed to be a matter of whether and how a sentence can be verified by observation, then it seems that sentences along the lines of 'Being is presupposed by the intelligibility of the world in which attempted verifications are conducted' are a lost cause. Much the same conclusion can be reached if we adopt certain assumptions that are prevalent in current philosophical psychology and philosophy of mind, where there is a tendency to emphasize propositional attitudes as pivotal to our understanding of the world and of each other. A propositional attitude takes the form 'x believes that p' or 'x desires that p', where p could be any intelligible proposition, such as 'it is raining today', 'the cat is in the kitchen' or 'Paris is in France'. Attitude types include remembering, perceiving, desiring, hoping and fearing. It is the propositional attitude of 'belief' that is assumed to facilitate our appreciation of what is and is not the case. Propositional attitudes might be understood as

---

[9] As Polt (1999, p.122) remarks, '"What is Metaphysics?" led indirectly [via Carnap] to Heidegger's banishment from the world of Anglo-American philosophy, and for decades this banishment prevented most English-speaking philosophers from using Heidegger as food for thought'.

attitudes towards explicitly *linguistic* propositions, Believing that the cat is in the kitchen would thus involve believing the sentence 'the cat is in the kitchen' to be true. However, a sentential conception of propositional attitudes is clearly too restrictive. When I enter the kitchen and see that the cat is there, I *take a situation to be the case*, rather than explicitly assenting to the truth of a sentence that describes the situation in question. So the propositional attitude of belief is usually construed more liberally, as that of taking certain states of affairs (which are describable in propositional terms) to be the case.

Now suppose we think of the sense of reality in these terms. Taking something to be real is just a matter of taking it to be the case and taking it to be unreal is a matter of taking it not to be the case. Our sense of reality just becomes the sum total of what we take to be the case. This kind of thinking does not accommodate the possibility of an additional sense of reality or existence. And we certainly couldn't encounter the nothing, since the sense of 'nothing' is exhausted by what is taken not to be the case, what is 'not'. We could believe that 'p is' or that 'p is not' but there is no further question to be addressed regarding a sense of reality. And we can't look for evidence of 'unreality' or 'nothingness', given that the search for evidence is restricted to the realm of what is. The question therefore arises as to how the view I am developing might be defended against the simple charge that there is nothing more to be said.

In short, the answer is that careful phenomenological reflection does reveal a changeable sense of reality, which is associated with varying feelings of relatedness to the world. This is something that is possible to describe and something that people do attempt to communicate. Everyday language is not restricted in the way that some philosophical language is. Just as people talk about what is and what is not, they also talk about the changeable ways in which they find themselves in the world and of perturbations in the sense of reality. I grant that existential predicaments are usually very difficult to express and that such talk is therefore often vague or metaphorical. However, there are no good philosophical grounds for dismissing this talk as meaningless. There is only the dogmatic imposition of certain contestable assumptions and the consequent insistence that there is no question to be addressed.

But how can we make a positive case for existential feeling, rather than just trying to force a stalemate? One way to appreciate that there is a genuine question here is to consider some of the reports of changed existential feeling that people have offered. Perturbations of existential feeling are especially pronounced in some psychiatric illnesses and it is to autobiographical reports of the relevant experiences that I now turn, the aim being to illustrate how (a) feelings are inextricable from a sense of belonging to the world, (b) a sense of belonging to the world is at the same time a sense of reality and (c) changes in the sense of reality are intelligible and also quite different from changes in sets of propositional attitudes.

Existential feelings in autobiographical accounts of psychiatric illness

In his memoir *Darkness Visible*, William Styron (2001) recounts the experience of a unipolar depression that first struck him at the age of 60. Something that comes across throughout his account is the way in which changed feeling was closely associated with a radical and all-encompassing alteration in the structure of world-experience. The feeling in question is something that he reports as almost impossible to describe, stating that it was 'close to, but indescribably different from, actual pain'. It was 'a form of torment so alien to everyday experience', like 'drowning or suffocation' (pp.14–15). The reference to drowning or suffocation suggests something that is not experienced solely as an internal bodily state but also as an altered relationship with the world. One feels suffocated *by* something, rather than just having a particular kind of internal bodily feeling.

For Styron, the world no longer opened itself up as a space of practical possibilities that might be pursued; it was not imbued with any significance. Instead, experience was akin to 'being engulfed by a toxic and unnameable tide that obliterated any enjoyable response to the living world' (p.14). This 'tide' was not some specific thing that he found himself facing; it was not something in the world. Rather, it was his world, an inescapable way of being. In the context of this, all objects and situations appeared somehow different, diminished in a way that was inseparable from changed bodily feelings:

> …my surroundings took on a different tone at certain times: the shadows of nightfall seemed more somber, my mornings were less buoyant, walks in the woods became less zestful, and there was a moment during working hours in the late afternoon when a kind of panic and anxiety overtook me, just for a few minutes, accompanied by a visceral queasiness…. (p.41)

He later describes how his 'beloved farmhouse' took on 'an almost palpable quality of ominousness' (p.44). He also remarks on how his body was no longer a medium of activity, immersed in various projects. Instead it was thing-like and plagued by conspicuous feelings: 'nothing felt quite right with my corporeal self; there were twitches and pains, sometimes intermittent, often seemingly constant' (p.43).

Throughout the account, Styron oscillates between descriptions of (a) bodily feelings, (b) how objects and situations appeared different, and (c) how his relationship with the world as a whole took on a different tone. However, when it comes to interpreting the relationship between bodily feelings and changed world-experience, he does so dualistically. Persistent feelings of bodily changes are, he suggests, symptoms of a psychological state that is projected onto the physical body:

> ... unwilling to accept its own gathering deterioration, the mind announces to its indwelling consciousness that it is the body with its perhaps correctable defects—not the precious and irreplaceable mind—that is going haywire. (p.43)

I suspect that Styron's retention of a distinction between bodily feeling and world-experience itself contributes to his sense of the predicament he tries to describe as bordering on the ineffable. The descriptions he offers do not respect such distinctions. The horror, pain and utter isolation are all blended together as a stage is reached where 'all sense of hope had vanished'. At this point, his body is no longer apprehended as something through which he experiences, thinks and acts but as something somehow devoid of life, with the brain 'less an organ of thought than an instrument registering, minute by minute, varying degrees of its own suffering' (p.58). In describing his recovery, Styron contrasts two very different ways of experiencing the body: 'I felt myself no longer a husk but a body with some of the body's sweet juices stirring again' (p.75). This sense of being a 'husk', a lump of stuff bereft of the feeling of being, is bound up with a changed existential orientation. The significance that the experienced world is ordinarily imbued with ebbs away as the body becomes more conspicuous and object-like. The phenomenology of Styron's depression is neither bodily nor non-bodily. It is a changed way of belonging to the world that is describable in terms of both bodily and worldly changes.

The close relationship between feeling and altered world-experience is also conveyed by John Hull (1990) in *Touching the Rock*, in which he describes the depression that he fell into after the onset of blindness. Hull talks of intangible, unbearable feelings, from which sleep is the only protection, and refers to a feeling that is so strong that it cannot be put into words, other than to describe it as a 'poignant sense of loss' (p.153). Like Styron, he emphasizes the difficulty of conveying the existential significance of certain feelings, which are not just feelings of internal bodily changes: 'the deepest feelings go beyond feeling. One is numbed by the feeling; one does not experience the feeling' (p.168).[10]

---

[10] Solomon, in stressing the way in which emotions constitute the meaningfulness of a life, offers an account of depression that rejects an impersonal, medical stance towards it and regards it instead as an emotional change, a loss of the meaning structures in which a life is embedded. He offers a voluntaristic account of the existential predicament involved, stating that 'our depression is our way of wrenching ourselves from the established values

In both cases, there is an intimate relationship between feeling and world-experience. However, even if it is admitted that feelings are somehow associated with a changeable sense of *belonging to the world*, it could still be maintained that they have nothing to do with a sense of *reality*. After all, although Styron describes things as looking somehow different, he never claims to have experienced a loss of or change to the sense of reality itself, at least not explicitly. But this is not always the case. For example, autobiographical accounts of changed experience in schizophrenia frequently refer to a loss of the sense of reality. In addition, the existential changes described by people with schizophrenia appear to differ, in certain respects, from those that tend to occur in depression, thus serving to illustrate something of the range of existential feelings (although, as I will argue in Chapter 7, it is highly unlikely that differences in *kinds* of existential feeling will reliably track broad diagnostic categories such as 'schizophrenia' and 'depression').

Consider the account offered by 'Renee', in *Autobiography of a Schizophrenic Girl* (Sechehaye, 1970).[11] She describes her experiences during different stages of the illness, making clear throughout her narrative the close connection between feeling, a sense of reality and a sense of purposive, practical relatedness to things. To begin with, there was 'a disturbing sense of unreality' (p.21). There were distortions of space and time; everything seemed vast, infinite. And everything was somehow stripped of meaning. For example, the schoolyard appeared 'limitless, unreal, mechanical and without meaning' (p.25). She also describes a loss of connectedness to other people, who seemed like puppets or mechanisms, rather than purposive agents interacting in a meaningful, shared world:

> Everything was exact, smooth, artificial, extremely tense; the chairs and tables seemed models placed here and there. Pupils and teachers were puppets revolving without cause, without objective. I recognized nothing, nobody. It was as though reality, attenuated, had slipped away from all these things and these people. (p.26)

In the early stages of the illness, Renee was drawn back into the world through practical activities and routines. During these transient periods of

of our world, the tasks in which we have been unquestioningly immersed, the opinions we have uncritically nursed, the relationships we have accepted without challenge and often without meaning. A depression is a self-imposed purge' (1993, p.237). The kind of depression described by Styron and others does involve a loss of meaning structures that were previously inhabited. There may even be *some* truth in the claim that depression can be self-imposed, to the extent that how one thinks about and evaluates one's life contributes to its onset. However, one cannot choose one's depression and it is not a 'self-imposed purge'. It is something that one finds oneself *in*, rather than something that is willingly performed.

[11] See Sass (1992, chapter 2), for a detailed phenomenological discussion of Renee.

practical belonging, the sense of reality was restored: 'to move, to change the scene, to do something definite and customary, helped a great deal' (p.27). The warmth and taste of food also helped. But, on each occasion, she again 'lost the feeling of practical things' and 'sensed again the atmosphere of unreality' (p.29). The loss of practical belonging sometimes intensified to become what she calls 'real "fear"', where unreality, itself characterized by 'uneasiness', became an all-embracing feeling of impending 'calamity' (p.32).

It is clear from Renee's descriptions that the unreality which enveloped her as the illness progressed involved a loss of felt familiarity, the disappearance of a practical belonging that is ordinarily taken for granted as an experiential background. She remarks on how things lost their functionality and consequently appeared without context, without significance. They were not simply present-at-hand in some mundane way but utterly alien, without meaning. She called out their names in an attempt to recover a sense of what they were, but to no avail (p.56).

The madness that Renee later describes is not only a *loss* of reality; it is also the inhabiting of a radically different existential orientation. Madness, she says, is a 'country' that is 'opposed to reality'; 'madness was finding oneself permanently in an all-embracing Unreality' (p.44). This 'unreality' is not just a lack of something, an 'absence' of familiarity from experience. It is something that is experienced, an all-pervasive way of being. And it is certainly not to be accounted for in terms of a set of deviant propositional attitudes. Indeed, Renee indicates that 'believing', in the usual sense of taking something to be the case, was no longer possible. For example, she reports that she 'firmly believed' that the world was about to be destroyed but that she 'did not believe the world would be destroyed as [she] believed in real facts' (p.34). It was not a matter of her believing that p, believing that not p or even believing that possibly p. The structure of belief had changed. The sense of conviction, of what it is for something to be or not be, had been altered. Hence the delusions and hallucinations that she later describes did not simply involve taking something unreal to be real:

> I cannot say that I really saw images; they did not represent anything. Rather I felt them. It seemed that my mouth was full of birds which I crunched between my teeth, and their feathers, their blood and broken bones were choking me. [...] I did not hear [cries in the head] as I heard real cries uttered by real people. (pp.58–9)

Rene was not presented with non-veridical experiences, whose contents she mistakenly took to be real due to the formation of mistaken propositional attitudes. One cannot maintain that p is the case or that p is not the case, when the sense of what it is for something to be the case has itself been eroded. One can utter 'it is the case that p' as much as one likes but, without a sense of reality, such assertions are empty.

That there is a sense of reality, integral to experience and presupposed by any assertion to the effect that some entity is real, is vividly conveyed by Renee's account of a short-lived return to reality, where she contrasts the existential orientation of unreality with that of mundane everyday experience:

> Instead of infinite space, unreal, where everything was cut off, naked and isolated, I saw Reality, marvelous Reality, for the first time. The people whom we encountered were no longer automatons, phantoms, revolving around, gesticulating without meaning; they were men and women with their own individual characteristics, their own individuality. It was the same with things. They were useful things, having sense, capable of giving pleasure. Here was an automobile to take me to the hospital, cushions I could rest on. With the astonishment that one views a miracle, I devoured with my eyes everything that happened. 'This is it, this is it,' I kept repeating, and I was actually saying, 'This is it—Reality'. (pp.105–6)

Again, we see how experience of 'reality' is at the same time experience of purposive, practical belonging, of being harmoniously entwined with a world that offers up possibilities for activity. As Renee goes on to say, 'for the first time I dared to handle the chairs, to change the arrangement of the furniture. What unknown joy, to have an influence on things' (p.106). To have a sense of reality is not to posit something in thought; it is an orientation that one takes for granted before positing anything. When the relevant sense of belonging is altered or diminished, the result is not an experience of 'self' and of 'world', decoupled from each other. Finding oneself in a world is more fundamental to the structure of experience than self in isolation from world or vice versa. When the relation between the two is changed, both are changed along with it.

There are significant differences between the existential orientations that Styron and Renee describe. He became entombed in a mechanical, thing-like body, painfully suffocated by a diminished world that no longer offered up possibilities. The phenomenology that Renee conveys is not so much a matter of being trapped in a world bereft of significance, as of falling away from an insignificant world and coming to inhabit a different existential realm. Whereas he yearns to escape, she longs to return. However, both cases draw attention to the close connection between feeling and world experience. Changed feelings are, at the same time, changed ways of finding oneself in a world. In Renee's case at least, the change is such that a background sense of reality, which we ordinarily take for granted, is rendered conspicuous by its absence.

Existential feelings in literature and everyday life

Changes in existential feeling are not restricted to psychiatric illness. In fact, I think that more subtle changes are commonplace. They are often only vaguely alluded to but are sometimes described in detail. Although existential feelings do not appear in nice, tidy lists of emotions and feelings, they are often communicated by literary narratives. Consider the following passage from Sebastian Faulks' *The Girl at the Lion d'Or*:

> She thought of the landscape of her childhood and the wooded slopes around the house where she was born. They seemed as alien to her now as these anonymous fields through which she passed. Since she felt she belonged to no part of it, she could make no sense of this material world, whether it was in the shape of natural phenomena, like woods and rivers, or in the guise of man-made things like houses, furniture and glass. Without the greeting of personal affection or association they were no more than collections of arbitrarily linked atoms that wriggled and chased each other into shapes that men had named. Although Anne didn't phrase her thoughts in such words, she felt her separation from the world. The fact that many of the patterns formed by random matter seemed quite beautiful made no difference; try as she might, she could dredge no meaning from the fertile hedgerows, no comfort from the pointless loveliness of the swelling woods and hills. (1990, p.243)

The predicament that Faulks describes involves an altered relationship between self and world, which affects the way in which both are experienced. A certain kind of feeling is at the same time a lack of connectedness to the world, an absence of warming familiarity, of significance, of belonging. Objects, when stripped of the usual familiarity that surrounds them, appear alien and without meaning. It is not a matter of self feeling a certain way plus world feeling a certain way; it is an altered sense of belonging, which frames experience of both.

Here is another example, this time from Margaret Atwood's *The Robber Bride*:

> Tony felt safe this morning, safe enough. But she doesn't feel safe now. Everything has been called into question. Even in the best of times the daily world is tenuous to her, a thin, iridescent skin held in place by surface tension. She puts a lot of effort into keeping it together, her willed illusion of comfort and stability, the words flowing from left to right, the routines of love; but underneath is darkness. Menace, chaos, cities aflame, towers crashing down, the anarchy of deep water. She takes a breath to steady herself and feels the oxygen and car fumes rushing into her brain. Her legs are wavery, the façade of the street ripples, tremulous as a reflection on a pond, the weak sunlight blows away like smoke. (1994, p.35)

The feeling described here differs from that related by Faulks. Tony is not detached from the world in the way that Anne is. The world does not offer up nothing for Tony, with everything appearing distant, insignificant, meaningless. A feeling of safety, a warming sense of belonging to a dependable world, is gone. It is substituted for a feeling of everything as contingent and unpredictable, an unsettledness where nothing is taken for granted and what remains is an all-embracing awareness of threat. The change in existential orientation is experienced as something bodily, as the wavering legs. But it is also a way in which things in the world appear, such as the rippling façade of the street. Bodily and worldly aspects reflect the same existential orientation, which shapes both experience and thought. Imagined scenarios such as 'cities aflame' and 'towers crashing down' are not identical with it but they are still symptomatic of it.

It is important to stress that existential feelings are not only constitutive of our relationship with an *inanimate* world. As suggested by Renee's account, a changeable relatedness to other *people* and to the *social* world is central. One can feel as though one belongs to the social world or one can feel cut off from it. One can feel close to other people or estranged from them, isolated. (As the case of Renee illustrates, it is even possible to lose the sense of others as *people*, something that Chapter 5 will discuss in detail.)

Certain existential feelings constitute an insurmountable isolation from others, as is beautifully conveyed by Sylvia Plath's *The Bell Jar*. The novel charts the progressive estrangement of the semi-autobiographical protagonist (Esther) from social life, culminating in a form of psychotic depression. Esther is in trouble even at the beginning:

> I wasn't steering anything, not even myself. I just bumped from my hotel to work and to parties and from parties to my hotel and back to work like a numb trolley-bus. I guess I should have been excited the way most of the other girls were, but I couldn't get myself to react. I felt very still and very empty, the way the eye of a tornado must feel, moving dully along in the middle of the surrounding hullabaloo. (1966, pp.2–3)

Already, there is isolation from the social world, an inability to experience anything as significant, captivating, worth pursuing. In conjunction with this, her activities are regulated by monotonous routines in a world that offers up no possibilities for spontaneous action. Later on, she finds herself in an apartment with an amorous couple:

> The two of them didn't even stop jitterbugging during the intervals. I felt myself shrinking to a small black dot against all those red and white rugs and that pine-panelling. I felt like a hole in the ground. [...] It's like watching Paris from an express caboose heading in the opposite direction—every second the city gets smaller and smaller, only you feel it's really you getting smaller and smaller and lonelier and lonelier, rushing away from all those lights and that excitement at about a million miles an hour. (1966, p.15)

She is physically *in* the room but she is not *in* a shared social situation. This sense of detachment, of not belonging, of not being part of a situation, is a way in which she *feels* and also a loss of relatedness that structures all her experiences of self, other people and impersonal objects. The 'bell jar' of the title is the metaphor used by Plath to express the culmination of this deadening of feeling, which takes the form of a suffocating, paralysing, pathological estrangement from the social world:

> I knew I should be grateful to Mrs Guineau, only I couldn't feel a thing. If Mrs Guineau had given me a ticket to Europe, or a round-the-world cruise, it wouldn't have made one scrap of difference to me, because wherever I sat—on the deck of a ship or at a street café in Paris or Bangkok—I would be sitting under the same glass bell jar, stewing in my own sour air. (1966, p.178)

It might be that all these narratives describe highly unusual experiences, which arise only in cases of diagnosed or undiagnosed psychiatric illness. These are to be contrasted with a normal, everyday way of encountering things, a consistent grasp of reality and a sense of belonging to the world that most of us take for granted almost all of the time. However, certain remarks suggest that the manner in which we find ourselves in the world during the course of everyday life is actually quite variable. Although the existential shift is especially pronounced in a case like Renee's, a diverse range of lesser changes in existential feeling are reported outside of psychiatric contexts. Maher (1999, p.552) notes that people sometimes refer to a '"feeling of awareness", "mood", "atmosphere", "feeling of significance", "feeling of conviction"'. But there are many other ways in which existential feelings are described. People sometimes talk of feeling alive, dead, distant, detached, dislodged, estranged, isolated, otherworldly, indifferent to everything, overwhelmed, suffocated, cut off, lost, disconnected, out of sorts, not oneself, out of touch with things, out of it, not quite with it, separate, in harmony with things, at peace with things or part of things. There are references to feelings of unreality, heightened existence, surreality, familiarity, unfamiliarity, strangeness, isolation, emptiness, belonging, being at home in the world, being at one with things, significance, insignificance and the list goes on. People also sometimes report that 'things just don't feel right', 'I'm not with it today', 'I just feel a bit removed from it all at the moment', 'I feel out of it' or 'it feels strange'.

Such talk suggests general existential orientations that are bound up with feelings. Some, like feeling 'settled', 'at home' or 'part of things', are quite mundane. Others, such as 'feeling estranged from everything', convey less frequent and sometimes pathological forms of experience. Once the variety of existential feelings that people express in everyday life is acknowledged, perhaps reports of existential changes in psychiatric illness will not seem quite so removed from certain everyday experiences, even though the changes involved in the former are of course more extreme.

It might be the self, the world, a situation, other people or the self–world relation that is described as *feeling* some way. However, that different objects feature in descriptions does not imply that some of these feelings concern *self and not world* and others *world and not self*. Descriptions can be changed without implying different kinds of experience. Consider the remark 'I feel strange'. The same feeling might be conveyed by 'it feels strange' or by 'everything feels strange'.

That there are numerous different descriptions of existential feeling does not entail that there are many such feelings. Different words might be used to communicate similar phenomena, with 'strangeness' amounting to the same thing as 'unfamiliarity', which might be much the same as a 'diminished sense of reality'. Although I do not attempt to offer a comprehensive taxonomy of existential feelings here, I will at least suggest that they are many and diverse and, in Chapter 7, I will distinguish some of the different variants. It is also worth keeping in mind that most of the more subtle changes in existential feeling will not be remarked upon at all. Such feelings are seldom explicit objects of reflection and they are, in any case, very difficult to express.

Propositional attitudes and the sense of reality

The language used to express existential feelings does not always clearly distinguish them from propositional attitudes. Even so, although statements such as 'the car looks blue' and 'the world looks strange' have the same superficial linguistic form, what they express is quite different. 'The world looks strange', in some cases at least, does not communicate a propositional content, which includes an object (the world) that is experienced as being a certain way (strange). The 'world', as the term is employed here, is not an object of experience at all, like a cup or a table but a lot bigger. Rather, it is something that is presupposed by such objects.[12]

Although the sense of reality is not describable in propositional attitude terms, the question of what our sense of being, reality or existence consists of is, I suggest, quite intelligible and can be communicated clearly enough. Consider a propositional attitude, such as that of 'believing that there is a cat on the table', where one takes a particular state of affairs (there is a cat on the table) to be the case. One might instead believe that there is not a cat on the table, that there might be a cat on the table, that there is most likely a cat on the table, that there is something on the table that might be a cat and so on. However, in order to adopt any such attitude, one must already have a sense of what it is for something to *be the case*. This cannot take the form of a 'belief',

[12] See Ratcliffe (2007, especially chapter 7) for a detailed critique of the view that propositional attitude psychology is central to human social life and for a discussion of what is actually meant by the term 'propositional attitude'. See also Sass (2004*a*, p.75) for some criticisms of the emphasis that is frequently placed upon propositional attitudes.

construed in propositional attitude terms, given that the distinction between being and not being the case is presupposed by the possibility of belief. Even if we believe that p is not the case, we must at least have a sense of what it would mean for p to be the case, in order to be able to adopt such an attitude.

So what does this sense consist of? It is surely something integral to experience, rather than something inferred on the basis of experience. In the ordinary case, we take the reality of things for granted in our experience, rather than first experiencing something and then judging whether or not it is real. I do not look down to see the pair of shoes on the floor next to me and only then adopt the belief that they are really there. To quote Husserl (2001, p.66), there is a 'believing inherent in perceiving'. Now it might conceivably have turned out that there was no way of addressing the question, that whenever we turned to it, we ended up with nothing more than the primitive, unanalysable assertion that certain things 'are' and others 'are not'. But, in practice, things are much more interesting than this. There are all sorts of subtle permutations in our feeling of belonging to the world, which are, at the same time, changes in the sense of reality. In contemplating these, we can gain at least some insight into the phenomenological structure of our sense of reality. Experience is not merely an input into a belief system, which offers up specific contents that may or may not be accepted in the form of beliefs. It also incorporates a background sense of belonging to a world through which all specific experiences, beliefs and thoughts are structured. Disturbances in this background reshape the modalities of belief, the sense of what it is for something to be or not be.

As Husserl observes, the natural attitude of believing in the existence of the world is not a matter of propositional believing. It is founded in a pre-articulate, practical dwelling. The world of everyday experience is not an intentional object. Both Husserl and Heidegger take it to be a practical, social world in which we are purposively immersed, rather than the totality of entities that we contemplate theoretically:

> In ordinary life, we have nothing whatever to do with nature-Objects. What we take as things are pictures, statues, gardens, homes, tables, clothes, tools, etc. These are all value-Objects of various kinds, use-Objects, practical Objects. They are not Objects which can be found in natural science. (Husserl, 1989, p.29)

I want to depart from both of Husserl and Heidegger in one crucial respect. Husserl talks of *the* natural attitude and Heidegger likewise indicates that there is an ordinary, everyday way of being attuned to the world. However, I do not think that there is a unitary, constant sense of reality that is integral to all ordinary living and susceptible to only a few permutations in exceptional circumstances. The sense of reality and belonging embedded in the natural attitude is changeable, not just in intensity but also in character. There are many different variants, some fleeting, some sustained and some that pervade an entire life. These seldom feature as explicit objects of reflection but they are phenomenologically accessible. The changes that Styron and Renee describe are unusually intense manifestations of more subtle changes that we all experience.

Matters are more complicated still. So far, I have used the terms 'reality', 'existence' and 'being' without distinguishing between them. However, although they are sometimes used as synonyms, they can take on quite different meanings and can even be used contrastively. Renee recollects that:

> When […] I looked at a chair or a jug, I thought not of their use or function—a jug not as something to hold water and milk, a chair not as something to sit in—but as having lost their names, their functions and meanings; they became 'things' and began to take on life, to exist. (Sechehaye, 1970, pp.55–6)

This experience of 'existence' is contrasted with a more familiar appreciation of the 'reality' of things. Objects 'existing' in this way amounts to a loss of practical connectedness to them, an absence of their availability, utility, tangibility and familiarity. Renee's altered relatedness to things is at the same time a change in the modalities of being. The 'is' of familiar things, which is constituted by practical relations with them, is gone. It is replaced by a different sense of the 'is'; things appear as just 'present' in some strange, wholly detached way, stripped of all practical significance. Thus there is no single, simple sense of existence/reality, which we either have or do not have.

We find something strikingly similar in Sartre's novel *Nausea*. Take the well-known passage where he describes the experience of a chestnut root, which becomes stripped of its everyday familiarity:

> Knotty, inert, nameless, [the root] fascinated me, filled my eyes, repeatedly brought me back to its own existence. It was no use my repeating: 'It is a root'—that didn't work any more. I saw clearly that you could not pass from its function as a root, as a suction-pump, *to that*, to that hard, compact sea-lion skin, to that oily, horny, stubborn look. (1963, p.186)

> …all of a sudden, it became impossible for me to think of the existence of the root. It had been wiped out. It was no use my repeating to myself: 'It exists, it is still there, under the bench, against my right foot'; it didn't mean anything any more. Existence is not something which allows itself to be thought of from a distance; it has to invade you suddenly, pounce upon you, weigh heavily on your heart like a huge motionless animal—or else there is nothing left at all. (1963, p. 189)

All familiarity is gone, the root being a focal point for what becomes an all-enveloping experience.[13] In referring to this as 'nausea', Sartre implies that the

---

[13] See also Sass (1992, pp.48–9, 66–7) for a comparison between Renee's experience of 'Mere Being' and the experience of 'the brute fact of existence itself' that Sartre describes in *Nausea*.

experience involves a kind of feeling. It is a *feeling of defamiliarization*, which culminates in an experience of the root as 'existing'. The existence of things, in this sense of 'existence', is not something that is ordinarily experienced. It is an unusual and unpleasant feeling of the utter *contingency* of things that have lost their usual familiarity. As Sartre remarks, you cannot conjure up this feeling of existence by assenting to the proposition that something exists. However many times you say 'it exists', you cannot recover the relevant sense of existence once the feeling has receded. Sartrean nausea is very like the predicament Renee describes, a detachment from oneself, other people and the everyday world that culminates in the experience of contingent, meaningless existence, as something revolting, horrifying. Individualized objects, with distinctive identities and purposes, dissolve away, leaving only what Sartre, in *Nausea*, describes as 'soft, monstrous masses, in disorder—naked, with a frightening, obscene nakedness' (1963, p.183).

An analogous point applies to reports of experiencing 'non-existence'. These too are rare and they are quite different from the many everyday experiences that might lead us to assert that an entity does not exist. Just as the experience of something as existing is not exhausted by the recognition that some entity currently occupies a spatial location, so too the experience of non-existence need not be a matter of its failing to do so. Experience of 'non-existence' can be very different from the sense of 'unreality' that I discussed earlier. A profound sense of utter absence is not the same as a feeling of something being present but somehow unreal. Consider this description of experience following spinal anaesthesia, offered by Oliver Sacks:

> If one is given a spinal anaesthetic that brings to a halt neural traffic in the lower half of the body, one cannot feel merely that this is paralysed and senseless; one feels that it is wholly, impossibly, 'nonexistent', that one has been cut in half, and that the lower half is absolutely missing—not in the familiar sense of being somewhere, elsewhere, but in the uncanny sense of not-being, or being nowhere. [...] [Patients] may say that part of them is 'missing', 'evacuated', 'gone': that it seems like dead flesh, or sand, or paste; devoid of life, of activity, of 'will'; devoid of the organic, of structure, of coherence—without materiality or imaginable reality; cut off or alienated from the living flesh. (1987, p.564)

This is not just an experience of a thing as somehow lacking but an experience in which the most salient element is a sense of absence. Experience of absence is not the absence of something from experience—the 'nothing', as Heidegger recognizes, is 'there'.

In exploring existential feelings, it is therefore important to recognize that terms such as 'reality' and 'existence' are not always synonymous and that they can both be used in a number of different ways. Heidegger observes that much of our talk about 'reality' is restricted to present-at-hand things:

> In so far as Reality has the character of something independent and 'in itself', the question of the meaning of 'Reality' becomes linked with that of whether the Real can be independent 'of consciousness' or whether there can be a transcendence of consciousness into the 'sphere' of the Real. (1962, p.246)

If we prioritize a subject–object perspective, reality becomes a matter of what resides in an objective, mind-independent world. But the way in which we find ourselves in the world is not describable in such terms. We are not set apart from it, gazing upon it from elsewhere and wondering what it consists of. Indeed, such an experiential standpoint has more affinity with the experience of 'unreality' that Renee describes than it does with our more commonplace relationships with things.

An account of what 'external reality' consists of cannot itself address what it means for something to be real. Hence, in discussing existential feelings, it is important to recognize that the relevant sense of 'unreality' is not just something that applies to some posited external realm. It applies to where we are already, before we construe ourselves as detached onlookers and set ourselves up in opposition to an external world. It is not restricted to the present-at-hand but involves a changed relatedness to all things, a diminishing of practical significance and belonging. I appreciate that the term 'unreality' is not always employed in such a way but at least *some* uses do attempt to communicate variants of changed existential feeling, as exemplified by Renee's descriptions.

Whenever we state that something is real or unreal, our ability to distinguish the two possibilities presupposes a sense of reality. Hence references to the 'sense of reality' need to be distinguished from specific judgements as to what is 'real'. It is also worth keeping in mind that the term 'real' can be used in a range of different ways. Austin (1962) recognizes that it is a rather treacherous term, which does not have a single, consistent meaning.[14] 'Real', he says, is quite an 'exceptional' word (p.64). In fact, the negative use 'not real' is more commonplace and best serves to specify what would be meant, in a given context, by claiming something to be real:

> …with 'real' […] it is the *negative* use that wears the trousers. That is, a definite sense attaches to the assertion that something is real, a real such-and-such, only in the light of a specific way in which it might be, or might have been, *not* real. (1962, p.70)

For instance, saying that something is 'a real diamond' usually means that it is not a 'fake diamond'. In this case, there is nothing more to being a 'real diamond'

---

[14] See also Morris (2002) for a brief discussion of Austin on the term 'real' and its relevance for discussions of the sense of 'unreality' in psychiatric illness.

than being a diamond. An 'unreal' diamond is a different kind of entity, which is intentionally produced so as to look like a diamond. Austin suggests that 'real' is used in many other ways too and that an explicit, comprehensive account of its uses cannot be formulated. Instead, we have to work out how the term is being used in each particular case.

It is important to be aware of such issues when exploring existential feelings. Suppose that someone says 'everything looks unreal' and qualifies this by saying 'it all looks fake somehow'. What is meant by this? The judgement that a specific entity, which appears to be of type x, is a fake x need not imply any phenomenological difference between a real x and a fake x. The difference might be something that only laboratory tests could determine. So 'looking fake' is not the same as being fake. A specific entity might 'look fake' due to various tell-tale observable properties but, again, this sense of 'fake' does not capture an experience where *everything* looks fake. Such experiences are not specific to individuals or types. References to everything seeming 'not real' or 'fake' are not just about some present-at-hand entity or group of entities. The world as a whole seems somehow different, intangible, unfamiliar and strange.

In order to understand this sense of unreality, it will not do to analyse what is meant by the word 'unreal' in this context. Conceptual analysis alone will not give us an understanding of the experience in question. Instead, a phenomenological description is required of what it is that people attempt to convey when they refer to everything looking 'fake' or 'not quite real'. Renee at least offers us a clue, when she says that 'objects are stage trappings, placed here and there, geometric cubes without meaning' (Sechehaye, 1970, p.44). The claim that things look *fake* indicates that they do not appear usable in the way that real things of that kind do. A stage trapping might look like an entity of some type but it cannot be used in the same way. Thus everything looking fake is suggestive of an all-enveloping loss of experienced functionality and practical significance. I will discuss the structure of the relevant experience in more detail in Chapters 5 to 7.

Another concern that needs to be addressed is that the occurrence of feelings of 'unreality' does not imply that there is also a feeling of 'reality'. Again, this is something that Austin's work draws attention to. That something could be an unreal x does not imply that there is such a thing as a real x. In some cases, a real x is just an x. Could the same apply to feelings of unreality? I don't think so. First of all, people not only talk of feelings of unreality but also of heightened feelings of reality. And second, feelings of unreality are consistently expressed in terms of something being *missing* from experience. This missing element is not an absent 'object' of experience but a practical connectedness that only becomes phenomenologically conspicuous when it is disturbed.

A feeling of unreality is not something added to experience; it is a change in the structure of experience and a change from structure p to structure q, regardless of whether or not it is described as a 'loss' of something, implies that there is such a thing as structure p. It is also worth reiterating that it is not a case of there being a simple phenomenological contrast between 'reality' and 'unreality'; there are many different existential orientations rather than two alternatives.

That 'real' and 'reality' are used in many different ways lends support to the view that a priori assertions regarding what is meant by them, which might preclude discussion of existential feeling, are unwarranted. It cannot be maintained that a sense of 'unreality' is unintelligible on the basis that 'this is the way in which the terms *real* and *unreal* are used', as the terms are not univocal. The same goes for 'non-existence'. Such terms are indeed used in some contexts to express changed existential orientations. What about 'being'? This too is used as a synonym for either 'existence' or 'reality' in some cases and can also be used in other ways. I will adopt only one of these uses in what follows, which maps roughly onto Heidegger's use of the term 'Being' [*Sein*] in early works such as *Being and Time*. Unlike 'unreality' and 'existence', 'being' does not depend upon a specific existential feeling. Rather, there are different ways of 'being'. By the 'sense of being', I mean the 'structure of background existential orientation in general', rather than some specific orientation. So, strictly speaking, being is never wholly lacking from experience. What we have in each case is a *changed* sense of being. Nevertheless, the loss of a habitual orientation, involving an eradication of significance, familiarity and belonging, might well be described by someone as their ceasing to 'be' or as a feeling of 'no longer being'. Hence it is important to be sensitive to different uses when interpreting reports of changed experience.

Chapter 3

The phenomenology of touch

In the last chapter, I described the *role* played by existential feelings. I now turn to their *nature*. It might seem that existential feelings cannot be bodily feelings. A bodily feeling is surely an experience of the body and of nothing else, whereas an existential feeling is a background sense of belonging to the world, which structures all experiences rather than just experiences of the body. In this chapter, I challenge such assumptions by showing how something can be a bodily feeling and, at the same time, a way of perceiving something else. To do so, I explore the phenomenology of touch. This is a slight detour from the topic of existential feeling. However, as will become apparent towards the end of this chapter, and also in Chapter 4, reflection upon the nature of tactile experience can contribute in several ways to an understanding of the nature and role of existential feelings in everyday life and in psychiatric illness.

I begin by suggesting that the tendency to impose a clear distinction between bodily feelings and world-experience stems in part from over-emphasis upon a questionable conception of visual perception. This emphasis is closely associated with the tendency to think of experience as a spectatorial, detached affair, which I criticized in Chapter 2. Then I show that the phenomenology of touch does not respect the distinction between bodily feeling and world-experience. Touch is a matter of relatedness between body and world, rather than of experiencing one in isolation from the other. In touching something, a bodily feeling is also a perception of something other than the body. I go on to distinguish cases of localized touch, such as picking up a pencil or being prodded on the arm by somebody, from the tactile background that we tend to take for granted. The latter partly comprises the setting for all our experiences and activities. When it undergoes significant changes, so does our sense of belonging to the world. So certain kinds of tactile feeling are not just analogous to existential feeling but also contribute to it, although they are not its only constituents.

Vision and touch

I think that many (but perhaps not all) of the phenomena referred to as 'bodily feelings' are not solely perceptions of our bodily states, distinct from the perception of our surroundings. The commonplace assumption that bodily feeling is distinct from world-experience stems in part from a tendency to characterize the latter primarily or even exclusively in terms of *visual* perception, which is sometimes construed in a curiously disembodied fashion. Several authors have commented on the privileged phenomenological and epistemic status that is generally assigned to disembodied vision. For example, Heidegger refers to 'the remarkable priority of "seeing"' in philosophical enquiry, conceived of as a 'pure beholding' of objects that is abstracted from our bodily, practical relationship with the world (1962, p.215). This, he says, is not a recent trend but something that has been engrained in philosophical thought from 'the beginning onwards' (1962, p.187).[1]

In what follows, I will explore the structure of world-experience by focusing on the sense of touch, rather than on vision. My aim is not to argue for the 'primacy' of touch over vision but to draw attention to aspects of world-experience that are easily missed if all the emphasis is placed upon vision. The reason why touch is a better starting point than vision from which to explore these aspects will be made clear towards the end of the chapter.

Touch is perhaps unlike vision in certain important respects and the same applies to the other senses. So it should not be assumed from the outset that the structure of all experience conforms to what might apply to the visual modality. Merleau-Ponty (1962, p.316) notes that vision is more objectifying than touch. It offers a view of the world that is seemingly uncorrupted by the body and thus fuels the tendency to separate subject from object, internal from external and the body from the rest of the world. Of course, what is seen depends upon where one's body is physically located. However, this is quite compatible with the assumption that visual perception is wholly divorced from perception of various bodily states, that how the body 'feels' does not determine how a scene is perceived visually. If we think of vision and of world-experience more generally in this way, the outcome is a clear distinction between perception of self and perception of world. Vision, it seems, is an externally directed sense, which is distinct from internally directed proprioception or 'body-sense'. The subject *looks out* upon a world of objects and views them in a way that is uncorrupted by bodily feeling.

As Merleau-Ponty recognizes, a crisp distinction between perception of self and perception of non-self does not characterize tactile experience. In touch, perception of the body and perception of things outside of it are tied together.

---

[1] See also Jonas (1954) for a discussion of how philosophers have long regarded sight as 'the most excellent of the senses' (p.507). Some have argued that this emphasis on disembodied, objectifying vision is androcentric, serving to marginalize certain more feminine approaches to philosophical and scientific enquiry. See, for example, Young (2005, pp.63–96) and Keller and Grontowski (1996) for discussions.

The division between embodied subject and perceived object, which might be thought to characterize at least some instances of visual perception, does not apply: 'as the subject of touch, I cannot flatter myself that I am everywhere and nowhere; I cannot forget in this case that it is through my body that I go to the world' (Merleau-Ponty, 1962, p.316). A description of bodily feeling and world-experience that takes its lead from touch thus draws attention to the relatedness between them.

Merleau-Ponty goes on to state that spectatorial accounts of visual perception fail to appreciate that all experience involves a background sense of belonging to the world. Like more localized tactile experiences, this background cannot be cleanly partitioned into perception of subject and perception of object:

> [Objective thinking emphasizes] visual qualities, because these give the impression of being autonomous, and because they are less directly linked to our body and present us with an object rather than introducing us into an atmosphere. But in reality all things are concretions of a setting, and any explicit perception of a thing survives in virtue of a previous communication with a certain atmosphere. (1962, p.320)

The way in which the feeling body constitutes this 'setting' is, I will suggest, better illustrated by the phenomenology of touch than by that of vision. However, although vision is sometimes thought of as divorced from proprioception, it is important to note that it need not be construed in this way. Merleau-Ponty (1962, p.316) refers to a tendency to 'forget' the role of the body in perception and also to the 'illusion' of 'being situated nowhere', implying that visual perception is not quite so detached after all. As will become clear in what follows, this is indeed so. Nevertheless, I will suggest that certain characteristics of touch still make it a better starting point from which to explore the manner in which we belong to the world.

Touch and proprioception

In recent Anglophone philosophy of mind, very little has been written about touch. To my knowledge, the two authors who have addressed the topic in most depth are O'Shaughnessy (1989, 1995, 2000) and Martin (1992, 1993, 1995), and I will explore the phenomenology of touch through a critical discussion of their work. Both emphasize the differences between vision and touch. Even so, I will argue that they impose upon tactile experience a misleading distinction between perception of body and perception of world.

What are the principal differences between vision and touch? According to O'Shaughnessy, touch, unlike vision, usually has a diachronic structure. We explore the world through touch, whereas 'the contents of a visual field are simultaneously presented to view' (1989, p.44). We can see that an edge is straight just by looking at it but, in order to perceive its straightness through touch, a temporally extended pattern of feelings and movements is required.[2] There is also no tactile analogue of the visual field. Furthermore, touch relies on bodily awareness in a way that vision does not—through touch, we use the properties of our own bodies to investigate the tactile properties of other bodies. I will focus on this last claim.

O'Shaughnessy acknowledges that bodily feelings are not always a conspicuous feature of tactile experience. In some cases, there is only a bodily awareness. But, in others, attention is not directed at the body; it 'unambiguously goes beyond our own body and we perceive the object which actively we explore' (1989, pp.43–4). However, he maintains that there are two perceptions at play in all cases of touch. There is a feeling of the body as it comes into contact with an object and there is also a tactile perception of the object. He claims that touch and proprioception are 'mirror-image senses', which work together in relations of mutual dependence, 'one sense leading us outwards beyond ourselves, the other taking us back into ourselves' (2000, p.674). Why distinguish the two, given the extent of their interdependence? O'Shaughnessy acknowledges that they 'depend inextricably' upon each other (2000, p.630); but he also lists several differences between them, which rule out their identity. For example, proprioception facilitates an immediate awareness of bodily position and movement, whereas all tactile perception is mediated by bodily awareness. They also have different objects. The objects of touch can be any number of things, whereas proprioception has only one object, the body. And there are various structural differences between the two. For example, proprioception does not ordinarily involve an appreciation of properties such as shape (1995, pp.176–7).

Hence touch, according to O'Shaughnessy, differs from vision in a number of respects, a central difference being the extent to which it is dependent upon proprioception. However, it is arguable that the two are not quite so different. One option is to maintain that touch is, after all, much like spectatorially construed vision. Another is to argue that spectatorial models of vision, which take it to involve the synchronic, passive, detached presentation of experiential contents, are mistaken and that vision is actually more touch-like than that.

---

[2] O'Shaughnessy (2000, pp. 667–8) claims that tactile perception of edges and the like is, sometimes at least, representational. By this, he means that we can intuit the shape of an object through the pattern of corresponding limb movements that occur as we actively explore it via touch. He notes that this is not the case when we touch complicated objects but suggests that representation still holds 'piecemeal'. In other words, although the pattern of movements as a whole does not correspond to the shape of the object, individual movements mirror parts of that shape.

The first approach is adopted by Scott (2001), who claims that vision and touch 'are both image processing systems that extract information from two dimensional sheets of receptors' (p.151). He acknowledges that proprioception and action facilitate both vision and touch but claims that they are *associated* with both senses, rather than being *constitutive* of them (p.152). He adds that touch does not rely upon proprioception to the extent that O'Shaughnessy indicates. This view is, I suggest, mistaken. A contrasting approach is required, which recognizes that neither vision nor touch is separable from proprioception. Consider, first of all, the relationship between touch and proprioception. It is possible to individuate and distinguish perceptual modalities in a number of ways. One might appeal to proper objects, phenomenological character, stimuli or organs, amongst other things (Gray, 2005). If we adopt a phenomenological conception of touch, as I do here, a distinction between proprioception and touch is untenable. Touch without proprioception would be so diminished as to bear little resemblance to the rich and heterogeneous phenomenology that we associate with tactile experience. For example, touch surely includes a phenomenological distinction between the feelings of actively touching something and of being passively touched by something. If touch is removed from proprioception, this distinction is lost. Without a sense of where the body is located and of how it is moving, the feeling of actively touching could not be distinguished from that of being passively touched. This is not to say that all touch would then be 'passive' but, rather, that the experience would involve neither the category 'active' nor the category 'passive'.

Furthermore, we make much more fine-grained tactile discriminations than that between active and passive, all of which would be lost in the absence of proprioception. Merleau-Ponty notes that passive point contact with an object facilitates only a somewhat impoverished tactile experience:

> [Passive touch] tells us hardly anything but the state of our own body and almost nothing about the object. Even on the most sensitive parts of our tactile surface, pressure without movement produces a scarcely identifiable phenomenon. (1962, p.315)[3]

In contrast, through exploratory activity we perceive characteristics such as smoothness, sharpness, softness, wetness, roughness, stickiness and oiliness. We do not experience an assemblage of synchronic tactile atoms, one following on from the next, from which properties such as smoothness are then inferred. Perception of these properties is diachronic in structure. It is a matter of how patterns of changing sensation correspond to patterns of

---

[3] See also Jonas (1954) for the claim that passive point contact is devoid of information.

bodily movements. A sense of what one's body is doing is inextricable from how the surface feels:

> Smoothness is not a collection of similar pressures, but the way in which a surface utilizes the time occupied by our tactile exploration or modulates the movement of our hand. The style of these modulations particularizes so many modes of appearance of the tactile phenomenon, which are not reducible to each other and cannot be deduced from an elementary tactile sensation. (Merleau-Ponty, 1962, p.315)

The range of subtle tactile discriminations that we make is nicely conveyed by the following passage from John Hull's book *Touching the Rock*:

> As a blind person, sitting on the beach, I have poured a fistful of sand upon the palm of my other hand, allowing it to trickle through my fingers. I have rubbed the sand between my finger and thumb, wondering at the various textures. Some of the grains are coarse and sharp, filing the skin in such a way that every little speck stands out. Some are so smooth and silky that it is almost impossible to tell the grains, the sand disappearing like water. (1990, p.70)

The textures are revealed through patterns of activity; a sense of what the body is doing is inseparable from the ability to discriminate them.

Scott makes the following point, in support of the claim that touch and proprioception are distinct senses:

> The fact that awareness of one's body commonly occurs without tactual experience, such as when one feels the position of a limb that is not in contact with an external object, tells in favour of the view that bodily awareness and touch are distinct experiences. (2001, p.152)

But it is by no means clear that this is so. It would be a mistake to limit the scope of touch to cases where the skin is in direct physical contact with some object. As recognized by Merleau-Ponty, an absence of tactile contact can also contribute to the experience:

> ...if I touch a piece of linen material or a brush, between the bristles of the brush and the threads of the linen, there does not lie a tactile nothingness, but a tactile space devoid of matter, a tactile background. (1962, p.316)

Touch is not simply a matter of 'touching'. 'Not touching' is often a very real part of the experience and sometimes the most conspicuous part of it. This not only applies to cases of active touch, such as the above, but to passive touch too. The touch of one's clothes is not ordinarily at the forefront of awareness but its absence can be. If one takes off one's clothes and walks around the room (even a warm room), the sense of not being touched can be quite pronounced, at least for a short time. There is a feeling of something being 'missing'. Indeed, I am not sure that there is ever a complete 'absence' of touch. Much of the human body is covered in fine hairs, which are sensitive to air currents, amongst other things. It is also arguable that a sense of hot and cold should be considered part of touch. It is possible to lose this whilst retaining tactile feeling more generally (Gallagher, 2005, chapter 2). However, this need not imply that the two are distinct senses. By analogy, visual perception of colour can be lost, whilst perception of shape, depth and movement are retained. All the same, colour perception is certainly part of vision.

No part of the body is ever in a tactile 'nowhere'. The absence of physical touch does not amount to an absence of tactile experience and there are numerous different tactile relationships, in addition to that between, say, a fingertip and an object. When all this is taken into account, it is not clear that awareness of bodily position and movement is ever fully separated from touch. Given that most, if not all, of the tactile discriminations that we make depend upon proprioception, it makes most sense to maintain that touch incorporates proprioception. O'Shaughnessy is quite right to note that they are not identical; there are indeed differences between them. However, it can be accepted that proprioception always *participates* in touch without any commitment to the stronger view that every aspect of proprioception is implicated in touch or that it is exhausted by its contribution to touch.

My emphasis here is on the *phenomenology* of touch. This leaves open the possibility that non-phenomenological methods for individuating sensory modalities might distinguish touch from proprioception. Sensory modalities can no doubt be individuated in many different ways and perhaps there are various, equally legitimate accounts of what a perceptual system is. Nevertheless, any account that failed to accommodate most of the perceptual discriminations that are ordinarily associated with a particular sense modality would surely be seriously deficient. Touch without proprioception would be stripped of almost all its phenomenological structure. Thus, if it were construed in such a way, a further account would be required of what it is that *does* enable us, by means of touch, to discriminate a wide range of different properties. So, although touch might be defined so as to exclude proprioception, this would just involve moving all the interesting questions elsewhere.

Scott's account of touch presupposes a particular characterization of vision. He claims that touch, like vision, is an image-processing system that has, as its input, patterns of sensation on a two-dimensional sheet of receptors. Models of vision based on such premises have a distinguished history and continue to be widely endorsed. For example, Marr's highly influential 1982 account treats vision as an information-processing task, which transforms a retinal image into a three-dimensional object representation. In taking the retinal image as the sole input for the process, Marr assumes that the visual system can be fruitfully investigated in isolation from the other world-directed senses, from proprioception and from an organism's active exploration of its world.

However, there is growing scepticism regarding such approaches. Gibson (1979) famously suggested that visual perception is dependent upon proprioception and patterns of bodily activity, and numerous authors have taken their lead from this view. Noë (2004), for instance, explicitly appeals to the similarities between vision and touch in order to challenge certain models of vision.[4] He is critical of approaches that construe vision in terms of static pictorial representations of the world, derived from retinal images. According to Noë, an organism does not passively observe a visual scene in its entirety but perceives it through a process of active exploration. Visual perception is a skilful activity, involving a largely tacit appreciation of how bodily movements correspond with changing patterns of sensory stimulation. He claims that the extent to which visual perception depends upon bodily activities is such that a loss of integration between patterns of sensory input and bodily activities would amount to what he calls 'experiential blindness' (2004, p.5), an unstructured experience bearing little resemblance to the organized environment revealed through visual exploration. So vision, like touch, is something that is bound up with our activities. In both cases, we perceive objects in virtue of our appreciation of how their appearances change in relation to patterns of bodily activity.

Acceptance of some such view need not entail that there are no significant differences between touch and vision. As I will suggest later in this chapter, one such difference renders touch a better guide than vision to the phenomenological structure of our relationship with the world. Nevertheless, regardless of what applies to vision, the term 'experiential blindness' certainly sums up the experience of touch without proprioception. Stripped of all the structure that enables the variety of tactile experience, touch would amount to little more than undifferentiated sensation. If anything, it would be an absence of perception, rather than tactile perception cleansed of contamination from bodily awareness. So, given that vision need not be conceived of in isolation from proprioception, there are no grounds for imposing such a view upon touch, where it is even less plausible.

Aspect shifts

Even if touch and proprioception are not distinct senses, the question remains as to how the relationship between bodily and non-bodily sides of tactile experience should be understood. Martin offers an answer. Like O'Shaughnessy,

---

4 Merleau-Ponty's later work also draws attention to the similarities between vision and touch. He even hints at the idea that vision is a kind of 'distance-touching' (see Cataldi, 1993, for a discussion).

he argues that vision and touch differ in important ways. For example, touch does not involve a tactile field akin to the visual field. Through vision, we not only see objects located in space; we also see the spatial relations between them and there is no tactile analogue of this.[5] As Martin recognizes, some experiences, such as pressing a warm coin onto one's palm and feeling its shape, do seem to involve a kind of tactile field. Conversely, there may be cases of vision where there is no field, such as extreme tunnel vision. However, he adds that tactile and visual fields differ in structure, the main difference being that the former has both inner and outer aspects. In touching the coin, one perceives a part of one's body in addition to perceiving the shape of the coin. Visual perception, in contrast, does not include this kind of bodily awareness. Unlike O'Shaughnessy, Martin suggests that the bodily and non-bodily sides of tactile experience are not distinct perceptions but aspects of a single, unitary perception. Attention can oscillate between them, in a manner analogous to perception of aspect-shifts. For example, when running one's finger around the rim of a glass:

> The sensation one feels in one's fingertip feels to be within one's body and at the limits of one's body, at the skin. One also feels one's fingertip to be pressing against an object, one which resists the further movement of one's finger down through the rim [...] We should think of this case not as one in which we have two distinct states of mind, a bodily sensation and a tactual perception, both of which can be attended to; but instead simply as one state of mind, which can be attended to in different ways. One can attend to it as a bodily sensation [...] or attend to it as tactual perception of something lying beyond the body but in contact with it...
> (Martin, 1992, p.204)

Martin claims that the body is always the 'proper object' of tactile feeling; 'anything which one feels in this way is taken to be part of one's body'. However, tactile feelings are felt to occur at bodily *boundaries*, at the places where the body meets the world. Hence they provide a sense of the limits of the body and, by implication, of there being a space outside of those limits (1992, pp.201–2). They fall within the boundaries and so are felt to be events within one's body, at the skin, but it is possible to attend to either side of a boundary (1995, p.270). Thus, by means of touch, we explore entities through the ways in which they come into contact with our boundaries: 'One measures the properties of objects in the world around one against one's body. So in having an awareness of one's body, one has a sense of touch' (1992, p.203). The body acts as a kind of 'template' that perceives things external to it through the

---

[5] Martin adopts a phenomenological conception of the 'visual field', rather than one that is explicitly based upon a specific philosophical theory of perception. He notes that O'Shaughnessy's account of the field presupposes a sense data theory (Martin, 1992, p.197).

ways in which they impress upon its boundaries. An organism can explore the world by sensing its body, where it can move, where and how it is impeded.[6]

Although I agree that bodily and non-bodily sides are aspects of a single perception, rather than being two distinct perceptions, I suggest that Martin's account of boundaries is phenomenologically incomplete and potentially misleading. He claims that the body is encountered as an object, situated amongst other objects, and does not indicate that it can be felt in any other way:

> ...awareness of one's body as one's body involves a sense of its being a bounded object within a larger space, and that just is to locate it within a space of tactual objects. The two kinds of awareness are [...] interdependent. (1993, p.213)

O'Shaughnessy (2000, p.628) similarly indicates that the body is perceived in an object-like way. He notes that, in touch, 'the body does not appear to consciousness as a rival object of awareness as we actively engage with our surroundings'. Even so, he adds that the background bodily awareness that we have when focusing upon an object external to the body is no different in quality from a bodily awareness that occupies the experiential foreground. The difference is only one of intensity—during tactile contact, the body can be felt to a greater or lesser degree. O'Shaughnessy offers the example of a game of tennis and claims that:

> Even though one's attention is focused primarily on the path of the ball, and doubtless also though to a much lesser extent on the path of the racquet, some small measure of attention must be left over for the movement of the arm. (2000, p.632)

Although the arm is perceived to a lesser extent than in certain other scenarios, it is still perceived in the same manner. He appeals to phenomenology in support of this, suggesting that we can reflect upon tactile exploration, whilst engaged in it. In so doing, we can attend to the hand as an object of awareness and, at the same time, to the object that it touches (1989, p.46).

However, the body can be *felt* in quite different ways and recognition of this is essential to an understanding of tactile experience. Proprioception (understood in a general way as an awareness of bodily position and movement that is unmediated by other senses), need not be an awareness of the body or some part of it as an *object* of experience. Indeed, it seldom is. One problem with reflecting upon experience is that the act of reflection can itself alter the experience. As Gallagher (2005, pp.30–1) cautions, 'any experimental situation that places the subject in a reflective attitude in order to ascertain something about prereflective experience is questionable'. This methodological concern applies

---

6 Martin does not think of an organism as having only one boundary. There are boundaries within boundaries. For example, a bone stuck in the oesophagus presses against one boundary but this boundary is internal to another boundary (1992, p.272).

equally to phenomenological reflection. For example, when reaching out to take a cup of hot coffee from someone, my hand is not conspicuous as an object; it is experienced as that through which an object is to be grasped. But, if I reflect on the act whilst performing it, my hand might become more conspicuous, object-like, and an exchange that would have been routine and effortless then becomes distinctly awkward. I strain to grasp the cup; the way in which my hand is felt now impedes the smooth movement of reaching. My hold on the cup is insecure, not dependable. I don't feel the cup so much as my own cumbersome fingers.

The question therefore arises as to whether the distinct bodily feeling that O'Shaughnessy finds always accompanying tactile perception, and the body-object that Martin emphasizes, are both artefacts of reflective exercises; exercises that may be influenced by debatable philosophical presuppositions about experience. How do we arbitrate between conflicting intuitions on this matter? A well-known example offered by Merleau-Ponty (1964b, 1968) serves to make clear (a) the way in which reflection can alter the structure of an experience and (b) how the body, during the course of tactile exploration, is not felt in an object-like way. Merleau-Ponty considers the experience of touching one's left hand with one's right hand:

> ...the moment perception comes my body effaces itself before it and never does the perception grasp the body in the act of perceiving. If my left hand is touching my right hand, and if I should suddenly wish to apprehend with my right hand the work of my left hand as it touches, this reflection of the body upon itself always miscarries at the last moment: the moment I feel my left hand with my right hand, I correspondingly cease touching my right hand with my left hand. (1968, p.9)[7]

When one hand touches the other, the two hands are 'felt' in very different ways. One is an organ of perception, whilst the other is an object of perception. When a hand is engaged in active tactile exploration, it is not encountered in a thing-like way at all, as illustrated by the contrast between how it feels and how the other hand is simultaneously felt. One might object that the relevant feeling is lurking in the background somewhere and can be attended to. However, when we try to attend to it, we end up changing the structure of the experience. The touching hand is no longer that which feels but that which is felt and there is a switch between the roles of the two hands, between perceiver and perceived. The touched hand, itself being an organ of perception, now becomes what does the touching, and the previously touching hand becomes the perceived object. There is a subtle 'reversibility' in the roles of the hands. When the touching becomes the touched, the bodily side is not felt in the

---

[7] Merleau-Ponty's discussion develops themes that are addressed by Husserl (1989, chapter 3).

same *way* that it was previously. In making the bodily aspect of touch available as a perceptual object, we change how the body is perceived. It cannot be made conspicuous without altering the way in which both the hand and the object it is in contact with are experienced.

Of course, the touched hand, although it is an object of experience, is not experienced in the same way as an object of experience that is not part of one's body. The hand is something that is itself capable of active perceptual exploration, and its potentiality to reverse the situation by becoming the perceiver participates in the experience. However, there is still a difference in the way the two hands are felt, with one being apprehended in at least a *more* object-like way than the other, even though it is not experienced merely as a passive object that is revealed to the touch of the other hand.

The example is effective because it serves to distinguish two ways in which one's body can be felt by presenting them both at the same time, thus inviting comparison. The touching hand is not just a recessive object of perception. It is what *does the feeling* rather than what is *felt* and it performs this role precisely insofar as it is *not* an object of experience. The body, as it touches, is not the conspicuous, awkward, uncomfortable, uncooperative, clumsy, pleasured or painful body. It is in virtue of its not feeling any such way that it falls into the background of awareness and plays the role of perceiver rather than perceived.

The term 'bodily feeling' therefore turns out to be equivocal, and this point is crucial to my account of existential feeling. In one sense, a bodily feeling is *a feeling that has the body as its object*. In another, it is *a feeling done by the body that has something other than the body as its object*. In routine tactile activities and the like, bodily feelings are feelings of something other than the body and, in other situations, they are principally feelings of the body. So far as the body is concerned, what we have is neither the perception of two objects (O'Shaughnessy) nor of one object that can be attended to in two different ways, facilitating perception of 'inside' and 'outside' (Martin). Instead, touch is a relationship between touching and touched. How the touching body feels is inextricable from how an object is felt. When the body is itself an object of experience, it is felt in a very different way from the feeling body.

As the example of the touching hands suggests, it is possible to reflect on the phenomenology of the feeling body. There are two risks though. By attending to it, we might inadvertently change the experience and reveal a body-object where there was not one before. And we might also pick up on the feeling body but then misinterpret it as an object, the felt body. However, could it be that, in those cases where the body is that which feels rather than an object of feeling, it is not actually felt at all? Or perhaps it is felt but only weakly?

A distinction between strong and weak feelings does not accommodate the phenomenological difference between perceiver and perceived. Consider again the example of the numb hand, which was mentioned in Chapter 2. When normal feeling returns to the hand, it is not a perception *of the hand*. The renewed feeling manifests itself *as* the perceptual disappearance of the hand, in its being an organ of perception, rather than a perceived object. Something surely *returns* to the hand but this does not consist in its becoming a more salient object of perception. Indeed, it was more conspicuous in its numbness, when it was experienced as lacking something. As the transition from an unfeeling, numb hand to an effective organ of tactile perception illustrates, the feeling body is phenomenologically accessible precisely as a *feeling* rather than felt body, so long as the temptation to reconstruct it as an object of experience, by altering or misinterpreting the experience, is resisted.

Of course, one could conceive of 'touch' in a non-phenomenological way, as simply a matter of one object (the body) physically touching another. Given this, it could be maintained that a numb hand is still an instrument of touch. For example, O'Shaughnessy (2000, p.662) claims that 'tactile sensation is inessential to tactile perception', as you can sense an object impeding your path even with a numb arm. But such claims are based on a misconception of touch. Touch is not a matter of one object colliding with another; it is a sense of relatedness between the two that is quite variable in structure. It is only when the body is felt as an organ of perception that something other than the body can be an object of perception. If the body neither feels nor is felt, all we have is a collision of bodies that does not amount to perception.

In addition to misconstruing the perceiving body, O'Shaughnessy and Martin also impose an overly strict division between the bodily and non-bodily aspects of tactile experience. The example of the two hands touching might suggest that tactile experience does indeed have a dual perceiver–perceived structure. But things are not so simple. The categories of passive, momentary tactile contact and active tactile exploration do not exhaust the varieties of touch. There are many other kinds of tactile perception. The bodily and worldly sides of the tactile relation can take up the experiential foreground to varying *degrees* and in different *ways*. As O'Shaughnessy (1995, p.176) rightly says, touch 'encompasses extremely heterogeneous phenomena'. Consider the following:

Visually guided manipulation of an object in a routine situation.

Exploratory touch.

Being in long-term bodily contact with a familiar object, such as a garment.

Being scraped by a branch whilst walking.

Feeling the cold wind against one's face.

Being touched expectedly or unexpectedly by another person.

The feeling of having clammy hands.

The feeling of not being touched; perhaps of not being wrapped up in clothing.

And the list goes on. In some cases, the body is more conspicuous and, in other cases, an object external to the body is more conspicuous. The aspect that occupies the experiential foreground can be experienced in different ways. One's body can feel clumsy or conspicuous, and one might also dwell on pleasurable bodily sensations. Turning to the other side of the relation, objects can solicit all manner of tactile feelings; something can feel slimy, rough, hard, smooth or soft. Tactile perception also seems to have an intrinsic valence to it; things can feel pleasant to the touch, soliciting further exploration. Or they can feel unpleasant in a variety of ways. Parts of the body can likewise feel pleasant or unpleasant during tactile contact with things.

However, there are also plenty of cases that do not involve a clear distinction between perceiver and perceived. In contrast to active tactile exploration of one hand by another, consider putting one's palms together, as if to pray. There is no touching–touched structure here. Indeed, it is not clear quite where the feeling is. It does not seem to be 'located' in one hand, the other or both; there is just the 'touch' that unites them. As I will now show, there are many such cases. They serve to challenge (a) an emphasis on bodily boundaries and (b) the assumption that touch always has two clearly distinguishable aspects, a bodily and a non-bodily aspect.

Boundaries

What is seen is not located in the same place as the organs of sight and what is heard is not experienced as residing in the ears. In the case of touch too, although the body perceives, it is not usually the object of perception and what is perceived need not be in physical contact with the body. There are plenty of cases where the objects of touch are not located at the physical boundary between body and world. An oft-quoted example is the blind person's cane, which is an organ of perception, rather than an object that is encountered by the hand. One feels through the cane, rather than encountering it as a perceptual object (Hull, 1990).[8] There are many other examples. A medical practitioner recently informed me that 'I have recurrently been struck by how the stethoscope vanishes: it is just the heart sounds. Despite me

---

[8] See also Merleau-Ponty (1962, p.143).

holding and manipulating a tool to access that sound'.[9] Ihde offers the example of running a pencil along a desk and perceiving the texture of the desk. He notes that the skin–object boundary, the feeling of pressure against the finger, cannot be brought to the forefront of awareness without altering the experience:

> ...by conscious effort you can [...] make this finger-pencil aspect of the experience stand out. But when it does, the pencil-desk aspect tends to fade and vice-versa. While both aspects are present one tends to stand in the centre of the [f]ocus while the other fades to a fringe awareness. (1983, p.96)

Once we discard the assumption that what feels must be what is felt, it becomes clear that touch need not have a bodily boundary or an entity in direct contact with a boundary as its object. The relevant 'boundaries' are not fixed and in some cases they extend beyond the skin. This view becomes all the more plausible once it is acknowledged that we have quite a lot of hair. Many tactile experiences do not involve something coming into contact with the skin but with body hair. Consider cat's whiskers or 'vibrissae'. These are connected to several nerves, under limited muscular control and extremely sensitive. The cat uses its whiskers to explore its environment and one of their roles is to perceive the width of an opening relative to the width of the cat's body. For whiskers to be effective, what is perceived must not be the surface of the skin where the relevant nerves are located but objects located a certain distance from the skin. The term 'perceive', as used here, need not be understood in a phenomenological way. Indeed, I have no idea what a cat's tactile phenomenology is like, but such examples at least suffice to show that touch is not always a matter of registering the properties of objects and events at bodily boundaries. And phenomenological reflection is, of course, possible with regard to our own body hair, which, when disturbed, does not always generate 'feelings of the skin'. For example, when having the hair on one's head caressed, one feels the touch of another person but not as a pattern of changing sensations situated on one's scalp. The feeling is much more diffuse than that, spread out beyond the skin and lacking a precise location.

When touching, we often do not distinguish our bodies from the entities we touch. When a skilled tennis player holds a racquet during a game, her hand is not experienced as perceptually 'confronting' the racquet. Boundaries become blurred during such activities and it is not wholly clear where the touching ends and the touched begins. Cases like the racquet and the cane, which involve an extension of bodily boundaries, also involve a diminution or loss of certain other bodily boundaries. In feeling *with* the cane, rather than feeling the cane, the boundary between body and cane disappears. Some ways in

---

[9] Thanks to Matthew Broome for this example.

which the body *feels* thus involve a lack of differentiation between the body and an object that it is in contact with.

The diminution or loss of boundaries also occurs in some experiences of passive touch, where the feeling–felt distinction is blurred or altogether absent. Many such experiences involve the tactile background, rather than episodes of localized touch. There is a tendency in the literature to emphasize instances of active touch that are in the foreground of experience. However, touch is much more pervasive than this and touches that fall into the experiential background do not distinguish boundaries so cleanly. Taking another of Ihde's examples, consider the way in which boundaries between body and object fade when lying on a really comfortable sofa or bed:

> I find that the cloud-like couch-me experience is so vague that not even any clear distinction between me and where I end and couch is capable of being made. Inner and outer, subject and object are here not at all clear and distinct. (Ihde, 1983, p.97)

Whilst I was making notes, in preparation for writing this chapter, I tried to reflect on my tactile experience at the time. There was a cool breeze on my left forearm from a draft coming through the open window. I felt the grip of the pen, with my hand more salient than usual, as it was tiring. I felt my sweaty finger slipping on the pen and, as it happened, that part of my body, rather than the pen, becoming the object of awareness. Did I feel my clothes? Most of my body was in contact with them and yet I did not draw a firm boundary between them and me. In fact, the light breeze on my arm was a much more conspicuous aspect of the experience, with clearer boundaries. On reflection, I could feel the rub of my collar on my neck and a slight tightness where I'd done my belt up one notch too far. But my tactile relationship with my clothes was not a salient part of my experience, as touching or as touched. There was no firm experiential boundary between me and them.

When we are habituated to active or passive tactile contact, when something becomes familiar, we do not fully differentiate between the bodily and non-bodily sides of the experience. Hence touch is a relation in which one side, the other or neither may be conspicuous and it includes varying degrees of self–world differentiation. There is nothing mysterious about this, once it is recognized that sensation at a boundary need not be feeling of a boundary and also that, even when what is felt does happen to be a bodily boundary, it need not be felt *as* a boundary. Touch is often a sense of diffuse or absent boundaries and, where boundaries are perceived, they need not correspond to the physical boundaries of the body. The body–world or inside–outside distinction is not an essential ingredient of tactile experience and the assumption that it is stems from the unwarranted a priori imposition of an internal–external contrast upon it.

Being in touch with the world

We are now in a position to reflect upon the relationship between tactile and existential feeling. By appealing to the phenomenology of touch, I have argued that certain feelings do not have the body as their object but are relations between body and world, in which body, world or neither appear as the experiential foreground. Chapter 4 will suggest that the same goes for 'feelings' more generally, which are seldom if ever just perceptions of internal bodily states. However, there is more than just an analogy between existential feeling and touch—the tactile background contributes to our sense of belonging to the world, structuring more localized tactile experiences and our experiences more generally. Thus it is partly constitutive of existential feeling.

O'Shaughnessy (1989, 2000) claims that touch is our most fundamental or 'primordial' sense. Although it is eclipsed by vision in most of our experiences, it is essential to the animal condition. Tactile contact with the world is bound up with the having of an animal body. Agency and touch work together; we could not have motor control without touch and vice versa. I do not want to endorse any claims regarding the overall primacy of one sense over another. For one thing, it is not at all clear what the criteria for making such comparisons ought to be. Even so, I do think there is something right about this emphasis on the centrality of touch to our *relationship* with the world. Touch, I suggest, is partly constitutive of the sense we have of being in a world. It is not a localized phenomenon that occurs only in hands or fingertips. Once we take into account all the varieties of touch, it becomes clear that the whole bodily surface is always involved. Certain touches are inconspicuous but it is precisely in virtue of their inconspicuousness that they contribute to our phenomenology. As I write this, the feeling of my body touching the chair is not a salient part of my experience, and my experience does not incorporate a clear distinction between my bodily boundaries and the cushion of the chair. It is this inconspicuousness and lack of differentiation that constitutes a sense of comfort, of being situated in an environment in such a way that my attention can be directed at other things. When I feel an itch or an ache and adjust my position, this is not simply a transition from a lack of feeling to a feeling. Once we stop thinking of bodily feelings as perceptions of a body-object, it is possible to appreciate that the body or part of it can be felt *as* inconspicuous, *as* undifferentiated from its surroundings, *as* comfortably belonging. There is no doubt that the nerve endings in my fingers are more concentrated and, as I type, more active than those in the skin that rests upon the seat. But the difference between the two feelings is not just due to differing levels of neural density and activity. These are not reliable indicators of the extent to which a body part is phenomenologically conspicuous or of the *way* in which it is felt.

Recall the example of the numb hand again. It is conspicuous because normal responsiveness is diminished or absent.

We might think of the whole skin as a tactile field (although I do not wish to suggest that this 'field' is isomorphic in any illuminating respect with the visual field). Montagu (1986, p.127) observes that 'the very phrase "sense of touch" has come to mean, almost exclusively, feeling with the fingers or hand'. However, it is misleading to emphasize only one aspect of tactile perception, such as a hand resting on the rim of a glass, and then wonder whether the sensory receptors in that hand alone comprise a field. By analogy, it would be a mistake to investigate the visual field by considering only a small part of the retina that happened to be where ambient light from an especially conspicuous object was falling. So why take only a slab of skin that is most proximal to an object at the forefront of awareness? We should at least consider the skin as a whole, the entire organ that, in conjunction with proprioception and movement, facilitates touch.

Ihde (1983) suggests that the tactile field as a whole becomes phenomenologically conspicuous on those occasions when the entire skin is simultaneously affected in the same way by the environment. He gives the example of jumping in a lake, where one feels one's whole body coming into contact with the cold, wet environment. Then, upon stepping out of the water and experiencing the warm sun upon one's body, there is another all-encompassing bodily feeling, which might be described as a sense of bodily exhilaration. He also indicates that this touch-field is integral to a sense of connectedness between self and world, of belonging to the world:

> ...when the whole of my touch field touches and is touched by the surrounding world, I realize how intimate is the I-world relation in touch. Through touch, I am constantly 'in touch' with that which surrounds me. But also in these states it is difficult to say just where I end and the world begins. All the specific touches found in focal attentiveness are never separate from the total Touch as the constant field in which I live. (1983, p.99)

The structure of our relationship with the world cannot be adequately conveyed in terms of any account that imposes a clear boundary between self and non-self or bodily and non-bodily upon all experience. The connectedness integral to touch provides a better clue. It is curious that so many accounts of perception emphasize the self–world boundary, the distinction between subject and object or the separation between bodily and non-bodily. Granted, we do distinguish between self and world but this is not to say that every aspect of our experience conforms to the distinction. Indeed, a sense of being situated *in* a world, rather than being cut-off from it or viewing it from some strange, detached, dislocated standpoint, is partly constituted by those tactile relations that do *not* cleanly differentiate self from non-self.

When we are comfortably passive or absorbed in a smooth context of bodily activity, neither the body nor the physical boundary between the body and everything else is especially salient. Body and world are, to some extent at least, undifferentiated. Take the example of typing, which I appealed to in Chapter 2 when explaining Heidegger's distinction between readiness-to-hand and presence-at-hand. As I type these words, I do not feel my fingers as objects and neither do I perceive the keys as a series of isolated objects. When the typing progresses smoothly, the keyboard is not cleanly differentiated from my manipulation of it. My attention is not focused on the bodily activity or on the keyboard but on the project of writing that my bodily activity is purposively directed towards. So the readiness-to-hand/presence-at-hand contrast is complemented by a description of our tactile phenomenology. Experiencing things as wholly ready-to-hand is often a matter of their disappearing into our tactile activities, of the body becoming inconspicuous and of the object that it is in contact with becoming phenomenologically indistinguishable from it. The experience involves a relation where neither side is salient in an object-like way. In addition, it is often a matter of distance-touch. What one feels is not the ready-to-hand tool that is touched but what that tool comes into contact with, such as the desk that the pencil scrapes. Heidegger famously offers the example of using a hammer, remarking that the less we 'stare' at it and the more we 'seize hold of it and use it, the more primordial does our relationship to it become' (1962, p.98). We are most at home with the things that we do not fully distinguish ourselves from. Fluent practical manipulation is at the same time a loss of boundaries between body and equipment. The experience of the hammer involves a sense of connectedness to it, rather than the estrangement that would be characteristic of staring at a broken tool.

Now consider tactile experiences where the body or the contrast between bodily and non-bodily is especially conspicuous. The cold, wet body that warms as it leaves the water becomes conspicuous in a pleasant way. But there are many other cases of bodily conspicuousness that are best characterized in terms of a failure to touch, to make contact with the world. Bodily boundaries and body–world duality often feature when things go wrong or of when we engage with something unfamiliar and perhaps threatening. In a scene from the film *Flash Gordon*, some characters have to undergo a trial, which requires inserting an arm into one of several holes in a tree stump. Inside lurks a 'tree beast', whose sting will result in an agonizing death. What would the experience of touch be like in this case? A feeling of the boundary between the hand and everything else would surely be unusually pronounced. Everything that brushed against it would be immediately felt as distinct from the body, as alien, disruptive, hostile. The hand itself would feel very conspicuous, standing out against its surroundings. As it moved through the stump, activities would be timid, awkward and very much at the forefront of awareness, a far cry from the practical familiarity, fluidity and integration between perceiver and perceived that characterize the experience of typing, from the sense of being rooted in an environment, not wholly separate from it, that the latter experience involves.

Not all cases where the body, an object and the distinction between them become conspicuous involve impediments to activity. There is novelty and there are various pleasurable sensations, often involving contact with other people. However, all of these are distractions from habitual activity, which are not indicative of our more general tactile relationship with the world. What characterizes rootedness in a familiar situation, belonging to a context, is the extension and diffusion of boundaries, a blurring of the self–world distinction. In touch, conspicuousness of the body is, at the same time, a failure to perceive the world, a loss of connectedness. Hence only a minority of tactile experiences have the kind of structure that O'Shaughnessy and Martin take to be typical of touch.

Turning again to the tactile background as a whole, suppose that one's body were experienced as a bounded object, ending at the skin. What would the experience really be like? It is important to note that any such change in background tactile feeling would also have a significant effect upon foreground tactile experience. When I type, I do so against the backdrop of undifferentiated belonging. I am anchored in a world and it is in the context of this background that I orient myself towards the computer and immerse myself in the project of writing. But if that background of belonging were not in place, if my body were conspicuous and experienced as something object-like, distinct from its surroundings, all my activities would be somehow less fluid, less 'natural'. One cannot disappear into a particular pattern of practical activity if all of one's experience is structured by an absence of practical belonging, if one does not feel 'in touch' with the world.

As I will discuss in Chapter 7, phenomenologically-minded psychiatrists have pointed out that an experiential structure much like this features in conditions such as schizophrenia. Diminished bodily feeling is, at the same time, an object-like conspicuousness of the body. In conjunction with this, there is a loss of relatedness to the world, a failure of the body as a 'feeling' rather than 'felt' entity, a lack of practical belonging and a feeling of estrangement. In Chapter 2, I noted that the feelings in question are often referred to as 'affects', suggesting emotional rather than tactile feeling. However, it seems plausible to maintain that various 'affective' feelings incorporate tactile feelings.[10] After all,

---

[10] See also Cataldi (1993) for the view that tactile feelings participate in affective feelings.

we often talk of things that 'make our hair stand on end', 'make our skin crawl' or 'send a shiver down the spine'. It is also worth noting that emotionally charged situations are often described metaphorically, using tactile vocabulary such as 'sticky' and 'delicate' (Cataldi, 1993, p.134). People also talk of being 'out of touch with reality' and of being in touch with things and with each other (Montagu, 1986, p.11). Surely tactile feelings contribute in some way to the forms of bodily conspicuousness and inconspicuousness involved in existential feelings. Could the body as a whole really *feel* conspicuous without any change in the tactile field? I suggest not. Awareness of one's body is, at least in part, a tactile awareness. As I will suggest towards the end of Chapter 4, it is no accident that we often express our relationship with the world by invoking the language of touch, such as 'things seeming intangible', 'feeling out of touch with the world' and 'losing one's grip on things'.[11]

Touch thus serves to illustrate something important about our relationship with the world: it is a matter of belonging and connectedness, rather than of full-scale confrontation between body and object. Touch is at least partly constitutive of the relationship. This is not to suggest that the self–world relation simply is 'touch'. Rather, it incorporates touch and its overall structure is touch-like, in so far as it involves a sense of relatedness between self and world, where the two are variably differentiated and one or the other can occupy the foreground of experience to different degrees and in different ways. Accounts that emphasize a bounded body-object misconstrue connectedness as alienation.

The intimate connection between existential and tactile feeling also indicates that there will be a variety of existential feelings, given that there are many different kinds of tactile experience. It is an open question as to which kinds of bodily state contribute to existential feeling and I will offer some suggestions in Chapter 4. However, given the range of feelings facilitated by touch alone, I think it is safe to say that relevant bodily states and the ways in which they are experienced are diverse enough to allow for many subtly different kinds of existential feeling.

The tactile background that sets the scene for localized tactile experiences is not impervious to feedback from these and other experiences. An overall feeling of bodily conspicuousness might gradually fade as one becomes first of all effortfully involved but eventually unthinkingly immersed in an activity. Conversely, the body as a whole might become more pronounced as a particular

---

[11] It is also worth noting that level of affective arousal is usually measured by monitoring skin conductance response. Conductance increases with arousal, due to increased perspiration. It seems doubtful that this and numerous other changes that might affect the skin as a whole are merely symptoms of affect, which do not themselves contribute to experience in any way.

activity fails, as one clumsily reaches for the glass and it smashes on the floor. So there is commerce between focal touch and the tactile field as a whole. Nevertheless, the tactile background frames all specific activities. Even though it can be reshaped by them, some variant of it always underlies them.

Through our various activities, we change and manage our 'boundaries'. For example, in taking hold of someone's hand, you might at first experience a clear boundary between yours and theirs. But, if you continue to hold it for a prolonged period, perhaps whilst walking together, the boundaries may well fade. Opposition between bounded bodies diffuses, to be replaced by a sense of connectedness. Given the extent of tactile contact between people and the many different ways in which people touch each other, it is curious that studies of interpersonal experience and understanding almost always emphasize visual perception of one person by another. Merleau-Ponty (e.g. 1964a) is an exception, in maintaining that touch is foundational to intersubjectivity. When you touch one of your hands with the other, you experience their oscillation between subject and object positions. And, he claims, when your hand is held by someone, there is a similar appreciation of that person's hand as something that can take up the position of subject or object.[12]

We often use tactile metaphors to describe other people. Montagu (1986, p.10) lists some of these: people can 'rub' each other up the wrong way and have 'prickly' or 'abrasive' personalities. They can get 'under one's skin' or be only 'skin deep'. We talk of 'getting in touch' with people, of people being 'hard' to deal with and needing to be 'handled carefully', of people being 'touchy' and 'thick/thin skinned'.[13] It is telling that the metaphors used to describe difficult people invoke those tactile experiences that involve confrontation and boundaries, such as encountering a hard, abrasive or prickly object. Experiences like these, where boundaries are pronounced and the subject–object distinction is clearest, are precisely those that disrupt our relatedness. They certainly do not typify it. I wonder whether at least some allegedly *metaphorical* talk about 'touch' can in fact be understood literally (a view that will be further explored and supported towards the end of Chapter 4). Perhaps some of the same tactile feelings that we have when touching certain kinds of object actually occur in interpersonal experiences. Keep in mind that touch need not involve physical contact with the skin. Indeed, as the example of the 'tree beast' illustrates, the tactile field can be primed in a particular way in advance of physical contact.

[12] See Stawarska (2006) for a discussion of Merleau-Ponty on touch, vision and intersubjectivity.

[13] Montagu (1986) also emphasizes the extent of the contribution made by tactile contact to interpersonal development.

The main reason why touch provides a better starting point for the exploration of existential feeling than vision is that, unlike vision and the other senses, it involves routine reversibility—bodily and worldly sides frequently oscillate between foreground and background, between perceiver and perceived. Most experience incorporates a taken-for-granted sense of relatedness to the world, of not being wholly separate from it. This remains presupposed when we carve ourselves off from it in theory or pit ourselves against part of it in practice. I suggest that the structure of touch, with its reversibility and varying degrees of differentiation between the two sides, can serve as a guide to this aspect of experience and circumvent some of the pitfalls that occur when world-experience is modelled upon vision, abstracted from its bodily context.

Vision does not so obviously manifests this reversibility, and the comparative lack of reversibility in vision is a key difference between the two senses. However, it does seem that vision is susceptible to at least some degree of reversibility. Merleau-Ponty (1962, p.315) contrasts the 'exploratory gaze of true vision' with perception of a dazzling light. The latter involves a reversal that is analogous to touch but rare in vision, where the organ of sight becomes an object of perception. This reversal, he suggests, amounts to a breakdown of the practical orientation that ordinarily structures visual perception. Hence it is arguable that the differences between vision and touch are less pronounced than is often assumed.

Vision is often construed in terms of the perception of a synchronic world of unchanging objects, in contrast to touch, which is diachronic and change-orientated. For example, Jonas remarks that:

> ...the simultaneity of sight, with its extended 'present' of enduring objects, allows the distinction between change and the unchanging and therefore between becoming and being. All the other senses operate by registering change and cannot make that distinction. (1954, p.513)

However, accounts of vision as 'enactive' (e.g. Varela *et al.*, 1991; Noë, 2004) emphasize the manner in which visual perception too is bound up with skilful activity and with proprioception. It is not a matter of passive registration of synchronic experiential contents but of active exploration. There is plenty of evidence to support the view that proprioception and bodily activity structure visual perception (see Gallagher, 2005) and, in Chapters 4 to 7, I will further describe the role played by bodily feeling in experience, including visual experience. This role, I suggest, is better appreciated if vision is regarded not as a matter of passively registering things but as an active process, which involves the various sensory and motor dispositions that constitute our sense of belonging to the world.

Even so, there are of course phenomenological differences between vision and touch. It is indeed plausible to suggest that the former facilitates a phenomenology of objects, whereas the latter offers only a phenomenology of patterned changes. For example, Hull (1990, p.82) contrasts the world of the sighted with the world of the blind, stating that 'mine is not a world of being; it is a world of becoming. The world of being, the silent, still world where things simply are, that does not exist'. He also describes himself as feeling 'enclosed' in his body, without vision to reach out into the world and escape from himself (1990, p.156). Another difference is that the role of the feeling body in visual perception is usually hidden, allowing one to forget the intimacy of self and world. Belonging falls into the background as experience directs itself towards a realm of objects that might seem, on the basis of superficial reflection, to be decoupled from one's situatedness in the world. So there is a tendency to overlook the sense of belonging and to construe experience in terms of the detached gaze that seemingly takes in a world which is unadulterated by one's being part of it.

A question I have not yet addressed is that of the extent to which vision and touch are phenomenologically interrelated. Both, I suggest, are shaped by a common background of bodily feeling, which includes a sense of bodily position and of actual and potential bodily movements. Hence they share some common structure. Merleau-Ponty claims that vision and touch are also intermingled in certain ways. Objects, as presented visually, incorporate a sense of salient tactile possibilities. Experience has a background structure that does not respect distinctions between the senses: 'these distinctions between touch and sight are unknown in primordial perception [....] We *see* the depth, the smoothness, the softness, the hardness of objects' (1964a, p.15).

Ihde (1983, p.100) similarly comments on the artificiality of an emphasis on touch, conceived of in isolation from the other senses. When I see textures, he says, I also 'feel' them. The point that they both make is not that the boundaries between *actual* tactile experiences and *actual* visual experiences are blurred but that actual *visual* experiences incorporate tactile *possibilities* and vice versa. The same goes for other senses. The objects that we see appear to us as things that might be touched, tasted, heard or smelled in various salient ways. So an object is, as Merleau-Ponty says, an 'inter-sensory entity'. Perception of it by one sense includes a range of salient potentialities for perception by other senses and for bodily activity:

> The sensory 'properties' of a thing together constitute one and the same thing, just as my gaze, my touch and all my other senses are together the powers of one and the same body integrated into one and the same action. (Merleau-Ponty, 1962, pp.317–8)

Regardless of whether we see, touch, smell, taste or hear something, all our perception is structured by a background bodily orientation: 'I perceive in a total way with my whole being; I grasp a unique structure of the thing, a unique way of being, which speaks to all my senses at once' (Merleau-Ponty, 1964a, p.50). Thus the phenomenology of perception does not ultimately submit, in its entirety, to compartmentalization into discrete senses. Its underlying structure is unitary.[14]

I have argued in this chapter that touch without proprioception is an abstraction from the richness of tactile experience. And I have suggested that conceiving of the body solely as a perceived object is an abstraction too, which extricates the perceiving body from a context of relatedness and misconstrues connectedness as estrangement. This is hardly a good point of departure for any conception of our relationship with the world. However, if Merleau-Ponty's phenomenological claims are plausible, a further word of caution is in order. The phenomenology of *touch* is itself an abstraction from the structure of experience, a structure that should not be interpreted exclusively in terms of discrete sensory modalities. In Chapter 4, I will support this view and offer a phenomenological account of how it is that inter-sensory possibilities shape experience of an object that is perceived through any one sense. In so doing, I will propose that all perceptual experience has a background structure that might best be described as a 'space of possibilities'. It is this space that existential feelings constitute.

---

[14] See Gallagher (2005, chapter 7) for a discussion of how the senses communicate and of how they are held together by a common, underlying framework of proprioception.

Part II

Varieties of existential feeling in psychiatric illness

Chapter 4

Body and world

In Part I, I suggested that all experience includes a background existential orientation, which is variable in structure, and that this aspect of experience is often overlooked. I also argued that existential orientations are bodily feelings. I did so by appealing to the phenomenology of touch, which does not conform to distinctions between perception of the body and perception of everything else. In this second part of the book, I fine-tune my account and then put it into practice, through an examination of the phenomenology of certain psychiatric conditions. In so doing, I seek to facilitate a better understanding of the relevant experiences by describing the contribution made by existential feelings, to gain further insight into the nature of existential feeling in the process, and to distinguish some of the variants of existential feeling.

The current chapter is mostly preparatory in nature and puts the last pieces of the phenomenological account into place. I begin by showing that what applies to tactile feeling applies to other kinds of feeling too. As in the case of touch, bodily feelings in general are seldom, if ever, just perceptions of internal bodily states. The distinction between localized and background feeling, which I made in the case of touch, has more general application too. I go on to note that the bodily nature of existential feeling serves to challenge any clear line that might be drawn between changed existential orientations in those illnesses that are labelled as 'mental' and in others that are labelled as 'somatic' or 'bodily'. Following this, I further discuss the constituents of existential feeling and suggest that what unites them is that they all contribute to a sense of salient *possibilities* for acting and being acted upon, which structures all experience. To convey the way in which world-experience incorporates possibilities, I appeal to the concept of a *horizon*, as employed by Husserl and Merleau-Ponty. The chapter concludes by indicating how an appreciation of the *horizonal structure* of experience might be applied to interpret some of the experiential changes involved in psychiatric illness. This sets the scene for a more detailed discussion of existential feelings in psychiatric illness, which will occupy Chapters 5 to 7.

The feeling body

Consider the following phenomenological characteristics of tactile feeling, which were discussed in Chapter 3:

1 What feels need not be what is felt. Thus a feeling of the body need not have the body as its object.

2 A feeling is a relation between body and world, rather than a perception of one in isolation from the other.

3 One or the other side of this relation might take up the foreground of awareness, to varying degrees and in different ways.

4 Bodily and worldly aspects of feeling do not respect a clear subject–object distinction. The relatedness between the two need not involve a boundary between them.

5 The object of feeling need not be in physical contact with the body.

6 Many tactile feelings have a diachronic structure.

Touch surely shares some or all of these characteristics with many other states that are referred to as 'feelings'. If it is admitted that tactile feelings do not respect a sharp body–world divide, why assume that other kinds of feeling do, when phenomenological reflection, everyday discourse and descriptions of pathological experience all suggest otherwise? It might be objected that the body–world duality of tactile feeling is applicable only to feelings of bodily boundaries. As Martin (1992, 1993, 1995) argues, it is because tactile feelings occur at a boundary that they can be perceptions of body or of world. However, (5) provides a response to this. What is felt through touch need not be in direct contact with the skin, as illustrated by examples such as running a pencil against a rough surface, where the surface rather than the pencil is the object of feeling. That there is sometimes a physical distance between what feels and what is felt allows for the possibility that feelings internal to the body, such as visceral feelings, structure experience of things outside of the body. One might have a visceral feeling, such as a sinking feeling in the stomach, but the areas of the body in which that feeling is phenomenologically localized need not be the primary object of the feeling, what is *felt*. It is the body or parts of it that *do* the feeling.

The phenomenology of feeling is often construed in terms of levels of awareness, a spectrum of intensity where feelings can be more or less pronounced *objects* of experience. For example:

> As I see matters, awareness of one's feelings can range from full reflective and attentive awareness, through dim and confused awareness, to total or almost total unawareness, including what in psychoanalytic terms is said to be preconscious or even unconscious. (Stocker and Hegeman, 1996, p.22)

But interpreting feeling in such a way misses out an important distinction. Some feelings reveal parts of the body in an object-like way but others operate as a medium through which something else is experienced. In addition, it is important to distinguish 'within-world' bodily feelings from those feelings that constitute a sense of belonging to the world. Whenever we experience an itch, a mild pain or a tightening of the chest, we already have a background sense of being in a world, regardless of whether the foreground feelings are perceptions of the body or of something else. This background also consists of feeling. The body, in so far as it sets up the world in which we find ourselves, is neither a medium of perception within an experienced world nor an object of perception within that world. It constitutes an aspect of experience that is presupposed by both.

The world-constituting role of the body is recognized by Merleau-Ponty, who contrasts the *lived body* with the body as an object of experience and thought. The lived body is what I have referred to as the 'feeling body'. It is never experienced in its entirety as an object of experience, even though it can undergo differing degrees and kinds of objectification. This is because it is the possibility of experiencing anything at all and therefore something that always remains, at least in part, in the background:

> In so far as it sees or touches the world, my body can [...] be neither seen nor touched. What prevents its ever being an object, ever being 'completely constituted' is that it is that by which there are objects. It is neither tangible nor visible in so far as it is that which sees and touches. (Merleau-Ponty, 1962, p.92)

For Merleau-Ponty, the lived body is not only directed towards things *in* the world. It also opens up the world as a space of purposive, practical possibilities, and thus shapes all our experiences, activities and thoughts. Hence an aspect of bodily experience and a sense of belonging to the world are one and the same:

> The reflex, in so far as it opens itself to the meaning of a situation, and perception; in so far as it does not first of all posit an object of knowledge and is an intention of our whole being, are modalities of a *pre-objective view* which is what we call being-in-the-world. Prior to all stimuli and sensory contents, we must recognize a kind of inner diaphragm that determines, infinitely more than they do, what our reflexes and perceptions will be able to aim at in the world, the area of our possible operations, the scope of our life. (Merleau-Ponty, 1962, p.79)

In tactile feeling, the hand can be a means through which something else is felt. Likewise, the feeling body more generally is a framework through which world-experience is structured. The body can play an experiential role without being an object of experience. For example, one can have a sense of 'up', 'down', 'left' and 'right' without reflecting upon one's bodily position. The difference between the lived body as a whole and a localized tactile experience or other specifically focused feeling is that the former is a medium that constitutes the sense of finding oneself in a world, whereas the latter is a medium through which one directs oneself towards objects when one is already in a world. Merleau-Ponty appreciates that the body plays both roles but his discussion does not always make the difference between them sufficiently clear.[1]

It is important to keep in mind that 'bodily awareness' need not be awareness of a 'body object', and that it seldom is. What might be described as a 'feeling' of the body or a 'perception' of the body often participates in experience of something else. However, there is a tendency to misconstrue these feelings, which stems from thinking of bodily experience as experience of a *thing* with which one is intimately acquainted. This mischaracterization of feeling is evident even in certain approaches that have emphasized the inextricability of bodily feelings and a sense of belonging. One such approach is that of Damasio (e.g. 1995, 1996, 2000, 2003, 2004) and it is worth considering here for three reasons. First of all, it acknowledges the existential role of background feeling. Second, it offers some indication of which brain areas and neurobiological processes might be implicated in background feeling, thus opening up the possibility of informative dialogue between phenomenology and the neurosciences. And third, it misconstrues the feeling body as the felt body, illustrating in the process how a distinction between the two can be put into practice to clarify a phenomenology that Damasio and others gesture towards but do not succeed in conveying.

Damasio proposes a theory of the nature and role of emotion, the principal element of which is his 'somatic marker hypothesis'. As discussed in Chapter 1, he takes emotions to be patterns of bodily changes and feeling to be an awareness of these changes. Emotions, he says, are bodily changes that arise in association with environmental stimuli and serve to 'mark' those stimuli. Their role is to guide decision-making and behaviour, by priming the body to respond in appropriate ways to features of the environment. Bodily changes might dispose one to attend to a stimulus, to pursue it, to ignore it, to steer clear of it or to flee from it. The relevant bodily changes, he says, 'arise in bioregulatory processes'. These can either take place in the brain and the rest of the body or circumvent the rest of the body by means of an 'as if loop', whereby the brain represents bodily changes without those changes actually occurring (1996, p.1415). He claims that several different brain areas are involved in generating emotional feelings:

> ...body-sensing areas such as the somatosensory cortices of the insula and of the second somatosensory region (S2), the cingulate cortex, and some nuclei in the brainstem tegmentum, show a significant pattern of activation or deactivation when normal

---

[1] See also Strasser (1977, chapter 7) for the view that not all bodily feelings are *internally* directed and for a distinction between specifically directed feelings and the background feeling of being in the world that they presuppose.

individuals experience the emotions of sadness, happiness, fear, and anger, and that, moreover, the patterns vary among the emotions. Of all regions receiving body signals the insula now appears to be the key cortical component in the process of feeling. (2004, p.55)

He suggests that other areas of the brain are involved in triggering the bodily changes that result in feelings. These include the amygdala, parts of the hypothalamus, the basal forebrain and the brainstem (2004, p.52).

Damasio draws a distinction between primary and secondary emotions. The former involve innate connections between stimulus types and bodily responses, whereas the latter arise through learned associations between stimuli and bodily changes. On some, but not all, occasions, we are aware of these emotions in the form of feelings. Both primary and secondary emotions are episodic responses to environmental stimuli. However, this is not to suggest that the body is emotionally silent on all those occasions when no such responses are occurring. All episodes of arousal take place against the backdrop of a fairly consistent bioregulatory background, which is experienced as 'background feeling'. As Damasio explains:

> The background feeling is our image of the body landscape when it is not shaken by emotion. The concept of 'mood', though related to that of background feeling, does not exactly capture it. When background feelings are persistently of the same type over hours and days, and do not change quietly as thought contents ebb and flow, the collection of background feelings probably contributes to a mood, good, bad, or indifferent. [...] I submit that without them the very core of your representation of self would be broken. (1995, pp.150–1)

It is interesting to note that he distinguishes background feeling from mood partly because moods involve recalcitrant feelings that persist over a period of time, whereas background feelings 'ebb and flow'. This complements my claim, in Chapter 2, that existential feeling is not simply a constant background hum that very rarely changes. Existential feelings are changeable in both subtle and more pronounced ways. Doubtless the 'ebb and flow' ordinarily occurs only within a limited range and so the changes are fairly inconspicuous, only minor tremors. In fact, Damasio suggests that it is the consistency of background feeling over time that facilitates a sense of being an enduring self in a changing world. It is clear from his discussion that he regards background feeling as more fundamental to our phenomenology than primary or secondary emotions:

> ...I am postulating another variety of feeling which I suspect preceded the others in evolution. I call it *background feeling* because it originates in 'background' body states rather than in emotional states. It is not the Verdi of grand emotion, nor the Stravinsky of intellectualized emotion but rather a minimalist in tone and beat, the feeling of life itself, the sense of being. (1995, p.150)

Despite claiming that background feelings make an indispensable contribution to experience and thought, and also offering an account of some of the relevant neurobiological processes, Damasio continues to think of these feelings as perceptions of bodily states. It is the body that is felt when we feel an occurrent emotion and, similarly, it is a background feeling *of the body* that constitutes 'the feeling of life itself'. He refers to background feeling as 'our image of the body landscape' (1995, pp.150–1) and elsewhere interprets feeling more generally as '*the perception of a certain state of the body*' (2003, p.86). The possibility that the phenomenology of feeling could be a phenomenology of anything other than the body is not explicitly entertained.

Damasio's failure to distinguish two quite different ways of feeling is remarked upon by both Sass (2003, 2004*b*) and Gallagher (2005, pp.135–7). As Sass rightly says, most emotional experiences are 'not representations of the objectified body image so much as implicitly felt experiences involving the body subject' (2003, p.171). Somatic markers should, he suggests, be construed as a 'medium' of perception rather than an 'object' of perception (2004*b*, p.134). It is far from clear how a consistent way of perceiving the body could amount to the 'sense of being', given that a sense of being surely includes a lot more than how one's body is feeling. However, once we think of the body as that which feels rather than that which is felt, it becomes apparent how background feeling can be *bodily* feeling and at the same time a way of experiencing something other than the body. Once we add a phenomenological characterization of 'existential feeling' to this, it also becomes apparent how a way in which the body feels can be a medium of perception that constitutes how one finds oneself in a world, rather than a medium of perception within a pre-given world.

The mistake that Damasio makes is commonplace. Given that the body is indeed 'felt' in some way (but not in an object-like way), the feelings in question can legitimately be described as 'bodily'. The mistake is to then assume that this is all they consist of, that a way in which the body feels must be a feeling that has the body as its object and as its sole object. A state that is described with reference to the body need not have an exclusively bodily phenomenology. Other equally legitimate descriptions of the same experience can usually be offered, which emphasize instead the world-side of the experience or the relatedness between body and world. This applies both to within-world and to world-constituting feelings. Let us consider the former first of all. Many such feelings are routinely described as an awareness of bodily states. For example:

> The state of affairs that a feeling alerts us to is most immediately a state of the self. Consulting our feelings is a good way to find out if we are tired, sick, thirsty and so on. (Sizer, 2006, p.122)[2]

---

[2] This is just one of many such remarks, selected at random, that can be found in the literature on emotion and feeling.

Sizer adds that feelings can also be *about* things other than the body, if they are reliably associated with those things, but the assumption remains that the relevant *phenomenology* is a bodily one. However, there are plenty of examples to indicate that imposition of a clear division between perception of the bodily and the non-bodily mischaracterizes a variety of bodily feelings. It is important to get out of the habit of drawing misleading conclusions about the nature of an experience, on the basis of contingent and partial descriptions that emphasize only one aspect of it. Feelings of the body and feelings towards objects in the world are two sides of the same coin, although one side or the other will often occupy the experiential foreground.

In the cases mentioned by Sizer above, it is not even clear that the bodily aspect of the feeling is always the most salient aspect. I might well be aware of my tired-ness, my sickness or my fatigue as states of myself, but I might equally be aware of them as states of the world. The unengaging, distant world can be what solicits sleep when one is very tired; thirst may be most conspicuous as the perceptual salience of a running stream; and various perturbations in the way the world appears might partly constitute the experience of illness. To quote Scheler:

> In the feeling of fatigue there is a warning that may be expressed in the language of common sense as 'stop working' or 'go to sleep'. The vertigo we experience when we stand before an abyss urges us to 'step back'. (1992, p.82)

What applies to touch applies here too—there is just the one feeling, which can be described in different ways. And, as with touch, it is often the case that reflection upon an experience changes its structure. The bodily feeling through which one experiences something else can become the object of a reflective awareness. Take Sartre's example of reading whilst having tired, sore eyes:

> ...this pain can itself be indicated by objects of the world; i.e., by the book which I read. It is with more difficulty that the words are detached from the undifferentiated ground which they constitute; they may tremble, quiver; their meaning can be derived only with effort ... (1989, p.332)

Before the eye strain is reflected upon as an object of perception, the feeling *is* the way in which the words on the page appear. The experience could be described as a feeling of the eyes or as a perception of words quivering on a page. But, whichever aspect is emphasized, there is a unitary experience here. The feeling of the eyes (or, rather, eyelids and eye muscles) is that through which the words are perceived. The eyes are what feel, rather than what is felt. Even if the experience is described with reference to the eyes, it must be distin-guished from a different experience where the relevant bodily feelings are the primary object of awareness. In the latter case, what we have is still more than just a feeling of the body. The conspicuousness of increasingly tired eyes is also a changed relationship with the world, which no longer solicits the activity of reading as it did before. Bodily conspicuousness is often, at the same time, loss of a feeling of practical connectedness to things.

The conspicuous body

Like within-world feelings, world-constituting feelings are a matter of relatedness between body and world. A helpful distinction is made by Leder (1990, pp.26–7), who notes that, when the body ceases to be an object of experience and disappears into the background, there is a phenomenological distinction to be made between 'focal' disappearance of a body part and 'background' disappearance of the body as a whole. As discussed in Chapter 3, when involved in an activity, parts of the body can become immersed in that activity and often do not feature as objects of experience. Alternatively, they can become conspicuous, sometimes disrupting the activity in question. What we have is a range of different ways in which parts of the body can be felt, all of which are tied up with practical activity or withdrawal from it. In addition to these localized changes in feeling, the body *as a whole* can be conspicuous to varying degrees. The body that falls into the background is not just the body that *acts*; it is the body that constitutes a sense of belonging, a context within which all purposive activities are embedded. And the increasingly conspicuous body is not just something that withdraws from a within-world activity; it is also a change in the sense of belonging. As with the tactile background, existential feeling (to which the tactile background contributes) is a way of inhabiting the world. Sartre comments on this in relation to the existential feeling that he calls nausea: 'The Nausea isn't inside me: I can feel it *over there* on the wall, on the braces, everywhere around me. It is one with the café, it is I who am inside *it*' (1963, p.35). It is a feeling of the body that takes the form of a relationship with the world as a whole, a changed sense of belonging and of being.

Even when the body as a whole is a conspicuous object of experience, the feeling in question is not *just* a feeling of the body. Bodily conspicuousness is a changed relationship with the world as a whole. That relationship can be quite different, depending on whether and how the body occupies the experiential foreground. When one feels 'at home' in the world, 'absorbed' in it or 'at one with life', the body often drifts into the background. It is that *through* which things are experienced. But it can enter the foreground in a number of ways. Consider, for example, the sudden realization that one is being watched by another, an experiential transformation that is vividly conveyed by Sartre's various descriptions in *Being and Nothingness*. Before becoming alert to the other, one is immersed in a set of projects. However, a rustle in the leaves, a creak on the stair or a pair of eyes pointing in one's direction can trigger an affective transformation that Sartre calls 'shame'. This is not a localized feeling.

It is a change in how the body as a whole feels. The body ceases to be an invisible locus of projects and is suddenly felt in an object-like way. Sartre claims that this feeling comprises our most basic sense that there are others. One can only feel oneself to be an object if one is an object *for* another. So to experience oneself as an object in this way is to recognize that there are others. He is quite explicit in stating that the experience involves a felt, bodily re-orientation:

> ...the Other is the indispensable mediator between myself and me. I am ashamed of myself as I *appear* to the Other. [...] this comparison is not encountered in us as the result of a concrete psychic operation. Shame is an immediate shudder which runs through me from head to foot without any discursive preparation. [...] shame is shame of *oneself before the Other*; these two structures are inseparable. (1989, p.222)

Shame, as Sartre conceives of it, is not something that we undergo having already evaluated our behaviour in relation to an interpersonal situation. Rather, it is an immediate, unreflective, inarticulate response that transforms a background of belonging into something quite different. It is a changed way of finding ourselves in a world. The body is no longer a medium of experience and activity, an opening onto a significant world filled with potential activities. It is thing-like, conspicuous, an object that takes its place as part of the purposive framework of another person:

> Pure shame is not a feeling of being this or that guilty object but in general of being *an* object; that is, of *recognizing myself* in this degraded, fixed, and dependent being which I am for the Other. (1989, p.288)

Something that Sartre's descriptions make clear is that forms of bodily conspicuousness and inconspicuousness are at the same time ways of belonging to the world. Whilst absorbed in projects, the world appears as a space of salient possibilities that reflect one's goals and purposes. As the body becomes conspicuous, this world falls away. One's relationship with the world is no longer configured in terms of what one is doing and of those things that one might do. The possibilities vanish and one's overall existential orientation takes on a more passive character. One is thing-like, an entity to be acted upon in the context of others' projects.

I do not want to suggest that the phenomenological change Sartre describes is something that characterizes all interpersonal relations.[3] Interpersonal relations are shaped by a variety of existential feelings. Even a sense of being watched by someone can take several forms, not all of which have the same phenomenological character. The sudden feeling of being stared at is different from the slowly dawning awareness that someone in a bar keeps glancing at you

---

[3] See Ratcliffe (2007) for further discussion of the phenomenology of interpersonal relations.

in an inoffensive manner. The former might well take the form of a swift, felt, existential reorientation, without any prior conceptualization of the situation, whereas the latter could be a much more 'within-world' affair, where an explicit conceptual appreciation of the situation precedes any of the associated feelings. Indeed, the existential feeling of being captured by the gaze of another is perhaps rare. Of course, Sartre does not want to maintain that all interpersonal encounters explicitly take the form of shame. Rather, he is claiming that a sense of being object-like before the other is phenomenologically foundational to a sense that there are people. Even so, as I will further discuss in Chapter 5, interpersonal relations generally involve a sense of familiarity and relatedness that is quite different in structure from the tension of Sartrean shame. Shame best captures those relations with others that are alienating and estranging. As Merleau-Ponty observes, the experiences that Sartre describes involve a breakdown of interpersonal relations, a feeling that something is lacking:

> …each of us feels his actions to be not taken up and understood, but observed as if they were an insect's. This is what happens, for instance, when I fall under the gaze of a stranger. (1962, p.361)

Nevertheless, Sartre does at least succeed in describing a distinctive kind of existential change, illustrating in the process that changed bodily feeling is inseparable from changed belonging.

Not all of the existential feelings involved in interpersonal encounters arise, like a Sartrean affective 'shudder', without any explicit, conceptual appraisal of an interpersonal situation. Take the example of giving a lecture. I might find, whilst doing so, that my body disappears into the background and that my words flow effortlessly. But suppose I become increasingly aware that students are giggling, yawning or passively staring at me with looks that indicate extreme boredom or confusion. The fluidity of my activities breaks down; words are summoned with effort; my gestures become strained and mechanical. My body as a whole gradually becomes more conspicuous and, although I remain *in* the room, my sense of being at ease *in* a situation breaks down. There is a different kind of relatedness, an unshakeable awkwardness and a feeling of failing to connect with the situation, which contrasts with the ease that previously permeated my world. To give another example, consider walking home on a dark evening, down a secluded path. As one becomes aware of footsteps behind, fast advancing, one's movements become more effortful, less natural. One trips and stumbles on the cobbles. The body that was previously absorbed in activity becomes conspicuous, cumbersome and vulnerable. A world that previously offered possibilities for activity now becomes oppressive. Experience as a whole is shaped by a pervasive feeling of vulnerability, fragility and lack of control. The world is no longer a safe context of belonging that offers opportunities for activity but something one is at the mercy of. Thus a conceptual appreciation of a situation, which is itself embedded in existential feeling, can serve to reshape the existential feeling in which it is embedded. Existential feeling is not impervious to the influence of experiences and thoughts.

The kinds of existential feeling that structure our relations with each other are not always momentary or short-lived. The body that is at ease in the world and seamlessly entwined with a range of projects can be an enduring way of being, as can the conspicuous, clumsy, thing-like body. For example, Young (2005) discusses the structure of female bodily experience in current Western culture and suggests that it is often characterized by an 'inhibited intentionality' (p.35); a lack of practical fluidity and an enduring inability to feel at home in one's activities. The body-subject is disrupted in its activities by an engrained, enduring sense of also being a body-object. Turning to the cause of this, she remarks on predominant voyeuristic attitudes towards women, who are objectified by the male gaze and come to live that objectification, through appreciating the constant possibility of being looked at in a certain way. A mode of being in the world, involving a bodily self-consciousness that is also an alienation from certain forms of effortless practical dwelling, is thus 'conditioned by [...] sexist oppression in contemporary society' (p.42).

A variety of changes in existential feeling are found in psychiatric illnesses and, in these cases too, what might seem to be an altered experience of one's whole body *plus* altered experience of the world is often in fact unitary. Forms of bodily conspicuousness and inconspicuousness *are* also ways of finding oneself in a world. The inextricability of the two is emphasized by van den Berg (1972), who offers a phenomenological description of 'the typical psychiatric patient' abstracted from many different cases. He notes that the patient does not complain of *psychological* changes but of changed bodily feelings and, at the same time, of the world being different. These seemingly distinct symptoms are, he suggests, different ways of describing the same phenomenon. A changed sense of body is also a changed sense of world and the experience can be described with reference to either side of a unitary self–world relation:

> His world is collapsing. Is he not saying the same thing when he states that his legs are failing him and he feels he is losing his sense of equilibrium! *World* and *body* are interrelated. Then the customary distinction of *world* and *body* is probably much too definite. (1972, p.56)

He goes so far as to say that being ill 'means first and foremost that the surroundings have changed' and relates this to the gloomy world of depression, the colourful world of mania and the world of the schizophrenic, which is permeated hy a feeling of impending disaster (1972, p.45). Elsewhere, he remarks that 'every pathological change of the body reveals itself originally in a new order of the "external world"' (1952, p.172). An appreciation of the nature of existential feeling shows how this can be so: a unitary body–world relation remains presupposed even by those experiences that might at first seem to be of one side of the relation in isolation from the other. In Chapters 5 to 7, I will offer detailed descriptions of some of the kinds of existential feeling that feature in psychiatric illness.

The phenomenology of sickness

We need not appeal to psychiatric cases or detailed phenomenological studies to appreciate the intimacy of bodily feeling and world experience. For example, a colleague of mine, when I recently asked how he was feeling, reported that he had an ear infection. This, he said, had enhanced his day, by amounting to an oddly pleasant feeling of being *dislodged from things* that made the large pile of work he was facing seem somehow less intimidating.[4] Remarks like this raise an interesting possibility. If it is accepted that certain 'bodily feelings' are also a sense of belonging to the world, it seems that there is no clear phenomenological distinction to be drawn between ailments that are 'bodily' or 'somatic' and others that are 'psychological', assuming that a sense of belonging to the world is to be treated as 'psychological'. I have indicated that at least some psychiatric illnesses involve significantly changed existential feeling. Given the extent to which other, non-psychiatric illnesses affect perception of the body as a whole, it would be peculiar if they did not include such changes too. And I think that they do. The narratives surrounding non-psychiatric illnesses tend to refer to bodily complaints and changed bodily feelings, such as pain, fatigue and nausea. I suspect that an emphasis on the bodily aspect is partly due to the fact that most diagnoses and treatments explicitly refer to, and attend to, the body. This emphasis has also entered into popular culture. However, the bodily feelings that are symptomatic of an illness can also comprise an existential orientation. As narratives of illness focus on the sick body rather than the changed world, these feelings are often difficult to express. Nevertheless, they feature in many illnesses, whether short-term, chronic, non-serious or terminal.

Van den Berg (1966) attempts to describe the existential phenomenology of illness and offers what he calls a 'psychology of the sickbed'. He focuses on the case of the chronic patient, for whom there is little hope of recovery. How does sickness affect existential orientation? Van den Berg claims that a peculiar feeling

---

[4] Thanks to Robin Hendry for this example.

of non-participation characterizes the experience of sickness. After being in the sickbed for a time, one still appreciates that all the shared routines that one used to take part in carry on much as before and so a sense of the practically significant world remains intact. However, one feels increasingly estranged from that world, disconnected, a non-participant spectator upon what one was previously immersed in. There is an awareness of the possibilities as still out there but they are no longer one's own. The possibilities that the world now offers are much more restricted: 'I have ceased to belong; I have no part of it. [...] The world has shrunk to the size of my bedroom, or rather my bed' (1966, pp.26–7). In a restricted world, where the usual purposive orientation no longer applies, the minor details come into view; patterns on the wallpaper or the texture of the bed sheets. In addition to this, the body that previously opened up the world now becomes unpleasantly object-like, an experiential content that consumes one's awareness:

> Now that I am ill, I become acutely aware of a bodily existence, which makes itself felt in a general malaise, in a dull headache and in a vague nausea. The body which used to be a condition becomes the sole content of the moment. (1966, p.28)

Van den Berg observes that a healthy person can be one with her body, insofar as she does not attend to it but attends to other things through it. The healthy body is not an instrument that is used but a feeling of being and belonging that underlies all dealings with instruments. In illness, however, the body becomes strangely foreign, like a defective tool.

In some cases at least, the alienation and estrangement that characterizes the phenomenology of illness is not a symptom of the bodily ailment alone. Knowledge of an illness can itself provoke changes in existential feeling. When faced with the diagnosis, there is a surge of feeling that is at the same time a falling away from the security of the familiar world. One is disconnected, lost, unsupported, without grounding. Van den Berg notes that a feeling of alienation can also be exacerbated by relations with other people, by a gulf between the orientation that visitors continue to take for granted and that which the patient has come to inhabit. The patient is, for them, someone who no longer participates in shared social routines, and they regard him in a somewhat voyeuristic, detached way. While he has to inhabit a world that is bewildering and frightening, they do not generally acknowledge this world. Instead, they offer platitudes, well-meaning insincerity and a false optimism that fails to connect with the place in which he now resides:

> [The patient] is certainly hurt when his wish to discuss the state of being ill as a form of life which is hard or impossible to bear, is declined with a trivial remark, or when his urgent questions about life and death are treated with a false optimism, as meaningless to the visitor as it is to him. (1966, p.45)

According to van den Berg, much the same applies to the relationships between clinicians and patients. If the patient is treated merely as a 'patient', whose existential predicament is inconsequential, an alienation that is integral to her sense of 'being ill' is further heightened. Being in the world is not just a matter of physical location. And being with others is not just a matter of proximity to them. Illness can be an eviction from the familiar world, a sense of detachment, strangeness and absence, exacerbated by the inability to communicate that predicament to others. In the sickbed:

> The world becomes an unusual, remote and strange place. And however near the visitor is to the patient, however much he is 'with him' and tries to reach him in his visit, he can never completely abolish the distance and the strangeness. (1966, p.120)

However, van den Berg also proposes that, existentially speaking, illness is not a wholly bad thing. In a state of consistent good health, there is a tendency to become engrossed in superficial pursuits, such as wealth and status, whereas the sick person, who is removed from all this, may find renewed significance in the 'little things'—the smallest details become significant, even breathtaking (1966, pp.68–74). Having no sense of one's own fragility itself amounts to a form of existential sickness, a forgetting of one's existential predicament; 'the really healthy person possesses a vulnerable body and he is aware of this vulnerability' (1966, p.74).[5]

Of course, different kinds of illness are experienced in a range of different ways, and two people with the same kind of illness can have very different experiences. Furthermore, friends, family members and clinicians do not always exacerbate a patient's feelings of alienation. Nevertheless, if we accept that descriptions such as van den Berg's apply to at least some 'somatic' illnesses, then there is at most a very fine line between the kinds of existential feeling found in psychiatric and non-psychiatric illnesses. Both can involve a sense of enhanced corporeality and alienation, which lies outside of the ordinary range of existential orientations. The world can seem not quite real, strangely unfamiliar and distant. Indeed, it may well be that there are kinds of existential feeling that are common to both and that the identification of a specific bodily ailment as causally responsible serves to exonerate the psyche from blame in one case but not the other.[6]

---

[5] See Tolstoy's *The Death of Ivan Ilych* for a vivid description of how sickness, coupled with gradual recognition of the inevitability of impending death, can dislodge one from absorption in a world of superficial social pursuits and awaken what Heidegger would call a more 'authentic' existential orientation.

[6] I will further discuss the relationship between diagnoses of psychiatric illness and the identification of bodily causes in Chapter 10.

All sorts of bodily symptoms are routinely implicated in psychiatric illness. For example, Kraepelin's original description of 'dementia praecox' (now known as schizophrenia) refers to headaches, widening and sluggishness of the pupils, various motor problems, facial spasms, seizures, circulatory problems, low blood pressure, increased saliva secretion, metabolic changes and fluctuating appetite (1919, chapter IV). Many of these surely affect world-experience in some way and some may even be inextricable from other 'psychological' symptoms. Hence cleanly distinguishing between the psychological and the somatic from the outset runs the risk of double-counting. If we interpret somebody against the background of a presupposed world to which we both belong, then we might well take certain within-world bodily and psychological symptoms to be distinct. But this fails to acknowledge the possibility that the person inhabits a different existential orientation and that it is in terms of this existential orientation that his various observed symptoms are to be interpreted. Where this is the case, seemingly distinct symptoms can turn out to be one and the same, as Chapters 5 to 7 will show.

So far, I have emphasized the contrast between estrangement and belonging. However, it is important not to over-simplify existential feeling. Experience is not a matter of *either* happily disappearing into one's projects *or* becoming unpleasantly aware of oneself as a thing. There are many ways in which one can disappear into the world or become aware of oneself as an object. Being at one with the natural world is not the same as feeling like part of a social situation or feeling at home in an environment of familiar artefacts. And the objectification of the body that sometimes occurs when being stared at by somebody is not the same experience as looking into the mirror for a long time and being confronted with a defamiliarized, utterly alien thing staring back at you. Neither is it like the injured or debilitated body that becomes an object of experience when it won't do what you want it to do. It is therefore highly doubtful that a contrast between the objective body and the body as a medium of activity adequately captures the range of existential feelings.

Some forms of bodily conspicuousness do not amount to alienation or a loss of practical belonging at all.[7] For example, Young (2005) reflects upon experience of the body during pregnancy and on the ways in which the pregnant body becomes conspicuous. She restricts her analysis to pregnancies of choice in the contemporary Western World. (Even given this restriction, bodily experience will of course differ markedly from person to person and

---

[7] As Leder (1990, p.91) remarks, there are many ways in which we 'experience or take action upon our body in the interest of enjoyment, self-monitoring, cultivating sensitivity, satisfying curiosity, or for no particular reason at all'.

will also change during the course of a pregnancy.) Young observes that, although the body becomes increasingly noticeable during pregnancy, it need not appear as something that one is alienated from or as something that disrupts projects and erodes a sense of belonging to the world:

> In attending to my pregnant body in such circumstances, I do not feel myself alienated from it, as in illness. I merely notice its borders and rumblings with interest, sometimes with pleasure, and this aesthetic interest does not divert me from my business. (2005, p.52)

Pregnant embodiment, Young suggests, does not involve experiencing oneself as a subject or as an object. There is more to it than that; the person becomes 'a source and participant in a creative process'. She is not passive before this process and she is not the agent of it either. Rather, she '*is* this process, this change' (2005, p.54).

Some of the authors I have referred to here also comment on the changeable relation between *body* and *self*, as exemplified by Young's statement that the person *is* the bodily process and van den Berg's description of experiencing one's sick body as an alien, defective instrument. Some such talk suggests that body and self are distinct, while some indicates that they are one and the same. A person can be at one with his body or feel somehow detached from it. He can inhabit his bodily activities or encounter his body as a broken tool.

I will not offer a comprehensive account of the phenomenology of 'self' here and I do not wish to suggest that the sense of self is wholly constituted by existential feeling. Nevertheless, I do at least want to maintain that existential feelings are *partly* constitutive of selfhood. When the self is described as detached from body or world, it can equally well be described as changed or diminished. The self that is felt to be disembodied does not remain wholly intact and at the same time disencumbered of body and situation. Reports of self being distinct from the body tend, at the same time, to emphasize something amiss with the self, something that has gone wrong or something that is lacking. Van den Berg (1966, p.66) states that 'the healthy person is allowed to *be* his body and he makes use of this right eagerly: he *is* his body. Illness disturbs this assimilation'. The outcome of this disturbance could be described as an experience of disembodiment but it could equally be described as a sense of incomplete, changed or even absent selfhood. What such talk expresses is a changed existential orientation, which can be referred to in terms of changes to self, body, world or the relationship between them, rather than the retirement of a disembodied self from both its environment and its contingent corporeal frame. In every case, some kind of body–world relationship remains, albeit one characterized by a feeling of distance rather than belonging. A sense of self is never wholly separated from this relationship. Talk of feeling detached from body and world might best express an all-pervasive feeling of estrangement but, importantly, that feeling is *itself* a way of experiencing the body–world relationship and so one has not actually escaped from body and world at all. In some cases, people refer to having *lost* all sense of self, indicating that the self is not something that survives every change in existential feeling. (I will discuss some such cases in Chapter 6.) Hence the phenomenology of self, whatever else it might involve, is not dissociable from existential feeling. It is a matter of relatedness, rather than of something pre-formed that then enters into a relationship with body and world. Any sense of self that we have is grounded in existential feeling, even though it might not be exhausted by it.

Existential feelings, bodily dispositions and possibilities

Existential feelings are seldom momentary occurrences and more usually have a temporal structure. They shape our dispositions to act and regulate our activities. When I type, my hands are what feel rather than what is felt. That mode of feeling is indissociable from my activity. As my hands tire, what was a background of ongoing activity enters the experiential foreground, becoming strained and awkward. Existential feelings are similarly bound up with our activities. For example, it is often in walking around and interacting with the world that the strangeness of things is most pronounced, perhaps when they do not solicit bodily responses in the usual ongoing, structured fashion. It is the whole context of practical relatedness that has changed, rather than *either* bodily experience *or* experience of objects and events outside of the body. Central to this change is an altered sense of the *possibilities* that a situation offers. A situation is not experienced as a detached, objective manifold, bereft of all purpose and significance; it appears as a space of salient possibilities. Some of these are actualized through our activities and, in the process, further possibilities appear. This process can proceed in a harmonious manner, constituting a consistent sense of belonging to the world. However, certain possibilities or kinds of possibility can be absent from experience, with the result that the world no longer solicits activities in the way that it previously did. In other cases, the possibilities might still be there but be changeable and disorganized, resulting in a fragmented existential orientation. Some of the relevant possibilities involve activities that one might pursue, but the structure of experience also incorporates a sense of possible happenings, possible activities of other people, and the ways in which these activities and happenings relate to one's own situation.

Existential feelings do not consist of the sum total of specific possibilities involved in an experience. Rather, they constitute the general *space* of possibilities that shapes ongoing experience and activity. In addition to changes in specific possibilities, the overall possibility space can be heightened, diminished, open or constrained. It can be fairly fixed in structure or changeable. It can involve a different overall balance of active and passive possibilities, taking the form of an arena of things to pursue or a realm of potential happenings. In conjunction with this, one can have an overall feeling of control, of belonging, of helplessness or of vulnerability. (Some of the variants will be further discussed in Chapter 7.)

My aim in the rest of this chapter is to develop a phenomenological account of how it is that possibilities can participate in an experience, rather than being non-actual states of affairs that are wholly distinct from what is *actually* experienced. In the remainder of the current section, I will indicate some of the likely constituents of existential feeling and address how it is that they contribute to experienced possibilities. Then, in the final section, I will show how the role of possibilities in our experience can be understood in terms of what Husserl and Merleau-Ponty refer to as *horizons*.

Existential feelings are a *phenomenological kind*, united by a distinctive experiential role. They play this role regardless of what their neurobiological underpinnings might be. Suppose that several people all described a particular feeling of strangeness in great detail and that no phenomenological differences were discernable from their descriptions. Now suppose that the neurobiological changes involved turned out to be different in each case. This finding would not warrant a re-classification of the feeling in question. If we are interested in the structure of the experience, this is the same feeling of strangeness in all cases. Neurobiological differences make no difference when there is no phenomenological difference. However, this is not to say that neurobiological findings are redundant when it comes to doing phenomenological research. Suppose that several people described what seemed to be the same existential feeling but it turned out that half of them underwent one set of neurobiological changes and the other half a completely different set. In this case, a phenomenologist could use the neurobiology as a guide and revisit their accounts, perhaps discovering in the process that there were indeed subtle differences in the descriptions offered by the two groups. It is also important to stress that an understanding of the neurobiological changes involved in existential feeling can play an important role in cases where medical or some other form of intervention is required. Phenomenology alone cannot dictate treatment method. If a kind of pathological existential feeling consistently involves the same changes, it might well be susceptible to a similar treatment in all or almost all cases. If it has diverse neurobiological underpinnings, this is less likely.

It might be argued that much of the neurobiology implicated in psychiatric illness is already understood and that further understanding can proceed quite happily without an appreciation of the relevant phenomenology. After all, this is what has happened to date. Hence the phenomenology makes no contribution to the science. However, there is also a need to understand what it is that one is seeking to explain in neurobiological terms. Phenomenology can supply explananda for scientific explanations, by offering clear descriptions of phenomena that neuroscience then sets out to explain. By providing more accurate and detailed descriptions than those currently employed, it can aid in untangling various confusions, such as the double-counting of somatic and psychological symptoms. It is also worth reiterating that no neurobiological account will be able to comprehensively 'explain' existential feeling. Neuroscience is concerned with what *is* and does not enquire as to what the sense of being, reality or existence consists of. As I argued in Chapter 2, no approach that takes the sense of reality for granted is equipped to fully understand the structure of existential feeling. Existential feelings set up the world that scientific explanations presuppose. Nevertheless, given that scientific study of the constituents of existential feeling will still have an important role to play, both in phenomenological enquiry and in medical intervention, it is important to provide at least some indication of what those constituents are likely to be.

Existential feelings, I suggest, have a variety of ingredients. They incorporate kinaesthesia (awareness of bodily movement), as they are inextricable from a sense of actual and potential bodily activities. They must also include at least some proprioceptive awareness of bodily position and orientation, given that a sense of potential activities and happenings involving one's body requires an awareness of where one's body is located. In addition, a range of visceral feelings are most likely implicated, including at least some of those that are commonly associated with emotional feeling. How one's body 'feels' is at the same time a sense of salient possibilities. Proprioception, kinaesthesia and an 'interoceptive' awareness of visceral feelings are phenomenologically inextricable aspects of existential feeling, rather than distinct components of experience. To accommodate all of them, we could perhaps understand 'proprioception' in a very broad way, as including visceral feelings, awareness of bodily position and experience of bodily movement. However, treating these three aspects of existential feeling as a single, unified 'body sense' would still lead to the imposition of misleading divisions between types of experience. In Chapter 3, I indicated that tactile background feelings also have a role to play in existential feeling. These incorporate proprioception (understood here as a sense of bodily position and movement), rather than being wholly distinct from it. Body sense, however broadly construed, is not a separate *sixth sense* that facilitates awareness of a *body-object*. It is something that participates in all experience, contributing to a feeling of belonging. Without a firm boundary between internally and externally directed senses, it is not possible to cleanly separate proprioception from perception of things outside of the body. So proprioception should not be thought of as something distinct from the other world-directed senses, which has the body as its exclusive object.[8]

That a range of ingredients are most likely involved in existential feeling presents a problem. A number of different bodily changes, all of which are 'felt' in some way, do not seem to add up to unitary existential feelings. But it would be a mistake to think of all these changes as occurring in isolation from each other. Existential feelings do not consist of lots of different things arising all at once and being felt independently of each other. The relevant bodily changes interact with each other in all sorts of ways and they should not be thought of as bundles of discrete occurrences. By analogy, the visual system does not consist of lots of different processes acting independently but of structured interaction between those processes. When I move my head or eyes, the objects I see do not move with them. However, if I poke my eye, the visual scene wobbles. The processes involved in initiating and monitoring eye movements can be distinguished from many other processes that occur when we see things but the constancy of the visual world when we turn our heads, bend down or move our eyes is not the achievement of any one of these processes operating in isolation from the others. Similarly, the suggestion that many existential feelings have neurobiologically diverse underpinnings does not detract from their phenomenological unity. Even when the relevant bodily changes are localized, these changes affect how other bodily processes and activities interact. And the feelings themselves need not be *of* any particular bodily change any more than vision is *of* the eye or of the neck muscles. What is felt is a changed relationship to the world as a whole, an alteration in the possibility space that one finds oneself in. To quote Leder:

> [A] relationship of exchange and intertwining characterizes all parts of the body, though one or another mode of function may predominate. The visceral depths always participate in ecstasis [intentionality]. [...] a hunger or hormonal mood colors the entire world. (1990, p.56)

---

8 Although I maintain that cleanly distinguishing proprioception, kinaesthesia and interoception is unhelpful when exploring the phenomenology of existential feeling, I do not wish to suggest that the same applies to all forms of enquiry. Such distinctions may be indispensable for certain non-phenomenological studies of body-sense. In addition, they may well be helpful when it comes to describing certain aspects of experience. They do not, however, apply to the background sense of how we find ourselves in the world.

The extent of interdependence between the bodily changes implicated in existential feeling becomes even clearer when the dynamic, *temporal* nature of existential feeling is emphasized. For example, a feeling of strangeness or unsettledness, which involves the world no longer soliciting coherent patterns of ongoing activity in the usual smooth, seamless way, might reflect a lack of temporal integration between bodily processes. Even those feelings that are sudden, fleeting and seemingly synchronic involve a changed sense of the possible activities that one *might* pursue and so have a temporal structure. I will further discuss this structure in Chapter 7.

The bodily changes involved in existential feelings are felt as changes to the overall shape of experience, to the kinds of possibility that it includes. For example, visceral and tactile feelings can both contribute to an experience of the whole body as conspicuous. The conspicuous body is, at the same time, a change in the sense of belonging to the world, often a retreat from a significant project in which one was previously immersed, a loss of practical possibilities that the world previously offered.

An obvious objection to all this is that experience does not incorporate the possible. We perceive only the actual. Even when we hallucinate, what we see is something non-actual that is experienced *as* actual. There is no sense in which possibilities are actually *present* in any experience, regardless of whether or not the experience in question is veridical. This kind of view is complemented by spectatorial models of experience, which take disembodied vision as the paradigm case of perception. A detached, voyeuristic perspective on the world does not involve bodily belonging or activity. Perception, construed in such a way, consists of the simultaneous revelation of perceptually accessible parts of the *actual* world. Jonas (1954) describes sight as follows:

> Sight is par excellence the sense of the simultaneous or the coordinated, and thereby of the extensive. A view comprehends many things juxtaposed, as co-existent parts of one field of vision. It does so in an instant. (p.507)
> With sight, all I have to do is open my eyes, and the world is there, as it was all the time. (p.512)

In Chapter 3, I mentioned a contrasting approach to visual perception, which treats it as inextricable from proprioception and activity. This kind of approach does accommodate experience of the possible. Detailed phenomenological descriptions of the role that possibilities play in experience, which emphasize the relationship between feelings, bodily dispositions and possibilities, are offered by Husserl and Merleau-Ponty. I will turn to these in the next section. By way of preparation, I will consider some complementary views that have been offered more recently, which draw on empirical science more so than on phenomenology.

Much recent empirical work on the role of bodily activity in perception is indebted to J. J. Gibson, who proposes that the ability to visually discriminate aspects of the environment involves associating patterned changes in the structure of the ambient optic array with kinds of bodily movement. For Gibson, proprioception (construed as a sense of bodily position and movement) is indissociable from the ability to perceive the world: 'I maintain that all the perceptual systems are proprioceptive as well as exteroceptive, for they all provide information in their various ways about the observer's activities' (1979, p.115). He rejects distinctions between subject and object, self and world, and internal and external, emphasizing instead that perception of our bodies and what they are doing is at the same time perception of how the environment is organized: 'The supposedly separate realms of the subjective and the objective are actually only poles of attention. The dualism of observer and environment is unnecessary' (1979, p.116). Gibson's doctrine of 'affordances' maintains that situations are perceived in terms of potential activities involving them. They 'afford' certain behaviours: 'the *affordances* of the environment are what it *offers* the animal, what it *provides* or *furnishes*, either for good or ill' (1979, p.127). To perceive an affordance is not to perceive something in the environment and only afterwards to recognize that it can be acted upon in a certain way. Potential activities involving an object are integral to perception of it. So the practical significance of things is something that we experience as belonging to them, in the form of activities that they afford.

As recognized by Gibson, in many cases we do not first perceive an opportunity and afterwards act. Rather, the situation summons the activity; it solicits it automatically and action is unreflective. This kind of 'motor intentionality' is something that Merleau-Ponty also draws attention to.[9] It does not involve a subject–object distinction or a distinction between understanding and activity; understanding is embodied in the activity. The world calls forth certain activities and it also appears as a space of possibilities involving others, which are not solicited in an automatic fashion but still appear as enticing. Unthinking doings and a sense of other possibilities that we could, if we wanted, actualize through our actions together anchor us to a world, giving us a sense of being *in* a situation.

A number of philosophers, psychologists and other scientists have taken their lead from Gibson. For example, as I discussed in Chapter 3, Noë (2004) draws on Gibson's work to argue that vision is like touch, in being a matter of active, skilful exploration of the environment. It is not the passive reception of visual images but something that we *do*. Integral to visual perception is an

---

[9] See Kelly (2002) for a discussion of Merleau-Ponty and motor intentionality.

'implicit practical knowledge' of sensori-motor couplings (2004, p.8).[10] In other words, vision relies upon a non-conceptual, bodily 'knowledge' of how kinds of bodily activity are correlated with changes in sensation. Noë adds that visual perception of an object incorporates a sense of how potential movements might transform its appearance. In seeing an object such as a chair, we see it as something that could be viewed from another perspective. So it is not just actual activities that enter into perception. Perception involves a host of practical dispositions, a sense of salient activities that *could* be performed. These are not simply experienced as internal reverberations of one's body, as felt inclinations to do one thing or another, but as potentialities embodied in the object as perceived. It appears *through* a set of practical dispositions, as something that might be approached from different vantage points so as to reveal hidden features. Hence, according to Noë, potential modes of perceptual access to things are themselves perceived.

I think that both Gibson and Noë place too much emphasis on the way in which possible *activities of one's own body* structure experience. The possibilities we perceive are more wide-ranging than that. The world is not configured solely in terms of what I can do with it. A sense of how I might act is tied up with a sense of what might happen, what might be avoided and what cannot be avoided. In addition, my possibilities are entangled with the possibilities that the world offers for others. I also sometimes experience an absence of the relevant practical possibilities, a sense of loss that pervades everything. So there is a lot more to be said here.

Activity and passivity are not wholly separate aspects of experience and this is something that Noë recognizes. Although he says that touch is primarily a matter of active *touching*, he also acknowledges that we can be *touched* and that some tactile experiences are not facilitated by bodily activities. He claims that a sense of bodily activities is equally necessary for the experience of passive touch, given that the ability to discriminate between being touched and actively touching depends upon an appreciation of the correspondence between bodily activities and changes in tactile feeling. However, even though a sense of passivity is dependent upon a sense of activity, there is no reason to emphasize the latter, as the dependence is mutual.

Experience of possible *happenings* involving a given entity can be inextricable from experience of possible and actual activities that are directed at something else. For example, the feeling of threat that structures perception of a fast-approaching object might involve a disposition to cover one's face with one's hands. The face may be what 'affords' protecting but, in addition to this,

---

[10] See also O'Regan and Noë (2001).

protecting oneself from an object rather than confronting it contributes to an experience of passivity before that object, the sense that it cannot be moved from its path and that something will happen regardless of what one does. This need not apply only to specific objects. A person's long-term practical disposition could be such that the world as a whole appears consistently dangerous and threatening. A feeling of vulnerability, consisting partly of a constant disposition to protect oneself, to hide, to curl up in a ball, might pervade all experience, in which case one's existential orientation as a whole takes on the character of threat. The interplay between activity and passivity also features in interpersonal experience. For example, certain feelings of passivity before the world, which sometimes take the form of a painful estrangement, are constituted by the sense that it is a world of possibilities for others but not oneself. Hence possibilities structure experience in a range of ways, rather than comprising a simple 'I can'.

At least some authors have indicated that, in addition to facilitating perception of specific objects and situations, felt bodily potentialities gives us a sense of being in the world. Shaun Gallagher proposes something like this in discussing the 'body schema'. He appeals to a substantial and diverse body of empirical evidence in support of the view that proprioception contributes to the structure of world experience in a variety of important ways. A range of body states comprise the implicit and explicit sense one has of one's body. This body sense contributes to the workings of the other perceptual modalities; 'perceiving subjects move through a space that is already pragmatically organized by the construction, the very shape, of the body' (2005, p.140). All experience is structured by a kind of tacit, background, bodily understanding. Proprioception is not a distinct sense but a background framework within which the 'externally' directed senses operate. For Gallagher, not all proprioception involves awareness of a body-object. He distinguishes phenomenal from pre-noetic body sense, admitting in the process that this distinction is a 'relative one' (2005, p.5). The phenomenal body is the body that we are aware of as an *object* of experience and thought. It can be a conspicuous or a marginal aspect of experience and Gallagher refers to it as the 'body image':

> The body image consists of a complex set of intentional states and dispositions—perceptions, beliefs, and attitudes—in which the intentional object is one's own body. (2005, p.25)

The pre-noetic body, in contrast, is not part of experience. It is an implicit background that underlies all experience, a set of capacities that shape experience but are not themselves experientially accessible. He refers to this as the 'body schema'. Although schema and image are distinct, Gallagher acknowledges that they interact in complex ways. He is not the first to adopt one, the other or both of these terms. But what he also offers is a detailed account of the distinction between schema and image, showing how the latter has been employed inappropriately to describe views such as that of Merleau-Ponty, where the role of the implicit body schema in structuring experience is what is really at issue.

Sometimes Gallagher's 'body schema' seems only to have a within-world role. For example, he states at one point that he is 'using the term 'body schema' to signify a certain collection of sensory-motor functions responsible for maintaining posture and governing movement' (2005, p.45). However, it looks as though there is more to it than this. Later on, he seems to suggest that the schema is how we find ourselves in the world, rather than something that contributes to perception only in the context of a pre-given existential orientation. For example, he refers to a 'pre-reflective bodily awareness that is built into the structures of perception and action, but that is not itself egocentric' and states that the pre-noetic body 'functions to make perception possible and to constrain intentional consciousness in various ways', by shaping it in terms of a range of practical possibilities (2005, pp.137–9). Thus, by acknowledging that bodily dispositions structure experience, as Noë and others do, we can accommodate a phenomenology of possibilities. And, by emphasizing a background body schema, as Gallagher does, we can also accommodate the distinctive role of existential feeling.

Gallagher claims that the body schema is not phenomenologically accessible: 'A prenoetic performance is one that helps to structure consciousness, but does not explicitly show itself in the contents of consciousness' (2005, p.32). I have suggested that existential feelings *are* phenomenologically accessible; hence the term 'feeling'. However, it is important to distinguish something that is accessible to casual reflection from something that can be made available to trained phenomenological reflection. Existential feelings are not 'objects' of everyday awareness but, as suggested earlier, they are indeed 'felt' in some way. As I illustrated via the analogy of feeling returning to a numb hand, it is possible to reflect on how something feels without turning it into something that is felt. Existential feelings are part of the structure of experience, rather than being wholly inaccessible goings on that serve to determine that structure. The feeling *is* the way in which one finds oneself in the world and, as such, it participates in all experience, albeit as something that is usually pre-reflectively taken for granted. There is, however, a fine line between what is phenomenologically accessible and what is not. It is primarily through changes in existential feelings that we can catch a 'glimpse' of them. For example, something like a 'sense of reality' is so deeply engrained in most experience that it seldom appears as an object of reflection. It is part of our experience but not something that we are usually reflectively aware of.

In offering accounts of the role played by the body in perception, Gibson, Noë and Gallagher all appeal to empirical scientific evidence, although Gallagher also makes use of phenomenology.[11] As I will now show, complementary claims have been made on the basis of phenomenology alone, unaided by scientific research. Nevertheless, the plausibility of these phenomenological claims should not be assessed in complete independence from scientific work, and the fact that they are supported rather than contradicted by a range of scientific findings serves to lend them further credibility.[12]

Horizons

The interplay between actuality and possibility in experience, the phenomeno-logical role played by existential feeling, and the relationship between possibilities and the sense of reality can all be understood in terms of the phenomenological concept of a 'horizon', as it is employed by Husserl (e.g. 1960, 1989, 2001) and later by Merleau-Ponty (e.g. 1962). Both appeal to the horizonal structure of experience in order to convey the way in which the body sets up the world and how it is then implicated in the various experiences that we have within that world.[13]

Husserl notes that experiencing an object, such as a table, requires more than perceiving what *actually* appears. One sees the table from a certain angle but the experience also includes a sense of other potential perceptions of the same object. One could walk round it and see it from another angle or look at it from above and reveal its hidden aspects. These possibilities are not inferred from what is actually perceived. Rather, they are integral to the experience:

> In the noema of the act of perception, i.e., in the perceived, taken as characterized phe-nomenologically, as it is therein an intentional Object, there is included a determinate directive for all further experiences of the object in question. (1989, p.38)[14]

---

[11] Varela *et al.* (1991), who coined the term 'enactive cognition', also bring together comple-mentary themes from both phenomenology and cognitive science. However, their approach remains distinctive, as it also incorporates themes from Asian philosophy.

[12] See Ratcliffe (2007, chapters 5 and 8) for a discussion of the ways in which phenomenology and cognitive science can interact fruitfully and for an account of how their interaction should be construed.

[13] The world that these possibilities set up is, in broad outline, much the same as the world that Heidegger describes in *Being and Time*; a teleologically organized possibility space. The relevant possibilities are implicated in experiences of entities as both ready-to-hand and present-at-hand. Thus, although there are many differences between the views of these phenomenologists, the points I draw from them do, I think, add up to a single, coherent view.

[14] See also Husserl (1960, pp.44–5).

What one experiences is an *object appearing in a certain way*, rather than just an *appearance*. As we move around it and its appearance changes, the object is not itself perceived as changing but as a 'continuity of appearance' that endures the changes. It is perceived as being 'naturally and simply there for us as an existing reality as we live naively in perception' (2001, p.35). Experience of something as an object consists of both its actual appearance from a particular perspective and the co-included space of possible appearances. Thus what is *actually* given in experience is not all that is given. A sense of the object as an enduring entity that is independent of oneself is a matter of its *not* being exhausted by the actuality that is revealed to one's current vantage point. The set of interrelated possibilities that surround an object are referred to by Husserl as its 'horizon'. He distinguishes between the inner and outer horizons of objects. The former consist of their hidden aspects, which are experienced as possibilities for further perceptual exploration. They also include potential activities involving the object, such as grasping it or eating it. The latter comprise the broader context in which an object is situated. For example, the outer horizon of my computer keyboard includes a range of potential interactions with other items of equipment.

Both Husserl and Merleau-Ponty make clear that a horizon is not constituted by a single sensory modality. When one perceives something visually, the possibilities that participate in the experience include perception by means of other senses, such as touch. The horizons of visual experience include salient possibilities for tactile manipulation, for practical engagement with an entity (Husserl, 1989, pp.42–3). Hence horizons should not be conceived of exclusively or even primarily as a matter of how things are experienced visually; 'any object presented to one sense calls upon itself the concordant operation of all the others' (Merleau-Ponty, 1962, p.318).[15] For example, when you look at the blade of a very sharp knife sitting on the work surface, you *see* that it is sharp, that it has the potential to cut you. The senses are intermingled in so far as actualities for one sense are presented alongside possibilities for that sense and for other senses.

Horizons are not static structures. Rather, they appear as potentialities for future activities and they unfold in organized ways:

> Everywhere, apprehension includes in itself, by the mediation of a 'sense', empty horizons of 'possible perceptions'; thus I can, at any given time, enter into a system of possible and, if I follow them up, actual, perceptual nexuses. (Husserl, 1989, p.42)

As certain possibilities are taken up by perception and actualized, further possibilities show up and experience of things takes on a harmonious, organized flow.

---

[15] Noë's (2004) view is very similar but he employs different terminology, with 'virtual perception' approximating what Husserl and Merleau-Ponty refer to as a 'horizon'.

The sense of what things are is constituted by this diachronic interplay between changing possibilities and actualities. Husserl uses the term 'passive synthesis' to refer to the binding together of appearances into structured, object-centred systems of perceptual unfolding. It is *passive* because it is not something we actively do but an aspect of experience that we take for granted. The objects are given to us in perception rather than actively constructed by us out of systems of appearances.

Like Merleau-Ponty, Husserl (1960, 1989, 2001) explicitly emphasizes the contribution made by *bodily* dispositions and activities to the structure of experience. The possibility space is, as he puts it, 'predelineated' in a way that reflects potential activities of one's own body and the bodies of others. When I look at something, only certain possibilities participate in my experience of it. The possibilities are always constrained and the different ways in which they are constrained partly constitute our sense of what different things are. A table is experienced as something that can be accessed from another vantage point, moved or touched in various ways. It is something upon which one might rest one's arms or perhaps place a plate. Integral to the experience is a sense of 'I can and do, but I can also do otherwise than I am doing' (1960, p.45). Things appear as what they are through a certain bodily connectedness to them, a non-conceptual, practical, habitual receptivity. The body is not just an object that is perceived but also that through which we perceive. Its dispositions are reflected in the things perceived: 'The Body [*Leib*] is, in the first place, the *medium of all perception*; it is the *organ of perception* and is *necessarily* involved in all perception' (Husserl, 1989, p.61). Horizons are not systems of possibilities to which we are indifferent. The thing, as Husserl says, 'calls out to us' (2001, p.41); it has an 'affective pull' (2001, p.98). He distinguishes between possibilities that are open and others that are 'enticing', acknowledging that there is a continuum between the two. An object may call forth an activity, present it as an especially salient option or simply accommodate its possibility. The extent to which a possibility is enticing *is* a matter of bodily feeling; it is through the feeling body that things show up as salient. The possibilities that structure perception are felt bodily potentialities, which Husserl refers to as 'kinaestheses'. The body is the inextricable counterpart of structured horizons; it is 'constantly there, functioning as an organ of perception; and here it is also, in itself, an entire system of compatibly harmonizing organs of perception' (2001, pp.50–1).

The possibilities that surround an entity take different forms. Some are *certainties* regarding what will happen. The certainty in question is not a propositional attitude of the form 'x will definitely happen' but a habitual, unthinking, bodily expectation. As you reach out for the cup, you take for granted that your hand will meet with a solid object. When these practical expectations are not fulfilled, there is surprise. However, horizons also include *uncertainty*. Not all possibilities take the form 'if I do x, characteristic p will definitely be revealed'. Some possibilities are less determinate, more general indications of how something will appear if manipulated or perceived from another vantage point, such as 'it will have a colour' rather than 'it will be light green'. And there can also be *doubt* regarding what one perceives, a feeling that it might not be as it seems and that potential activities could reveal it to be something different (Husserl, 2001, Division 1). All of these are integral to perception. For instance, the kind of doubt Husserl refers to is a *felt* uneasiness that shapes what is perceived, rather than a belief that is inferred from what is perceived. When possibilities that are actualized cease being perceived, those actualities do not simply re-enter the space of possibilities, taking on exactly the same form that they had prior to their actualization. Rather they are held 'retentially' and become 'abiding epistemic possessions' (Husserl, 2001, pp.45–6). They are grasped as re-accessible and can become incorporated into the system of habitualities that directs ongoing perceptual exploration. Of course, not everything we perceive is a solid, unchanging object and Husserl acknowledges that systems of appearances are harmoniously drawn together in other ways too, so as to constitute structured systems of change, for example; processes rather than enduring objects.

In addition to incorporating specific possibilities, experience has a general horizonal structure, an all-encompassing shape. As stressed by both Husserl and Merleau-Ponty, there is a kind of inarticulate background that delimits the possible forms that any experience might take. The world is, as Husserl puts it, a 'universal horizon' (1970, p.281) or, as Merleau-Ponty says, 'the universal style of all possible perceptions' (1964c, p.16). It is, I suggest, the world as 'universal horizon' that existential feelings constitute.

Consider the horizon of any particular object. Involved in this are possibilities such as 'its being touched', 'its being seen by someone else', 'its hidden aspects being revealed' and so on. Not all of these are involved in all experiences. A cloud, for example, does not appear tangible. However, the ability to distinguish intangible things like clouds from tangible things like cups presupposes the possibility of things being tangible. We encounter objects in the context of a pre-reflective background sense of belonging to the world and this belonging, this universal horizon, is a space of possibilities. All specific experiences are shaped by a sense of there being certain kinds of possibility, such as tangibility, usability, being accessed from other vantage points and so on. It is also important to emphasize that experience of the world is ordinarily experience of a *shared* world. The possibilities it offers are not possibilities for me alone. Possibilities for others are sewn into the horizonal structure of all experience. For example, when I look at the glass in front of me, I see it not only as something that I might drink from but something that is *for* drinking from. It is not just *for me* to drink from but *for anyone* to drink from. Its being is exhausted neither by my actual experience of it nor by the co-included possibilities involving me and it.

Husserl recognizes the difference between a background sense of belonging and specific experiences. He also acknowledges how difficult it is to reflect upon the former:

> ...natural life can be characterized as a life naïvely, straightforwardly directed at the world, the world being always in a certain sense consciously present as a universal horizon, without, however, being thematic as such. What is thematic is whatever one is directed toward. Waking life is always a directedness toward this or that, being directed toward it as an end or a means, as relevant or irrelevant, toward the interesting or the indifferent, toward the private or public, toward what is daily required or intrusively new. All this lies within the world-horizon; but special motives are required when one who is gripped in this world-life reorients himself and somehow comes to make the world itself thematic, to take up a lasting interest in it. (1970, p.281)

The contribution the body makes to world-experience is not restricted to how we experience specific objects. Husserl and Merleau-Ponty both acknowledge that bodily dispositions determine the shape of the universal horizon too, the orientation in which all experiences, thoughts and activities are embedded:

> To have a body is to possess a universal setting, a schema of all types of perceptual unfolding and all those inter-sensory correspondences which lie beyond the segment of the world which we are actually perceiving. (Merleau-Ponty, 1962, p.326)

The world, as Merleau-Ponty says, is 'the horizon of all horizons' and 'its counterpart within me is the given, general and pre-personal existence of my sensory functions' (1962, p.330). Changed bodily feeling can at the same time be a changed self–world relation and an altered sense of the being of things. But is the term 'feeling' warranted here? I think it is. According to Husserl and Merleau-Ponty, the relevant bodily dispositions are not objects of perception but, even so, they are phenomenologically accessible. They are modes of the feeling, rather than the felt, body.

As with horizons more generally, the structure of the universal horizon is not the accomplishment of any one sense. This raises an interesting possibility with respect to existential feeling. People frequently describe these feelings in terms of distance, closeness, tangibility or intangibility. It might seem that such language is metaphorical—we do not literally *see* that things are *intangible* or experience them as *remote* from us. However, an appreciation of the horizonal structure of experience suggests otherwise. If tactile *possibilities* were to be removed from visual perception of an object, then that object would indeed appear curiously intangible and remote. Distance, in the phenomeno-logical sense, has more to do with practical relatedness than geographical location. Someone can feel 'close' or 'far away', regardless of where they are. So some of the 'metaphorical' language used to describe experience might not be quite so metaphorical after all.

Now apply this to existential feelings. A world stripped of *all* tactile possibil-ities really would look remote and intangible. Similarly, 'losing one's grip' on the world could involve a loss of practical belonging, a failure to connect with things, where nothing appears manipulable anymore. One no longer inhabits a tranquil realm of organized, interrelated practical possibilities that mesh seamlessly with one's activities. Changes in existential feeling are often expressed in terms of an altered bodily relationship with the world. Consider the following:

> When we are in a state of deeply felt hope or expectation and what we have hoped for proves illusory, then the world—in one stroke—becomes radically 'different'. We are completely uprooted, and we lose our footing in the world. (Binswanger, 1975, p.222)

Once we allow for the role of perceptual and practical possibilities in experience, it is not difficult to understand what is meant by 'losing one's footing' or being 'uprooted'. The orientation that previously structured all one's activities, that connected one to the world in a practical, purposive way, is gone. One loses a feeling of belonging to the world, one's grounding in it. Binswanger suggests that, in disappointment, when we 'fall from the clouds', we '*actually* fall' (1975, p.223). Perhaps there is a sense in which this is true. In disappointment, certain possibilities disappear from experience; in losing a space of practical possibili-ties that connected us to a situation, we do lose our hold on it, our rootedness in it. A feeling not unlike slipping or falling away may indeed characterize the experience. As Binswanger puts it:

> In such a moment our existence actually suffers, is torn from its position in the world and thrown upon its own resources. Until we can regain our equilibrium in the world, our whole existence moves within the meaning matrix of stumbling, sinking, and falling. If we call this general meaning matrix the 'form', and the bitter disappointment the 'content', we can see that in this case form and content are *one*. (1975, p.223)

The falling in question is not an episode within the world. It is an alteration in the possibility space as a whole, in the structure of being in the world.

In certain other kinds of existential feeling, the world might be described as suffocating or as overwhelming. Here, the overall structure of experience takes on a different shape. One does not fall away from the world and lose a sense of belonging. Rather, one remains rooted there but the possibilities narrow and experience as a whole is characterized by a passivity before potential happenings. Things no longer appear as 'things to be dealt with' but as 'things that happen to me, over which I have no control'. It is not surprising that words such as 'drowning' and 'suffocating' are invoked to describe such experiences. One is immersed in them, rather than detached or estranged from them. No possibilities for efficacious activities show up and everything closes in. The world becomes an oppressive possibility space over which one has no influence, before which one is helpless.

In addition to being an all-encompassing way of relating to things, the universal horizon also constitutes the sense *that* things are. Again, the role of inter-sensory possibilities is pivotal. According to Husserl, when an object is perceived through one sense, 'intentions of other sense spheres' are 'co-constitutive of the objective sense' (2001, p.144). In other words, certain structured relationships between the possibilities offered by different sense modalities constitute the experience of an object's reality. Hence the *possibility* of those relationships applying in any given case is constitutive of the *sense* of reality. Merleau-Ponty (1962, p.324) remarks that 'the real lends itself to unending exploration; it is inexhaustible'. By this, he means that experiencing something as real involves a sense of there being an endless series of possibilities for perceptual and practical exploration by oneself and others. No perspective can fully actualize it and no inventory of concrete possibilities will exhaust what it has to offer. He also acknowledges that a sense of the 'real' is something that can be diminished or lost. For example, he says of hallucination in schizophrenia that it 'causes the real to disintegrate before our eyes, and puts a quasi-reality in its place' (1962, p.334). How can this be interpreted in terms of the horizonal structure of experience? Imagine an experience that is bereft of tactile horizons. Everything would seem intangible. Or consider an experience with no sense of practical connectedness to objects. Everything would seem somehow distant, not quite there. The sense of reality is not just a matter of perceiving an actuality through a particular sense. The feeling that something *is* involves a space of inter-sensory and practical possibilities that might be taken up by oneself or others. Without those possibilities, its sense of being is changed, diminished.

Jonas claims that touch adds something to the experience of reality that vision alone lacks:

> …touch is the sense, and the only sense, in which the perception of quality is normally blended with the experience of force, which being reciprocal does not let the subject be passive; thus it is the sense in which the original encounter with reality as reality takes place. […] external reality is disclosed in the same act in which one's

own reality is disclosed by self-action: in feeling my own reality by some sort of effort I make, I feel the reality of the world. (1954, p.516)[16]

Vision, in contrast, offers what he describes as a 'calmed abstract of reality denuded of its raw power' (1954, p.517). Such claims are, I think, misleading, given that visual perception incorporates tactile possibilities and thus also has the 'force' that he refers to. However, without these possibilities, things really would seem somehow not quite real, 'not really there'. A world without any tangible possibilities would appear curiously distant, detached. It is interesting to note that many hallucinatory experiences are, as Kraus (2007, p.105) observes, 'monomodal', whereas 'normal perceptions are usually multimodal, e.g. what we see we can also touch and smell'. A hallucination is not just a non-veridical perception. It is also an experience that lacks something of the sense of reality. However, the lack in question need not involve possibilities that are specific to a particular sense modality. For example, it could be that what is missing in many cases is a space of possibilities involving other people. To quote van den Berg, 'the sick person who hallucinates has some objects for himself alone. He has a world of his own that is founded in his isolation' (1972, p.107).

It is also possible that breakdown of experiential structure, rather than consistent absence of some aspect of it, plays a role in some cases. For example, Jaspers (1962, p.74) claims that hallucinations need not be monomodal and that, as with everyday perception, 'one sense supplements another'. However, he adds that there is still a significant difference, given that sensory integration is uncoordinated in the former case, resulting in a reality that is lacking in some way.[17] So the sense of reality is susceptible to various kinds of change. In Chapter 5, I will discuss one variant in more detail, an existential orientation where a sense of others as *people* is diminished or absent.

---

[16] Jaspers (1962) similarly states that 'what is real is *what resists us*' (p.94). He notes how touch can be used in the attempt to restore a sense of reality. In the words of one patient, 'all objects appear so new and startling. I say their names over to myself and touch them several times to convince myself they are real. I stamp on the floor and still have a feeling of unreality' (p.63).

[17] Hallucinations are usually distinguished from delusions, on the basis that the former are perceptual in character, whereas the latter are a matter of holding propositional attitudes. I doubt that things are this clear-cut and will argue in Chapters 5 to 7 that certain 'delusions' consist largely or wholly of altered experiences. Frith (1992) similarly doubts the applicability of a clear-cut delusion/hallucination distinction but for different reasons.

Chapter 5

Feeling and belief in the Capgras delusion

The aim of this and the next two chapters is to show how a phenomenological account of existential feeling can contribute to an understanding of anomalous experiences that occur in psychiatric illness. The current chapter is concerned with the Capgras delusion—the belief that one or more familiars have been replaced by impostors, who often take the form of 'robots' or 'aliens' (Ellis and Lewis, 2001, p.149). (For convenience, I will refer to the case of a 'replaced spouse' here.) In discussing recent explanations of the delusion, I draw out two assumptions that tend to characterize philosophical approaches to mental disorder more generally. First of all, experience or perception is construed as a kind of input system, through which perceptual contents are presented to a spectatorial subject. Second, it is maintained that conditions such as the Capgras delusion involve propositional attitudes with specific contents, which are formed by faulty or intact reasoning processes that act upon the products of perception. In contrast to such approaches, I argue that the delusion is a matter of changed existential feeling, involving a diminished sense of the *personal*. What might at first look like an isolated content (a replaced spouse) is in fact a much more encompassing change in the structure of experience. There may also be reasoning impairments but these too are embedded in a background of existential feeling, rather than coming *after* an anomalous experience.

Interpersonal relations

Before turning to the Capgras delusion, I will outline some assumptions about intersubjectivity that are commonplace in current philosophy of mind and cognitive science. These assumptions are, I will suggest, partly responsible for misinterpretation of the Capgras experience. The orthodox view in philosophy of mind and cognitive science is that interpersonal experience and understanding are enabled by a 'folk psychology'. Central to this, it is claimed, is the attribution of internal mental states on the basis of behavioural observations, principally the propositional attitudes of 'belief' and 'desire'. Debates are generally concerned, not with whether we do this but with how we do it. According to some, folk psychology is facilitated by a 'theory'. In other words, it rests upon a systematically organized body of conceptual knowledge concerning the relationships between kinds of mental state and behaviour. Others claim that it involves an ability to model or 'simulate' another person, rather than a theory. One puts oneself in her situation or psychological predicament, works out what one would do and predicts that she will do the same. Thus the attribution of mental states to people depends upon a practical *skill*, rather than a body of knowledge. One can know how one would behave in a given situation without having any understanding of the cognitive processes that generate the behaviour. However, theory and simulation approaches are not mutually exclusive, and most recent accounts maintain that folk psychology involves a combination of both theoretical abilities and simulation routines.

Discussions of folk psychology usually presuppose a rather standoffish, spectatorial conception of interpersonal understanding. One *observes* another person, assigns mental states to her and then explains or predicts her behaviour accordingly. The 'theory' view of folk psychology, or 'theory theory' as it is often called, implies that understanding another person is just a matter of postulating the internal ingredients of a very complicated object. As noted by Heal (1995, p.45), for the theory theorist 'people are just complex objects in our environment whose behaviour we wish to anticipate but whose causal innards we cannot perceive'; how we *feel* about these objects is beside the point. Some simulation theories allow a more substantial role for feeling in psychological understanding. In simulating another person, we might imagine ourselves in her situation and, in so doing, feel something of what we would feel if placed in that situation. Alternatively, we might try to put ourselves in the other person's psychological predicament, rather than just her physical situation, and feel what *she feels*, rather than what *we would feel* in the same situation. Either way, feelings assist interpretations of that person's psychological states; we understand how she feels by having similar psychological states.[1]

Nevertheless, simulation theories, like theory theories, presuppose a misleading detachment between interpreter and interpreted. Both theories take, as a starting point, an observer *watching* a third party and trying to interpret her by either theorizing about or modelling the internal mental causes of her observable behaviour. However, many, if not most, of our encounters with each other do not involve an observer–observed relationship but patterns of

---

[1] See Ratcliffe (2007) for a survey and critical discussion of various different 'theory' and 'simulation' theories of folk psychology, and of hybrid theories that involve aspects of both.

interaction (Gallagher, 2001, 2005; Ratcliffe, 2007).[2] An aspect of interpersonal understanding and experience neglected by accounts of so-called 'folk psychology' is the practical interaction and *relatedness* between people that typifies most social encounters. It is arguable that feelings structure and regulate interpersonal interactions in ways that are not acknowledged by theory or simulation theories. Gallagher (2001, 2005) suggests that relating to people is not usually a matter of *inferring* the presence of hidden mental states but of *perceiving* the meaning of behaviour in contexts of interaction. Perception of another's behaviour, he claims, incorporates one's own bodily dispositions, including affective dispositions.[3] Others have offered similar views. For example, Cole (1998) discusses the effects of facial problems on interpersonal relations and argues that problems such as disfigurement or paralysis of the facial musculature lead to breakdowns of ordinarily taken-for-granted patterns of affective interaction between people and to consequent disruption of mutual understanding. It is not a matter of failing to theorize or simulate but instead of losing a shared context of mutual, bodily attunement, which both parties are responsible for constructing and maintaining.

It is arguable that patterns of affective relatedness not only facilitate understanding between people but also contribute to experience of them as *people*. Drawing on developmental evidence from typical and autistic children, Hobson (2002, p.59) claims that 'to be emotionally connected with someone *is* to experience the someone else as a person'. Complementary views are offered by various authors in the phenomenological tradition, who emphasize that we have a distinctive sense of others as *people*. For example, Husserl states that the natural attitude incorporates what he calls a 'personalistic attitude', through which others are encountered as people. This is:

> ...the attitude we are always in when we live with one another, talk to one another, shake hands with one another in greeting, or are related to one another in love and aversion, in disposition and action, in discourse and discussion. Likewise, we are in this attitude when we consider the things surrounding us precisely as our surroundings and not as 'Objective' nature, the way it is for natural science. (Husserl, 1989, p.192)

---

[2] See also the essays collected in Hutto and Ratcliffe (2007) for a critique of orthodox approaches to intersubjectivity and of the pervasive emphasis on standoffish, observational stances towards other people.

[3] Some maintain that simulation is not an explicit exercise that people perform but a 'sub-personal' cognitive process. However, Gallagher (2007) argues that so-called 'sub-personal simulation' is better regarded as something integral to perception. Hence the perceptual, affective relatedness that he discusses does not depend upon an additional 'simulation routine'. See also Ratcliffe (2007, chapter 5).

For Husserl, experiencing someone as a person is neither a matter of spectatorial understanding nor of inferring hidden mental states. It is a practical attitude that is part of everyday experience and involves a pre-conceptual, bodily sense of relatedness between self and other. Schutz (1967, p.163) similarly claims that central to interpersonal experience is a 'Thou-orientation', a diachronic experience of bodily relatedness between an 'I' and a 'you', involving synchrony of gesture, expression and movement. This, he says, comprises our foundational sense of what people are. Sartre's (1989, Part III) discussion of shame, although very different in its emphasis on conflict and loss of purposive belonging, likewise suggests that feeling is constitutive of the sense that one is encountering another person. According to Sartre, it is through shame that others are revealed as 'others', as loci of experience and agency.

The claim that a sense of relatedness is constitutive of *personal* experience has also been proposed in the context of psychiatry. For example, Laing (1960, pp.19–25) discusses the difference between perceiving others in personal and impersonal ways, and likens the difference to a gestalt switch. A science of persons should, he emphasizes, remain personal throughout, rather that attempt to dispense with a personal stance altogether and construe the personal in impersonal terms. Personal understanding is not mechanistic understanding and it need not be misleadingly recast in mechanistic terms in order to give it scientific credibility. Indeed, Laing indicates that the practice of doing so is no more intellectually respectable than the pathological stance involuntarily adopted by schizophrenic people:

> ...we shall be concerned specifically with people who experience themselves as automata, as robots, as bits of machinery, or even as animals. Such persons are rightly regarded as crazy. Yet why do we not regard a theory that seeks to transmute persons into automata or animals as equally crazy? (1960, p.22)

Others have more recently argued that breakdown of interpersonal experience is central to understanding certain psychiatric conditions. For example, Stanghellini (2004) discusses the loss of felt interpersonal connectedness in schizophrenia. He proposes that a sense of self is bound up with a sense of others and that both are diminished in schizophrenia, largely due to the loss of certain kinds of feeling. Sass (2004b, p.128) similarly remarks on how, 'for normal individuals, affectivity provides a medium of connectedness' to other people, which is often lacking in schizophrenia. If a diminished or absent sense of the personal is indeed involved in various pathologies of experience, the failure of theory theorists and various others to even acknowledge that there is something distinctive about experiencing someone as a person will prohibit them from understanding the relevant phenomenology.

It should be noted that interpersonal relations are quite diverse. We experience, understand and relate to people in different ways in different contexts. The routine exchange between a shopper and a cashier in a supermarket is regulated largely by shared norms of conduct for such situations, applicable to all. *Who* the cashier is matters little to the shopper. Relating to a spouse in the environment of the family home is a very different matter; an appreciation of who a family member happens to be is, of course, central to one's relations with her. It is likely that the extent and perhaps also the nature of the contribution made by feeling to interpersonal experience, understanding and interaction will differ from case to case. Feeling is surely more central to relations with those to whom one is close. The Capgras delusion usually arises in relation to such people, and it is generally acknowledged that loss of affective response contributes to formation of the delusion. Hence this delusion can serve as a case study through which to explore at least some of the roles played by feelings in interpersonal experience and understanding. I will suggest that recent discussions of the delusion, like discussions of interpersonal experience more generally, are marred by spectatorial assumptions and by an overemphasis on propositional attitudes. Then I will draw on the concept of a 'horizon', which was discussed in Chapter 4, in order to argue that the delusion arises due to changed existential feeling, involving the diminution or absence of possibilities for interpersonal relatedness.

The Capgras delusion

The Capgras delusion is a monothematic, circumscribed delusion, meaning that its content is restricted to the impostor claim and that it is not usually elaborated in complicated ways. The belief that familiars have been replaced is resistant to change, despite appeals made by other people and sometimes the patient's own admission that his claims seem far-fetched. However, despite claiming that close friends or relatives have been replaced, patients often exhibit a lack of concern for the missing persons (Stone and Young, 1997, p.333). Thus it has been noted that the impostor belief is not always fully integrated into a 'coherent web' of beliefs and other mental states (Young, 2000, p.49). For example, one might expect such a belief to be associated with attempts to locate the missing spouse and with concern for her safety.

As discussed in the last section, accounts of interpersonal understanding tend to emphasize the structured interplay between beliefs and desires, through which people's actions are interpreted. Delusions are usually taken to be intractable, false *beliefs* (e.g. DSM-IV-TR, 2004, p.821). But interpreting them as such raises questions regarding their intelligibility, given that coherence with other beliefs is often taken as a necessary condition for something's being a belief. Davidson (2001) and Dennett (1987), amongst others, maintain that belief–desire relations are necessarily subject to a constraint of rationality. If beliefs, desires and actions did not relate to each other in fairly systematic ways, no inference from beliefs to other beliefs or from beliefs and desires to actions would be possible. So the whole framework of belief–desire psychology could not be applied to people in an informative or even meaningful way. As Campbell puts it:

> It is often said that rationality on the part of the subject is a precondition of the ascription of propositional attitudes such as beliefs and desires. One simple reason for thinking that rationality is critical here is that unless you assume the other person is rational, it does not seem possible to say what the significance is of ascribing any particular propositional state to the subject. (2001, p.89)[4]

Surely, if B believes that p, the belief that p should cohere with a range of other beliefs. However, lack of concern for missing persons and imperviousness to overwhelming contrary evidence both suggest that this does not apply in the case of the Capgras belief. If a person holds onto the belief 'A is not my spouse', whilst explicitly acknowledging its tension with a host of other held beliefs (such as 'A looks like my spouse', 'A sounds like my spouse' and 'A has all my spouse's memories'), its retention seems to be in tension with a presumption of rationality. And if rationality is constitutive of belief, then B cannot hold the belief in question. But this rests uneasily with the general acknowledgement that in the majority of instances 'patients should be interpreted as having the bizarrely false beliefs that their utterances seem to express' (Davies and Coltheart, 2000, p.7). Patients are not just talking nonsense or exaggerating another belief, such as 'my spouse's behaviour has changed' or 'I don't love my spouse anymore'. They do sometimes act on their beliefs. One person shot his impostor family members. Another, who believed her husband had died and been replaced, dressed in mourning clothes and ordered the impostor to leave. In one frequently reported case, a patient decapitated his robot stepfather to look for the wires. Hence, as Young (2000, p.53) remarks, 'if actions reflect the strength of one's convictions, there can be no doubting the sincerity of these patients'.

What could explain (a) the insistence that a person one cares about (or at least used to care about) has been replaced, (b) the oft reported indifference to the situation and (c) the imperviousness to contrary evidence? An influential recent account is offered by Ellis and Young (1990), who propose that the

---

[4] Davies and Coltheart (2000, p.2) similarly note that the problem with treating delusions as beliefs 'can be seen to flow from the fairly widely accepted idea that the attribution to people of beliefs is governed by a constraint of rationality or reasonableness'.

delusion is a 'mirror image' of prosopagnosia, the latter being a condition in which overt visual recognition of familiar faces is impaired, whilst affective response to those faces remains intact. They appeal to the hypothesis that visual recognition depends upon two distinct neural pathways: the ventral route is responsible for overt recognition and the dorsal route for covert, affective recognition. In prosopagnosia, the ventral route is impaired but the dorsal route remains intact. In Capgras, the converse applies. Hence, although the Capgras patient recognizes his spouse (in one sense of 'recognize'), perception is drained of affect, resulting in an experience of the spouse as 'unfamiliar'. There is, as Stone and Young (1997, p.345) put it, a loss of 'affective familiarity'.[5] This explanation is supported by the finding that, in Capgras patients, skin conductance response to familiar faces is lower than in a control group, indicating diminished affect (Ellis *et al.*, 1997; Ramachandran and Blakeslee, 1998, chapter 8). Capgras patients have a lowered response to all faces, rather than just to the faces of close relatives and friends. However, affect is likely to play a more significant role in perception of those to whom a person is close. In addition, the absolute decrease is greater for familiar faces, where affective response was higher to begin with and so has further to fall. So its absence is likely to be especially unsettling in such cases, thus accounting for the fact that the delusion is usually restricted to a small group of familiars (Ellis *et al.*, 1997, p.1091).

This neat account is not without its problems. Although the delusion is often said to be circumscribed, monothematic and restricted in scope to familiar people, things are not quite so tidy. The content can also include animals, household objects and places (Ellis and Lewis, 2001, pp.149–50).[6] In addition, it is not always an isolated complaint and often occurs in conditions such as paranoid schizophrenia.[7] Even when schizophrenia is not present, patients tend to report other unusual experiences, such as auditory hallucinations and feelings of depersonalization and derealization (Ellis and Young, 1990, p.241; Fine *et al.*, 2005, p.149). Furthermore, the Capgras delusion is not always specific to the visual modality. Young and de Pauw (2002. p.58) report that some blind people have it in relation to voices and that some sighted

---

[5] See Ratcliffe (2004) for a discussion of 'affective familiarity'.

[6] As Bayne and Pacherie remark, 'monothematic delusions do not have quite the monothematicity that they are often presented as having' (2004, p.8).

[7] Malloy *et al.*, (1992) distinguish 'primary' from 'secondary' Capgras delusion. The former occurs in patients with a psychiatric history, often involving paranoid schizophrenia. The latter has an identifiable neurobiological cause and, unlike primary Capgras, does not usually involve other psychotic symptoms, paranoia or violence.

people also have it in relation to voices but not to visually perceived faces.[8] Ellis *et al.* (1997) observe that lowered affect is found in visual face recognition but not in response to auditory tones. It is thus 'to some extent circumscribed' (1997, p.1091). But it is unclear just how circumscribed it is or whether its scope varies from person to person. Hence the term 'Capgras delusion' perhaps encompasses a mixed bag of variably similar experiences and convictions, rather than a condition that, in all cases, has the same neurobiological cause, involves the same perceptual processes and has the same content. Nevertheless, there is at least a common theme. The primary content of the delusion is that a person, animal or other entity to which the patient has a particular emotional attachment has been replaced by a duplicate or impostor. It is this content that I will focus on here.

Does an anomalous experience that is drained of affect suffice to explain the impostor belief? It is generally maintained that a further impairment is required. Although a spouse might look somehow different, this does not explain why the patient forms the recalcitrant belief that she is an impostor. There are plenty of other candidate explanations for the anomalous experience, one of which is that it arises due to a change in the perceiver rather than the perceived.[9] So why do patients settle on an implausible impostor belief, rather than opting for a more commonplace explanation of their changed perception?

Most accounts postulate a second 'cognitive' stage in order to explain why the impostor belief is ultimately adopted. There are several different views as to what this stage involves. One view is that it is a matter of normal reasoning processes acting upon altered experience. Although some, including Maher (1999), maintain this, others argue that the belief arises due to impaired reasoning. For example, Stone and Young (1997) suggest that Capgras patients have an attribution bias, which disposes them to explain perceived changes in terms of external rather than internal causes. Patients settle on something that is observationally adequate and fail to seek out more plausible alternative explanations. Hence they are not sufficiently cautious and conservative in their management of beliefs. Stone and Young add that the bias may be due to paranoia, which involves a disposition to assign external rather than internal

---

[8] Cutting (1991) also notes that Ellis and Young's emphasis on face recognition is problematic, given that some patients insist that objects and non-human animals have been replaced.

[9] It has also been suggested that some people have the same anomalous experience but do not develop the delusion. This is debatable though. A more detailed phenomenological study of the relevant experiences might well reveal differences in intensity or character. In addition, it may be that different brain areas are affected in the two cases (Davies *et al.*, 2001, p.145).

causes in order to explain changed experience. Davies *et al.* (2001) propose, as an alternative explanation, that a failure to reject a belief on the grounds of its implausibility is involved. Most of our beliefs are not explicitly inferred from experience. Rather, we take it as given that experiences are veridical. For example, when I see a cup in front of me, the content 'there is a cup in front of me' is part of the experience. In 'believing that there is a cup in front of me', there is no second stage where I infer that the contents of my experience are veridical and therefore adopt the belief that the cup really is there. I just take for granted that it is. The Capgras delusion, according to Davies *et al.*, arises from a failure to inhibit this default stance of credulity in cases where there are good reasons for doing so.

Hence there is debate as to whether the belief 'my spouse has been replaced by an impostor' is an *explanation* of an experience, arrived at via a process of reasoning, or an *expression* of an experience that is mistakenly accepted as veridical. And, regardless of which option is favoured, there is also the issue of whether a cognitive impairment is involved.[10] This latter issue is further complicated by the likelihood that reasoning strategies, dispositions and biases within the 'normal' population are quite diverse. It is debatable as to where the line should be drawn between 'normal' and 'anomalous' or 'impaired' reasoning.

Although so-called 'bottom-up' approaches, which claim that the delusion originates in experience, are most popular, a 'top-down' alternative has also been proposed. According to this view, anomalous beliefs influence perception, causing diminished affective response and altered experience (Campbell, 2001). After all, if you believed a person to be an impostor, your emotional response to that person would most likely differ from your emotional response to someone you took to be your spouse. Rather than arbitrating between these two approaches, I will argue that the conception of experience and cognition that they both work with is misleading. Experience is construed as an input system that gives us perceptual contents, and belief is construed as something that is separate from experience. What such conceptions fail to appreciate is that all beliefs presuppose an existential background, which is part of experience. I will suggest that the Capgras delusion arises due to a change in this background, a change in existential feeling.

The feeling of unfamiliarity

It is generally accepted that loss of 'affect' contributes to the Capgras experience. However, as discussed in Chapter 2, it is frequently unclear what is

---

[10] See Fine *et al.* (2005) for a survey of 'explanation' and 'expression' accounts, which further distinguishes between those that appeal to 'normal' and 'abnormal' reasoning.

meant by the term 'affect' In discussions of the Capgras delusion, it is sometimes used to refer to phenomenologically accessible feelings. For example,
Stone and Young (1997, p.327) claim that faces are 'perceived as drained of
their normal affective significance' and Ellis and Lewis (2001, p.155) note that,
in the normal case, there is an 'automatic concurrent "glow"' during recognition of familiar people and also certain objects to which one is emotionally
attached. However, others treat 'affect' as an unconscious physiological
response, the absence of which leads to an altered experience (e.g. Davies *et al.*,
2001, p.140). As discussed in Chapter 2, it is important to keep these conceptions distinct. Absence of physiological affect is not absence of feeling and it
does not entail absence of feeling. Indeed, many patients do not report a *loss of
the feeling of familiarity* but a *feeling of unfamiliarity*. The sense of there being
something missing, strange or not quite right is part of the experience:

> Capgras patients do not merely fail to experience the affect of familiarity when seeing
> their loved ones; rather, the normal feeling of familiarity has been replaced by a dis-
> turbing feeling of unfamiliarity and estrangement. (Bayne and Pacherie, 2004, p.4)

My aim here is to offer a phenomenological description of the *feeling of
unfamiliarity* involved in the Capgras experience and its relationship to the
content 'this person is not my spouse but an impostor'. So I will be concerned
with the phenomenology of feeling, rather than with associated changes in
physiological affect.

How could a 'feeling of unfamiliarity' contribute to the belief 'this person is
not my spouse'? As discussed in earlier chapters, feelings are often assumed to
be perceptions of one's own bodily states. Given this assumption, it is unclear
how altered feeling could contribute to the delusional content. As Campbell
(2001, p.92) remarks, a spouse is not ordinarily thought of as 'whoever it is
that produces that affective response in me'. However, even though one might
not *think* that feeling or affect (construed phenomenologically) is constitutive
of spouse-recognition, it might well turn out that it *is* constitutive of spouse-
recognition. After all, casual phenomenological reflection is not always
reliable. And, as argued in earlier chapters, feelings are not simply perceptions
of internal bodily states; they also shape experiences of things other than the
body. It is important to distinguish two senses of 'bodily feeling':

1 A feeling of the body that has the body as its primary object.
2 A feeling done by the body that has something other than the body as its
  primary object.

If our concern is with (2), it is indeed possible to maintain that the relevant
feelings contribute to interpersonal experience, rather than being perceptions

of internal bodily states that accompany the perception of other people. However, even if feeling does shape how other people are perceived, this need not imply that it participates in the recognition process. Someone can look different in all manner of ways without any doubt arising as to who she is. So how might feelings contribute to the belief that a spouse has been replaced by an impostor? In the remainder of this chapter, I will show how a feeling of unfamiliarity, which need not itself be directed at anyone in particular, can at the same time *be* the experiential content 'this person is not my spouse but an impostor'.

Relatedness and recognition

Discussion of the Capgras delusion has tended to emphasize propositional attitudes. It is generally assumed that the content of the delusion is a proposition, to which the person assents. Campbell (2001, p.90) takes the proposition to be 'that [currently perceived] woman is not that [remembered] woman'. This content could either be integral to the experience or arise following an experience with some other content, such as 'that woman does not look like that remembered woman' or 'that woman looks somehow strange'. Alternatively, it might be that the relevant experiential content is non-propositional in nature, a 'feeling of strangeness' perhaps, which somehow contributes to the eventual acceptance of a propositional content.

The emphasis on propositional content is associated with a rather impoverished conception of experience. Accounts of delusions often construe experience as an input system, which feeds into belief-forming mechanisms. For example, a recent discussion of delusions of alien control refers to a mechanism called a 'pre-potent doxastic response', which 'takes experiences and turns them into beliefs' (Hohwy and Rosenberg, 2005, p.145). Experiences are seemingly *presented* to a voyeuristic cognitive system, which either accepts or rejects their contents, thus generating propositional attitudes. If the relevant experiential content is indeed expressible as a propositional content, then it looks as though feeling and content are distinct. To quote Campbell (2001, p.96), 'the mere lack of affect does not itself constitute the perception's having a particular content'.

However, there are plenty of cases where feeling cannot be cleanly distinguished from content. Consider the belief 'this person is my friend'. It no doubt owes much to memories with propositional content, such as 'she went out of her way to help me when I was depressed'. But the recognition that someone is a friend also involves a sense of relatedness to her. Suppose that, when one meets one's 'friend', there are no feelings of happiness, ease or belonging and that she no longer solicits dispositions to smile, laugh or interject conversationally. Instead, encounters with her involve a pervasive feeling of unease, discomfort, unsettledness and bodily conspicuousness. The breakdown of felt relatedness, culminating in avoidance of her company, might best be expressed as 'she is not a friend' or, more specifically, 'we were friends but we've drifted apart'. The belief 'she is my friend' does not originate in an experiential content presented to a voyeuristic subject but in consistent feelings of relatedness and sharing that characterize interaction with her.

Recognizing that someone falls under the category 'friend' differs from recognizing a specific entity. In the latter case, one identifies a particular in a way that does not require an evaluative judgement. In asserting that 'B is not my friend', I still appreciate that B is B. Likewise, one's spouse is who she is, regardless of how one feels about her. Despite such differences, it is arguable that recognizing a person or other entity also involves feelings, sometimes at least. Consider Campbell's formulation again: 'that [currently perceived] woman is not that [remembered] woman'. This assertion is not suggestive of any feelings, whereas 'that [currently perceived] woman is not my wife' might well be. Different wording can indicate quite different experiences. Compare 'that person I perceive approaching me in the park is Bob Jones' to 'that person I perceive approaching me in the park is the village murderer'. The former might be a case of indifferent recognition. However, the latter implies a rather troubling relationship between one's own predicament and the other person's presence. Use of the term 'wife' is similarly suggestive of feeling and relatedness. The same goes for family members more generally. When a father announces 'I have no son', he implies the end of a relationship rather than a denial that there is a particular of the kind 'sons of person B'. And when Othello says 'I have no wife', having murdered Desdemona, he is not merely asserting that 'this individual, Desdemona, is dead' but conveying the loss of someone to whom he related in a unique way, blended with utter, unfathomable horror at his deed.

As the example of a decaying marriage serves to illustrate, an interpersonal relationship can change dramatically without the belief 'this perceived person is not that remembered person' arising. However, it seems unlikely that the change in feeling towards an estranged spouse is like that involved in the Capgras delusion. There may be quite pronounced feelings towards an estranged spouse, perhaps including anger, animosity, resentment, jealousy, loss and a host of others. In addition, a person would most likely retain something of the earlier sense of relatedness to the spouse, perhaps a disposition to smile, a sense of comfort, a desire to hug her. These might be deliberately suppressed or, alternatively, be eclipsed by stronger, more negative emotions.

In addition, estrangement usually involves a prolonged sequence of events, accompanied by a growing list of reasons (usually embedded in elaborate narratives) that account for the changed feelings. A loss of all or many of those subtle feelings that ordinarily constitute a background of relatedness between a person and her spouse, without any precipitating events or pronounced negative emotions, would amount to a very different experience. Could this background be partly constitutive of recognition?

I doubt that 'recognition' is a single, unitary phenomenological category. In other words, it does not have the same experiential ingredients in all cases, even if we restrict ourselves to a single sensory modality. Consider being shown a photograph and recognizing that the object depicted is the Eiffel Tower. If one had never been to the Eiffel Tower or attached any personal significance to it, one might recognize it with indifference. Contrast this with the case of returning to one's old home, a few years after moving. When I last did this, the house I once lived in appeared somehow different. Even though the exterior remained unchanged, it looked curiously unfamiliar, strange and distant. Although in one sense 'I knew' this was the house I used to live in, I had the 'feeling' that it was not. My old home was something very familiar, warming, safe and comforting, whereas I had no such attachments to this thing that I looked upon from across the street. To give another example, several years ago, my wife lost a unique ring, which she was very fond of, as the result of a burglary. Some years later, she found it in an antique shop in the same city, to which she had returned. When she initially came across it, she noted out of curiosity that it looked remarkably like the ring she once owned. Then she saw that one of the stones was cracked, in exactly the same way as the stone on her ring. So she recognized that the perceived object looked exactly like the remembered object but, although the chance of it being a different ring was, as she acknowledged, extraordinarily slim, she still did not identify it as her ring. She finally did so when she felt a growing sense of attachment to it, a while after she bought it.

It could be maintained that both these experiences are symptomatic of memory loss and also, in the latter case, of an unanticipated and unlikely encounter. But I doubt that this explains the feeling of uncertainty as to whether a perceived entity is really a remembered entity, given that similar experiences sometimes occur without a lengthy intervening time period. Recently, I was suffering from a cold and feeling rather tired when I went to give a lecture. I knew the lecture theatre very well and had given several lectures in it already that term. I knew the number on the door, the positions of the white board, the overhead projector and the upturned, slightly outdated table with a scratch on it, sitting in the corner. Even so, I was suddenly struck by a disorienting feeling of being in the wrong room. It felt strangely unfamiliar, not quite right. Even though everything looked just as it always did, it also felt different somehow. It was only after the first seven or eight—thankfully familiar—students entered that my sense of being in a familiar place was restored. Of course, it could have turned out that I had after all entered the wrong room in my fatigued state. As Maher (1999, p.554) notes, in everyday life it often happens that 'we begin with a "feeling" that something is different and then we try to find out what it is that has changed'. It may turn out that something is indeed different or, alternatively, that the feeling does not correspond to any real change. A person could come home one evening, be struck by a general feeling of unfamiliarity and later realize that the house had been burgled. Or she could have the same feeling but eventually come to accept that nothing had changed.

Hence feelings of familiarity, unfamiliarity, relatedness and estrangement do sometimes play a role in the recognition that a perceived entity is or is not a remembered entity. But there is still the question of how they do so. The examples I have offered seem to imply that a perceived entity can look identical to a remembered entity and yet look different at the same time. Indeed, it has been noted that the Capgras delusion involves just such a paradox and that it is not at all clear what the alleged difference between the perceived person and remembered person consists of:

> The patients often claim to be able to tell the difference between the original and the impostor, although they are unable to explain convincingly how they do this. (Stone and Young, 1997, p.334)

> The essential paradox is that patients with Capgras delusion simultaneously recognize a face and, at the same time, deny its authenticity (Ellis and Lewis, 2001, p.149)

Jaspers (1962) observes that this problem applies more generally when attempting to understand the phenomenology of delusional experience. There is he says a 'delusional atmosphere' or 'delusional mood', where experience is significantly changed but not in a way that involves concrete alterations in what is actually perceived:

> The environment is somehow different—not to a gross degree—perception is unaltered in itself but there is some change that envelops everything with a subtle, pervasive and strangely uncertain light. A living-room which formerly was felt as neutral or friendly now becomes dominated by some indefinable atmosphere. (1962, p.98)

Phenomenological changes of the kind that he refers to can, I will now suggest, be understood in terms of the contribution that *possibilities* make to the structure of experience.

Perceiving the possible

How can someone look exactly like one's spouse but, at the same time, appear so different that she is claimed to be an impostor? In offering an account of how people can look the same and yet different to the Capgras patient, I will propose that the delusion involves changed existential feeling, rather than a circumscribed experiential content. In *Nausea*, Sartre says of a shift in existential feeling that 'nothing has changed, and yet everything exists in a different way. I can't describe it; it's like the Nausea and yet it's just the opposite' (p.82). The reason why such shifts are so difficult to describe is that they are not changes in actual features of specific objects or of objects in general. However, we can accept that entities look exactly alike but also look different once we acknowledge that the *actual* is not all there is to experiential content. As discussed in Chapter 4, experience also involves possibilities. It is easy enough to describe perceived changes in the actual features of objects. For example, 'it is no longer red', 'it has shrunk' or 'it has had a part removed'. It is much more difficult to communicate changes in the co-included possibility space. Reports of an object's actual features may remain unchanged. Even so, it can still appear different, in so far as the experience does not include certain possibilities or beckon the usual bodily responses.

Focused feelings can involve changes in the possibilities surrounding a specific entity. For example, it no longer looks *nice* or *inviting*. But existential feelings are not specifically directed. A changed existential feeling, if it is describable as a 'loss' of something from experience, is not the loss of a specific, concrete possibility, such as 'this particular cup being grasped by me'. It is the loss of all possibilities of a certain kind, such as the possibility of things being experienced as 'real'. I suggest that, in the Capgras delusion, certain kinds of *interpersonal* possibility are absent and that this not only results in everything looking somehow different but also in an experience of particular people as 'impostors'.

The Capgras delusion is not just a matter of something being *absent* from experience. There is also a conspicuous feeling of unfamiliarity, the *feeling that something is absent*. This is something that an account of horizons can accommodate. In including salient possibilities, experience can also include *absences*. The sense that something or someone is *not there* is often a real part of an experience, rather than a propositional attitude that is inferred from the fact that the thing is not present. Imagine you are walking along the street and catch sight of a friend approaching. As you near her, everything else disappears into the background and the anticipated mutual greeting takes centre stage. However, when she is just a few feet away, there is the shock of realizing that this is not the friend but a stranger. There is a feeling of disorientation and unfamiliarity, of *her not being there*. Such feelings of conspicuous absence are not restricted to people. For example, there is the experience of suddenly realizing that you've forgotten something important or left a valuable possession on the train. The familiar world falls away momentarily, transformed by an absence which is, first and foremost, felt. The world *surrounds* the absence, a backdrop to a conspicuous void.

Sartre offers the famous example of waiting in a café for Pierre to arrive. Experience of the whole scene is structured by expectations, by the possibility of his arrival. When he fails to show up, the awareness of his absence does not simply consist in not perceiving him. The possibility of his appearing structures perception of the actual café, which becomes a setting for the central figure of Pierre:

> ...the ground is that which is seen only in addition, that which is the object of a purely marginal attention. Thus the original nihilation of all the figures which appear and are swallowed up in the total neutrality of a *ground* is the necessary condition for the appearance of the principle figure, which is here the person of Pierre. (1989, p.10)

Given that the perceived café is shaped by the anticipation of Pierre's presence, his absence is a very real part of it; there is a background without a foreground. The experience can be described as having the content 'Pierre is not here'. To pursue the example further, in addition to 'Pierre is not here', it can also include the content 'this person is not Pierre'. Suppose that, whenever someone enters the café, you look up and your expectations cluster around that person. But every time, it turns out to be someone else. Each person appears as 'not Pierre'. And sometimes the recognition that a person is not Pierre takes a moment or two. Perhaps he looks rather like Pierre and you scrutinize him, waiting for the feeling of mutual recognition. It fails to arrive though and again there is 'not Pierre'. Now suppose that you have been waiting for a long time, the experience 'not Pierre' becoming routine. Finally, someone arrives who looks exactly like Pierre. But, for a few seconds, he also looks rather strange, unfamiliar. The café remains as background to an absent foreground; the scene does not embrace the perceived person. Then he smiles and there is a feeling of recognition. You orient yourself towards him and smile, as he takes his place in the café. What happens if he fails to complete the scene, if the sense of absence remains, even though the approaching person looks just like Pierre? The expectation of meeting Pierre continues to structure the experience; the outer horizon is there. But Pierre fails to take his place. Perception of him does not incorporate the usual Pierre-specific possibilities and does not draw him into the wider scene in which those possibilities are embedded. Perhaps the experience 'this is not Pierre' would then remain, even though he is recognized as looking just like Pierre.

There are of course many other situations where one encounters a familiar person without expecting to do so. In such cases, a horizon of expectations is not set up beforehand; there is no place in the scene reserved for that person. Suppose I meet my wife on the street unexpectedly. As I recognize her, there is a feeling of warming familiarity and relatedness. Her presence solicits a smile, a greeting. Reaching for her hand and talking appear as salient possibilities. In the process, the way in which the rest of the scene is experienced changes. The street falls into the background, as do other people. The scene becomes, like the café, a background, with relatedness to my wife occupying the foreground. Recognition does not take place in a void; it sets up its context. If the perceived person did not fall into place within a framework of expectation or if a characteristic field of possibilities did not form around that person, even though her actual appearance were exactly like that of my wife, then the result would be an experience of her as identical in actual appearance to my wife but somehow very different. I will now propose that the Capgras experience has this kind of structure. What is absent from experience is not something specific to a particular person though. There is a change in existential feeling, a loss of certain *kinds* of possibility involving others. The relevant possibilities are partly constitutive of the sense of others as *people*.

Experiencing people

It is possible to feel a variety of different ways about an object on different occasions, whilst having no problem at all appreciating that these feelings all relate to the same object. However, this is not to say that *all* feelings shift from one encounter to the next. One can be angry that one's clock has stopped without losing a background sense of the clock as something familiar, connected to various concerns and practical routines. If this sense of familiarity were reduced or absent, things might look very different. Changes in existential feeling are quite different from changes in feelings that are directed towards a pre-conceived object in a pre-given experiential world, and the Capgras delusion should be understood in terms of the former. The delusion often arises in the context of schizophrenia, and it has been noted that general diminution of feeling in schizophrenia is associated with experience of familiar objects as stripped of their practical significance. Consequently, many of the possibilities that ordinarily surround them are absent (see, for example, Sass, 2004b; Stanghellini, 2004). As discussed in Chapter 2, Renee describes something like this in *Autobiography of a Schizophrenic Girl*. Without their practical significance, things appeared different to her; everything seemed 'artificial, mechanical, electric', somehow fake (Sechehaye, 1970, p.31).

The Capgras delusion consists of the conviction that only *certain* entities, principally people, have been replaced by impostors. However, many studies acknowledge that patients also report more general feelings of unfamiliarity and strangeness. For example:

> Although the impostor accusations may be directed at only one or two people, Capgras patients commonly report more pervasive feelings of strangeness, lack of affective response, and feelings that everything is somehow unreal or unfamiliar. (Stone and Young, 1997, p.337)

> Patients sometimes report that everything looks strange, for example, things may look painted or not natural and faces may look like masks or wax models or seem to have been changed by plastic surgery. (Ellis and Young, 1990, p.241)

The question arises as to how this diminution of feeling might affect experiences of people to whom one is emotionally close. Our relations with each other are quite different in structure from our relations with most, if not all, non-human organisms and inanimate objects. Indeed, I suggest that a sense of people as distinct from inanimate objects and most non-human animals is partly comprised of the distinctive kinds of possibilities for relatedness that they are perceived as offering. In looking at another person, one is not merely aware of her as an object that can be perceived from another angle or manipulated in certain ways. The experience incorporates an appreciation that there are many currently unactualized possibilities for conversational, gestural and expressive interaction, some of which can be solicited by one's own activities. Those *hidden aspects* that are distinctively personal are neither parts of an object that can be perceived from a different vantage point nor internal mental states locked inside the person's head, the presence of which can be inferred by means of a theory of mind or ability to simulate. As noted by Merleau-Ponty (1964*b*, p.172), when we experience another person, she is not actualized in her entirety but those aspects of her that are absent remain 'rooted in presence'. Experience of people as *people*, rather than as things to be manipulated, involves a distinctive space of *relational* possibilities, some of which can be actualized through interaction to reveal further possibilities (Ratcliffe, 2007, chapters 5 and 6).

Consider experiencing a table without co-included possibilities like seeing it from another angle, moving it or sitting on a chair in front of it. Without the possibilities of its being accessed from different perspectives or acted upon, it would appear strangely distant, intangible and incomplete. Perhaps it would look somewhat like a holographic projection or a two-dimensional model. Now let us assume that such perceptual and practical possibilities are still apprehended by the Capgras patient, at least to some extent. These would not be sufficient to allow a *personal* experience. To experience a person without sensing the possibilities for communication and relatedness more generally would be to experience her in a curiously impersonal way. Renee describes just this. She remarks of encountering a familiar person:

> I knew her name and everything about her, yet she appeared strange, unreal, like a statue. I saw her eyes, her nose, her lips moving, heard her voice and understood what she said perfectly, yet I was in the presence of a stranger. (Sechehaye, 1970, p.36)

She goes on to say that she perceived the person as 'a statue by my side, a puppet, part of the pasteboard scenery', who later seemed 'more a statue than ever, a mannikin moved by a mechanism, talking like an automaton' (Sechehaye, 1970, pp.37–8). Stripped of personal possibilities, someone would not appear as a person at all but as an impersonal imitation, a model, fake, waxwork, manikin or mechanism. Such experiences seem to characterize many instances of the Capgras delusion and possibly not just those that are associated with schizophrenia.

Not all Capgras patients are quoted as complaining that people in general look different or that everything has an aspect of strangeness. One possibility is that there are distinctive *kinds* of feeling that are specific to interpersonal relations and that these can be affected without any change to the horizons of inanimate objects; but this is at odds with the fact that many patients do report more general feelings of unfamiliarity. An alternative possibility, which I favour, is that certain feelings that are not person-specific play a more pronounced role in constituting personal experience than they do experience of inanimate objects. Furthermore, they play a particularly pronounced role in patterns of relatedness with family, friends and perhaps also certain non-human animals and possessions to which one is especially attached. Thus, when the impairment is less severe, it is most conspicuous as a changed experience of familiars. Even if everyone looks strange, unfamiliar or curiously impersonal, this will not be as troubling in the case of a shop assistant as in the case of a spouse. An appreciation of who or even what the shop assistant is need not impede the project of buying the weekly groceries. A sense of who a person is plays a much greater role when that person happens to be a spouse, where experience is characterized by a quite distinctive set of relational possibilities. In the absence of those possibilities, she would look somehow different, like a replica spouse.

It is likely that, in most cases of the delusion, a sense of the personal is *diminished* rather than *absent*. In the case of a spouse, where feelings of relatedness are most pronounced, the diminishment is still sufficient to make him appear somehow fake, not imbued with the full set of spousal possibilities. However, some instances of the delusion may involve something more extreme than this. Frequent references to 'robots', 'aliens' and the like in the literature suggest that it can involve the spouse not being experienced as a person at all. An impersonal object with all the actual characteristics of a spouse would strike one as a replica, a fake, a strangely impersonal duplicate. It would still appear as something that could be perceived from different angles, walked around and so on but the experience would be stripped of all those felt, relational possibilities that are distinctively personal.

It is sometimes claimed that the content 'this perceived person looks like my spouse but is not my spouse' is integral to the experience, rather than something that is inferred. For example:

> It is part of the representational content of a Capgras patient's visual perception that 'This is someone who looks just like my close relative but is not really her/him,' and the patient simply accepts this perceptual experience as veridical. (Davies *et al.*, 2001, p.153)

But what is not recognized is that someone's being an *impostor* or *replica* can also be part of the experience. An experience of the spouse that did not offer up the usual possibilities would involve her appearing somehow incomplete, lacking. If some sense of the personal remained, she might strike one as a person still but not as one's spouse. However, this is not to say that she would look just like an unfamiliar person, as experience of unfamiliar people would be altered too. The relevant diminishment of the personal, of certain possibilities involving others, would affect all interpersonal experience, but it would be most conspicuous in cases such as spousal experience. If a sense of the personal was diminished still further, the spouse would appear impersonal, and an impersonal thing with actual features matching those of a spouse would not just look like a *spouse* but like a *replica spouse*.

Merleau-Ponty (1962, p.334) remarks that the 'morbid world' appears 'artificial', lacking something 'needed to become a 'reality''. I suggest that it is a sense of artificiality that characterizes experience of the spouse. This interpretation is unavailable to approaches that focus solely on how *actual* experiential content fuels the formation of propositional attitudes, and construe recognition as a spectatorial achievement, rather than situating it in patterns of felt relatedness. It is often remarked that the impostor hypothesis is an odd one to come up with. As Fine *et al.* (2005, p.147) ask, 'of all the possible explanations of emotional hyporesponsivity, why is the impostor hypothesis the only bizarre hypothesis at which patients arrive'? However, if the relevant experience is anything like what I have described, then the impostor hypothesis is so widespread because it is an accurate expression of the experiential content, even though details such as whether aliens or robots are involved are not fixed by that content. Furthermore, the delusion is not, first and foremost, a specific experiential content. Rather, it is an all-encompassing change in existential feeling that has an especially pronounced effect on the way in which certain people are experienced.

It is possible that, in experiencing the perceived spouse as fake, the patient retains intact feelings of relatedness to the remembered spouse. But this need not be so. The strangeness or feeling of unfamiliarity that characterizes the experience does not require a comparison between the unfeeling way in which a person is currently experienced and the felt way in which someone is remembered. It might be that the patient has a memory of how his spouse used to look when the relevant feelings were intact, rather than having a memory of his spouse that continues to elicit those feelings. By analogy, one can feel physical discomfort without re-living a remembered state of comfort and one can feel sick without at the same time summoning up feelings of good health from memory. This fits better with the indifference towards the missing spouse that is often reported (Eilan, 2001, p.124). However, either scenario is compatible with the patient having the sense that there is something missing, that this isn't how things used to look, that this isn't how things are supposed to look.

It is also important to emphasize that relatedness goes both ways. It would surely be difficult for any person to retain her habitual feelings towards a spouse who consistently branded her an impostor and refused to interact with her in the usual manner. She would most likely depart from established routines and also modify her expressions, her gestures and the tone of her voice. So a consequence of the delusion could be that the spouse really does start to look different, perhaps further fuelling the delusion. Psychiatric conditions do not occur in a social vacuum. A patient's behaviour will affect others, often in ways that are hurtful and detrimental to relationships. Consequent changes in the behaviour of those others, changes that might themselves be symptomatic of altered existential feeling, may in turn have a further effect upon the patient.

Experience and belief

Most recent accounts of the Capgras delusion accept that two stages are involved, one involving anomalous experience and the other impaired reasoning. So far, I have only considered the former. Hence the question remains as to whether another stage is required. I have argued that the content 'this person is not my spouse but an impostor' is part of the experience and symptomatic of a more general change in the structure of existential feeling. This serves to undermine top-down approaches, which maintain that a delusional belief causes an experience that is drained of affect. One of the central motivations for such approaches is the assumption that an experience of anomalous affect cannot approximate the content of the delusion. I have argued that it can.

In showing how the content 'this person is not my spouse but an impostor' can be part of the experience, I have also dispensed with the need for an inference procedure to get us from experience to belief. So certain kinds of bottom-up approach are ruled out too. But there is still the question of why the experiential content is taken to be veridical. Thus a bottom-up model of the kind that posits a cognitive impairment in order to account for acceptance of the experiential content in the form of a 'belief' remains a possibility.

One problem with two-stage models is that they generally presuppose a simplistic conception of experience, which is construed as an input system for propositional attitude formation. Once we think of experience as involving a background sense of belonging, rather than just being the presentation of some specific content to a within-world subject, it becomes clear that the reasoning processes which generate beliefs do not *follow* experience but are embedded in it. Reasoning does not take place 'outside' of our sense of belonging to the world, in some mysterious elsewhere. Hence a shift in existential feeling may be what explains both changed perception of the spouse and any altered reasoning that occurs.

To add to this, there is considerable ambiguity over what is meant by the term 'belief' in this context (Bayne and Pacherie, 2005; Bortolotti, 2005; Ratcliffe, 2007). Suppose I assent to the proposition 'I will die one day'. I could 'believe' it in quite different ways. I might dispassionately affirm it. Alternatively, I might be filled with a sense of existential dread and helplessness when envisaging the all-too-real prospect of my non-being. Do I really *believe* it in the former case?[11] The linguistic description 'A believes that p' masks a range of different kinds of conviction.

Not everyone claims that delusions are beliefs. For example, Currie and Jureidini (2001) propose that they are imaginings that are mistaken for beliefs. They cannot be beliefs because 'representational states are beliefs in virtue of their occupancy of a certain functional role, which includes such things as roles in theoretical inference, practical reasoning, and the generation of action', and delusions do not fulfil the relevant criteria (2001, p.160). However, much of the debate over whether delusions are or are not beliefs is based on a very restrictive conception of belief. Once it is recognized that 'belief' picks out a heterogeneous range of phenomena, it is not at all clear that such things as mistaken imaginings can be clearly distinguished from beliefs.[12]

---

[11] I owe this example to Peter Goldie, who mentioned it at a 2006 conference in Bonn.

[12] See Ratcliffe (2007, chapter 7) for a discussion of some different ways in which the term 'belief' is used in philosophy, cognitive science and everyday life.

Why do Capgras patients assent to the proposition 'entity B is not my spouse but an impostor', when they can at least entertain the possibility that their experience is misleading? What kind of conviction is involved? It is worth reminding ourselves that existential feelings are tied up with a range of practical dispositions and, in the case of the Capgras delusion, it may not be possible to change or over-ride those dispositions, regardless of which propositions are uttered. By analogy, consider standing on the edge of a perceived cliff that you know to be a cleverly constructed illusion. However many times you tell yourself that if you jump you will land on a cushion a few feet below, you might still find yourself full of fear and unable to bring yourself to do so. In this case, it is debatable whether you believe that 'this is a cliff' or that 'this is an illusory cliff'. Perhaps what you believe is indeterminate. What about the belief that someone is not your spouse? If it were just like the cliff example, then patients would acknowledge the person to be their spouse but would respond to her as though she were not. And this is not what they do. However, given that all the felt dispositions constitutive of spouse-experience are absent, perhaps the utterance 'she is my spouse' would amount to an ineffective speech act, irrevocably divorced from all relevant experiences and behavioural dispositions. So the persistent and pervasive sense that the spouse is an impostor might be better expressed as the belief that she is, given that it resists all attempts by the patient to over-ride it.

A further problem for two-stage models of experience and belief is that, if the sense of reality is itself altered or diminished in some way, then the general *structure* of conviction will be affected too. One cannot believe that q is really the case, in any of the usual senses of 'belief', if one has lost the sense of reality that is ordinarily presupposed by beliefs as to what is or is not the case. Where experience p is itself a change in the modalities of belief, it is misleading to claim that B experiences p and then comes to believe q.

Are certain alleged 'second-stage' contributions attributable to changes in a non-conceptual sense of reality, familiarity and significance that is integral to perceptual experience? This may well be so. It is sometimes said that any reasoning impairment that contributes to the delusion is specific to the delusional content and that patients are otherwise rational (e.g. Davies *et al.*, 2001, p.150). However, there are many difficult questions regarding what it means to be 'rational'. For example, it is important to distinguish an ability to engage in abstract probabilistic reasoning from processes of evidence collection and evaluation in practical, everyday situations (Bermúdez, 2001). Even assuming that all reasoning occurs against the backdrop of the changed existential feeling, this does not entail that all reasoning will be affected by the change, given that there are different kinds of reasoning.

It might even be that the retention of a specific 'belief' despite overwhelming contrary evidence can be explained in terms of altered existential feeling without any appeal to abnormal reasoning. The Capgras delusion is in fact overwhelmingly *supported* by the evidence that is available to the patient. Every time she encounters her spouse, she experiences an impostor, a fake, a replica spouse. Whatever other people say, all of her own experiences of the spouse are consistent in revealing an impostor. And the weight of these cumulative experiences might well outweigh the evidence of testimony. If a sense of the personal is diminished or absent from all experience then there is no possibility of experiencing one's spouse in a way that does not corroborate the delusional belief. The changed existential feeling involved in the Capgras delusion is fairly consistent and long-term. And, without a change in this existential feeling, there is no possibility of any experience of the spouse conflicting with the delusional conviction.

However, a more general sense of others as strangely impersonal surely leads to a disinclination to seek or trust their testimony. So some of the counter-evidence needed to challenge the conviction that a spouse has been replaced is not available, this unavailability being a result of the same experiential change that gives rise to the delusional belief in the first place. If this is the case, then there is a reasoning impairment, which consists in failing to obtain or take seriously the testimony of others. Even so, this impairment is not separate from the experience but, rather, wholly symptomatic of the relevant existential changes. I certainly do not rule out the possibility that other reasoning impairments are involved too; changed existential feeling could potentially affect reasoning in all manner of ways.

Hence the concept of existential feeling casts new light on the delusion, by drawing attention to an aspect of experience that has been passed over by perception-belief models. A phenomenological account which acknowledges the role of possibilities in everyday experience shows how the content 'this person is an impostor' might be part of an experience. It also suggests that some of the confusion surrounding the nature of such experiences is due not to their strangeness but to misleading philosophical assumptions about the nature of experience. Regarding the delusion as a particular belief content that arises due to a particular experiential content is mistaken, as it involves abstracting these contents from the existential background in which they are both embedded.

It is worth noting that we do not ordinarily identify *kinds* of psychological state by their contents. For example, 'belief' is an *attitude* (albeit one I claim to be heterogeneous) that can have a diverse range of contents. For the purposes of philosophical and psychological enquiry, kinds of belief are not usually categorised in terms of contents like 'Eiffel Tower beliefs', 'beliefs about cats' and so on. Such categorisations would not be psychologically informative. Although the Capgras delusion is identified with a particular content, I have argued that a content-based approach is uninformative here too. What is involved is a way of experiencing, a kind of existential orientation. The impostor content is symptomatic of this, rather than being the essence of the delusion.

However, it should also be kept in mind that other kinds of delusion could well turn out to be beliefs that have specific contents. Indeed, it is at least conceivable that some cases of believing a spouse to have been replaced by an impostor do originate in irrational inferences from specific experiential contents. But given the nature of the descriptions offered by clinicians and patients, it is likely that all or almost all cases of the Capgras delusion involve the kind of phenomenology I have described here. If it were to turn out that certain other instances of the same 'belief content' required very different explanations, the right conclusion to draw would be that 'Capgras delusion' refers to at least two very different kinds of mental disorder, the explicit content being incidental and thus insufficient warrant for grouping them together. More generally, if some 'delusions' are within-world attitudes and others are changed existential orientations, then the term 'delusion' refers to at least two different kinds of 'mental disorder'. My emphasis in this book is upon the latter.

Chapter 6

Feelings of deadness and depersonalization

In the last chapter, I argued that the Capgras delusion, although usually taken to be the product of an anomalous experience with a specific content plus faulty reasoning, is better understood in terms of changed existential feeling. This chapter adopts the same approach towards the Cotard delusion, which is often referred to as the belief that one is dead, and then also to the closely related phenomenon of depersonalization. I begin by rejecting the view that the Cotard delusion is a propositional attitude and propose instead that utterances such as 'I am dead' and 'I do not exist' are expressions of existential changes. The existential orientation that patients inhabit renders them unable to see *outside of* their predicament and appreciate its contingency. This explains why the delusion is impervious to counter-evidence and therefore dispenses with the need to postulate an additional reasoning bias. I go on to address 'depersonalization' and suggest that this too should be understood in terms of existential feeling. Depersonalization is often regarded as similar in certain respects to the Cotard delusion but also importantly different, the former involving feeling but not believing. However, given that the Cotard delusion is not a matter of possessing a 'false belief', I suggest that the difference between the two is not so clear after all. In the process, I criticize the commonplace tendency to presuppose clear-cut distinctions between world-experience and belief, which can lead to a misleading double-counting of unitary symptoms.

The Cotard delusion

A defining feature of the Cotard delusion is harder to identify than the 'impostor claim' that is characteristic of Capgras. It is often said to consist of the belief that one is dead. However, this can take the form of 'emotionally dead', 'not real' or 'literally dead' (Davies and Coltheart, 2000, pp.30–1). Some patients claim that they are 'damned', 'disembodied' or 'non-existent', rather than actually 'dead', and one patient described herself as made up of 'mere fresh air' (Young and Leafhead, 1996, pp.153–7). Despite this diversity, there is a common underlying theme here: these assertions all refer to some kind of *nihilation* of self and often of world too. 'I am dead' and 'I no longer exist' might be regarded as analogous to 'my spouse has been replaced by a robot', in that they are more specific interpretations of the conviction that one has somehow been erased from the world. As with the Capgras delusion, utterances are not empty speech acts that have no effect upon behaviour, and they are not just colourful metaphors either. Young and Leafhead (1996) mention one patient who asked to be dressed in a shroud, another who felt guilty about claiming social security while dead and another who stabbed himself in the arm to demonstrate that he had no blood flowing through him.

The delusion is consistently associated with severe depression and tends to subside with the depressed mood. So it seems likely that depression is at least partly responsible. Severely depressed people sometimes express their predicament as that of feeling 'dead' inside or feeling nothing. Cotard patients make more extreme claims along the same lines, the difference being that a depressed person might assert that he *feels* dead whereas a Cotard patient will maintain that he really *is* dead or non-existent.

It is arguable that these utterances cannot be coherently interpreted as beliefs with the content 'I am dead' or 'I do not exist'. In Chapter 5, I discussed the rationality constraint that many take to be a prerequisite for the assignment of belief. It seems that the 'belief that p' cannot be meaningfully attributed to a person unless the attributor assumes that it is systematically interconnected to a host of other beliefs and desires, all of which contribute to the person's actions in predictable ways. Suppose I assert that I believe there to be a tiger loose in my office. I add that I am terrified of tigers, that tigers always eat people with whom they share rooms and that there is nothing in the world I would like less than being eaten by a tiger. Having just said all that, I casually stroll into my office without a care in the world. An interpreter would surely conclude that I do not really believe there to be a tiger in the room. It is not intelligible for someone to believe such a thing and then behave in that way. Even so, my utterance can still be regarded as a meaningful statement of belief. It is just a false statement—I do not really believe what I say I believe. However, there are other cases where it is not clear that anything is even meant by an utterance. Suppose again that I say there is a tiger in my office. When quizzed about this, I am adamant that the tiger's presence has no practical repercussions whatsoever for anyone. When asked what tigers are, I offer no information, other than to state that they are not mammals, that I don't know what colour they are, what they eat, where they live and so on. My 'tiger belief' appears to have no inferential connections with other beliefs and no effect on my activities, other than on the activity of repeatedly stating that there is a tiger in my office. So I don't really have a belief at all, given that my claims regarding 'tigers' are devoid of content.

Now, in order to regard the Capgras delusion as a propositional attitude, we could weaken the rationality constraint so as to accommodate indifference towards a missing spouse and immunity to counter-evidence. Bayne and Pacherie (2004, p.7), for example, concede that patients are not fully rational but add that their failings are not severe enough to warrant the conclusion that they have lost their grasp of the meanings of terms. However, the Cotard delusion presents a greater problem. Being dead surely implies not breathing but a Cotard patient might say that she is dead and at the same time freely admit that she continues to breathe. In fact, the belief 'I am dead' looks like a performative contradiction. In order to say 'I am dead', a person must be able to speak, and dead people cannot speak. Regardless of how much the rationality constraint is loosened, there is a point beyond which we cannot go. If we insist on taking the proposition 'I am dead' literally, this does not require a mere weakening of the rationality constraint but its reckless abandonment.

Such concerns hinge on the assumption that the utterance 'I am dead' or 'I no longer exist' communicates a propositional attitude adopted by the patient, which has a univocal content. This assumption is, I think, false. What the patient is expressing is a radically altered existential orientation, rather than a propositional content. A background sense of being part of the world, which most of us take for granted most of the time, is absent. The resultant existential predicament may well be best conveyed in terms of being dead, disembodied, non-existent, stripped of all that makes one a human self. This is not to say that the word 'dead' is being used in a non-literal or metaphorical way. It is worth keeping in mind that the word does not have a single, precise, literal meaning. As Bayne and Pacherie note, there are plenty of other meanings that the word takes on in different contexts:

> The semantics of a word may reflect the fact that it is part of several scientific or folk-psychological domains. For 'death' these domains include biology, the subjective realm of consciousness, religious beliefs concerning life after death, supernatural entities, etc. In his use of words, a delusional patient may break the rules governing one of these intersecting language games while retaining the meaning his words have in other language games. (2005, p.182)

A patient, in claiming that she is 'dead', may not be using the word in connection with strict criteria for biological death. Otherwise she would indeed be contradicting herself in the admission that she continues to speak and breathe.

Variations around the theme of the 'living dead' frequently crop up in popular culture. For example, many films have drawn on this theme and strike most people as quite intelligible. The rotting zombies that stagger around a chopping mall in Romero's *Dawn of the Dead* make noises, respond to various environmental stimuli and eat human flesh. Yet they are still dead and this is a premise that most viewers seem quite happy to accept. The term 'dead' is also frequently used to express a loss of feeling:

> We already speak of feeling *dead* or *deadened* when we sense a diminution of the normal emotional tonality of life. Why, then, should it be surprising that someone who feels an utterly undeniable, experiential alteration of this kind, might conjecture or even conclude that she must be dead? This need not imply, however, that such a person is using *dead* in quite the standard way this term might be used. (Sass, 2004a, p.73)

This is also something that some films seem receptive to. For example, *An American Werewolf in London* subjects viewers to scenes of progressively rotting corpses imploring the werewolf protagonist to kill himself and, in so doing, lift their curse of living death, which, we are assured, is quite painful. The film *La Morte Vivante* (*The Living Dead Girl*) is focused around the emotional desolation of 'being dead'. The protagonist, Catherine, is reanimated by a chemical spillage and returns to her former home. She looks through her possessions and is reminded of the life she once had; but she remains disconnected from all of it, inanimate, devoid of the feeling of life. When Catherine's former lover insists that she is not dead, all Catherine can do is repeatedly insist that she really is. Her body is physically located in the world but she is not *there* anymore; she does not belong. The world she sees is a distant memory, something she can no longer inhabit, no longer feel. All that remains is a painful sense of its absence.[1]

We should be wary of enforcing overly strict semantic boundaries and jumping to the conclusion that utterances to the effect that one is dead are meaningless. Indeed, if the Cotard delusion is interpreted in terms of altered existential feeling, I think it is fairly clear how someone could experience herself as somehow 'dead' or 'non-existent'. As emphasized in Chapter 4, the feeling of having a body is not an awareness of some conspicuous *thing* in the world with which one is intimately acquainted. Amongst other things, bodily feelings constitute a background sense of belonging to the world. The loss of bodily feeling is not just a matter of no longer having some object of experience, as illustrated by the description of experience after a spinal anaesthetic in Chapter 2. In the absence of normal background feeling, the affected body

---

[1] Something not unlike the Capgras experience features in some well-known films too. For example, in *Invasion of the Body Snatchers* (remade three times), familiars are replaced by aliens who, though identical in appearance, don't *seem* quite right. Confrontations with replaced relatives are understandably harrowing. Similarly, *The Astronaut's Wife* is based around an alien taking over a husband's body. He looks the same, sounds the same, but seems different somehow.

part can be experienced as conspicuously non-existent, strangely and unpleasantly absent. The Cotard delusion does not involve a complete absence of all bodily feelings. Nevertheless, diminution of certain kinds of feeling, such as those that participate in emotional responsiveness, could still have a profound effect on how the body is experienced and, consequently, on the sense of belonging to a world. An object-like body that is no longer solicited to act by the world might appear much closer in its phenomenological character to the dead flesh of a corpse. Coupled with this, the feeling of practical connectedness with the world, sustained by the animate, feeling body, would be absent and the sense of self would be consequently changed, diminished.

The sentence 'I have ceased to exist' might look like 'the tree in the garden has ceased to exist' but it expresses something altogether different. The experienced absence of oneself or one's body from the world is not the removal of an entity from the inventory of things that exist. What is lost is the *sense of existence* that ordinarily operates as a background to all experience; it is not that something no longer exists but that existence is no longer a possibility. As Sass (2004a, p.74), puts it, there is a 'transformation in what might be called the very framework of experience—in the normal, affectively grounded sense of existing as a living subjectivity'. A lack of feeling is at the same time an alienation from the world, an impoverishment of experience, a conspicuous, strangely inanimate body and a diminished self. The predicament is vividly conveyed by a description of extreme delusional derealization offered by Gerrans:

> ...the subject proceeds beyond reporting her rotting flesh or her death to the stage of describing the world as an inert cosmos whose processes she merely registers without using the first-person pronoun. In this type of case the patient conceives of herself as nothing more than a locus, not of experience—because, due to the complete suppression of affect, her perceptions and cognitions are not annexed to her body—but of the registration of the passage of events. She has effectively effaced herself from the universe: nothing which occurs is of any significance to her and, hence, she describes the world without implicating herself in the description. (2000, pp.118–9)

Ramachandran and Blakeslee similarly describe Cotard patients as 'stranded on an island of emotional desolation, as close as anyone can come to experiencing death' (1998, p.167).

The view that the delusion involves an existential reorientation rather than a specific content is supported by references in the literature to altered feelings, which are, at the same time, changes in the way *everything* is experienced. For example, Young and Leafhead (1996) observe that Cotard patients complain of 'feelings of derealisation', 'a lack of familiarity [...] especially buildings and people's faces' and 'more general feelings of unreality and being dead' (p.155). They quote one patient who said that she was uncomfortable at night because her 'body felt strange', that 'nothing feels real' and that she was 'just a voice' (p.157). Another reported 'feeling nothing inside' (p.160).[2]

Against two-factor accounts

It is arguable that changed existential feeling is not the only factor involved in the Cotard delusion. Although 'I am dead' serves to express a certain anomalous way of experiencing things, there is still the question of why the subject comes to genuinely *believe* that she is dead or non-existent, rather than making the weaker claim that it is *as though* she were dead or had ceased to exist. Young and Leafhead (1996) offer a two-factor account, according to which the delusion arises due to the combination of an anomalous experience and a reasoning bias. They claim that the same anomalous experience is common to the Capgras and Cotard delusions. A lack of affective response to familiar faces gives rise to a strange experience. However, the two conditions involve different reasoning biases and it is these that distinguish them. Capgras patients are generally paranoid and thus attribute the changes they perceive to external causes, whereas Cotard patients are extremely depressed and therefore prone to the attribution of internal causes. So the former assert that familiars have been replaced by impostors, whilst the latter seek out a change in themselves, concluding that they are dead.[3] The view that the two delusions are closely related is supported by the fact that some patients have alternating Capgras and Cotard delusions (Wright *et al.*, 1993).

In Chapter 5, I suggested that such explanations operate with an incomplete conception of experience, according to which the subject is presented with anomalous perceptual contents and then extracts beliefs from these via normal or aberrant reasoning processes. This leaves out a background sense of reality and belonging that is integral to all experience and also influences reasoning. Given a richer characterization of experience, it is not at all clear why a depressed mood should be distinguished from experience. A depressed mood, in so far as it is a matter of changed existential feeling,

---

[2] Berrios and Luque (1995) discuss the history of what is now referred to as the Cotard delusion and make clear that, whatever transformations the diagnosis has undergone, changed feeling has always been recognized as a key feature. In so doing, they challenge the claim that it is a 'delusional belief' and explore the view that it is a syndrome, which has anomalous moods and feelings as a key feature.

[3] Stone and Young (1997, p.338) likewise claim that 'there are many other ways a person might try to make sense of their anomalous percepts, but reasoning biases created by unusual moods lead some patients toward accounts of a certain type'. See also Young (2000, pp.64–5).

participates in all experience. So the anomalous experience and the reasoning bias are not distinct stages; they are symptomatic of the same existential orientation.

Why does the patient accept the experience as veridical; why does she move from 'I feel dead' to 'I am dead'? The reason, I suggest, is that no alternatives to her current predicament are able to present themselves. The changed experience does not take the form of being faced with some object of experience that might or might not be accepted as veridical. Instead, the patient comes to inhabit an all-encompassing existential orientation that is inflexible and closed to alternative possibilities. Something really has happened to her, something difficult to describe that is best expressed in everyday language by terms like 'dead', 'disembodied' and 'non-existent'. Assertions regarding her death or non-existence do not communicate the proposition 'it is not the case that some entity x (me) exists' but are expressions of changed existential feeling. She cannot contemplate the possibility of an alternative to this way of being because she has lost the sense of existence that is required in order to be able to envisage any such alternative. She can reflect back on when things were different and she can acknowledge that something she used to *be* has gone. She can also feel a sense of loss or absence; but a feeling of being part of the world is something she remembers experiencing rather than something that she is still able to experience. She does not merely *feel* her new existential orientation; she has become it. She cannot feel anything else.

Other more familiar kinds of experience involve a similar, although less pronounced, inability to appreciate the contingency of one's current predicament. For example, whilst I was writing this chapter, I was interrupted by a recent Durham graduate who wanted to apply for a place on our Philosophy MA course. He explained that he had not discussed the matter until this point because, throughout the academic year, he had been suffering from a chronic and serious throat infection, which had now been corrected by surgery. The infection, he said, had left him 'dead to the world'. He could not contemplate applying for an MA at the time because his sense of 'wanting anything' had been diminished. During his illness, he was unable to 'get outside' himself to figure out what he would want to do once he had recovered. To quote, 'I did not know how I would feel when I was better because I was not better'. The space of possibilities he required in order to make his decision was absent. Thinking of a scenario in which this was not the case did not allow him to think as he would if it were not the case. He could not see beyond the existential predicament of his illness.

An inability to appreciate the possibility of an alternative to how one currently finds oneself in the world is sometimes reported by people suffering from severe depression. For example, Lewis Wolpert recalls how his psychiatrist was:

> ...extremely reassuring, telling me again and again that depression is self-limiting and that I would recover. I did not believe a single word. It was inconceivable to me that I should ever recover. The idea that I might be well enough to work again was unimaginable and I cancelled commitments months ahead. (1999, p.154)

The Cotard delusion involves an extreme version of this inability. The patient is not in a position to contrast it with anything else and so is unable to construe it as a contingent mode of feeling rather than an all-embracing mode of being.

Jaspers (1962) construes the transition from feelings of derealization and depersonalization to a Cotard-like predicament as a continuum, rather than in terms of a contrast between *feeling* a certain way and *believing* oneself to be that way. In a less severe case, 'everything appears as though through a veil; as if I heard everything through a wall [...] I touch myself to convince myself that I exist' (1962, p.62). However, a point can be reached where all sense of reality is gone and the whole possibility space is shaped by a non-existence from which there is no possibility of escape:

> Terrified and restless, the patients begin to experience their feelings as the reality itself and are then inaccessible to reason. Now the world has escaped them. Nothing remains. They are alone in terrible isolation, suspended between infinities. They have to live for ever because time no longer exists. They themselves no longer exist; their body is dead. Only this fake-existence remains as their horrible fate. (1962, p.63)

The move from 'feeling dead' to 'believing one is dead' is not, therefore, a leap from affect to propositional attitude, for which some additional factor is responsible. Rather, the intensification of a certain way of experiencing is at the same time a diminished sense of alternative possibilities. The 'belief' that one is dead expresses a predicament that offers up no alternatives.

More 'everyday' existential orientations reveal the world as a realm of possibilities that are relevant to one's predicament and that might affect one in a variety of ways. An appreciation of these possibilities as self-affecting is at the same time a sense of one's current way of experiencing things being contingent, fragile and subject to modification. The contribution made by existential feeling to experience is not exhausted by 'how the world currently appears' or even by 'how the world consistently appears'. How the world actually appears points to possible ways in which it might be otherwise. The loss of practical significance in the Cotard delusion is at the same time a loss of those possibilities that might have revealed the contingency of the patient's experiential predicament. Without them, it is all-enveloping and closed to alternatives, a feeling of deadness without hope of reprieve. Without the feeling of alternative possibilities, one can make assertions about how things might change but can never really become convinced or moved by them.

Thus a separate reasoning bias is not required in order to explain why the 'belief' is impervious to revision. Even so, reasoning is likely to be defective in various ways. It is doubtful that practical or abstract reasoning would proceed wholly as before when the existential background has been altered so significantly. As pointed out in Chapter 5, much of our practical reasoning involves an appreciation of contextually relevant information and is regulated by the guidance of other people. So a loss of the significant, relevant world and an associated disconnectedness from other people would surely affect it.

In contrast to what I have proposed here, Young and de Pauw suggest that alternative explanations are available to the Cotard patient and that some account is therefore required of why she claims to be dead:

> Rather than concluding that they have died, a person experiencing a lack of emotional responses and feelings of depersonalization and derealization could offer one of many other possible explanations; they could say that they feel peculiar and they had better see a doctor, that they must have been drugged, and so on. (2002, p.57)

However, such assertions do not take account of the extent to which a patient's existential orientation has been altered. Suppose a person feels utterly estranged from the world, his body feels more like dead flesh than the purposive orientation that it once was, and a conspicuous sense of something vital being absent envelops everything. To say that he feels peculiar or needs to consult a doctor does not do justice to the relevant phenomenology. It is also worth keeping in mind that the assertion 'I am dead' is only one way in which patients communicate their predicament. The delusion is not characterized by a specific propositional attitude. As Young and Leafhead (1996, p.153) acknowledge, Cotard's original eight patients complained of not having a body, of not existing and of being damned. Only one said she was dead. In fact, Cotard's list of symptoms was very wide-ranging and included:

> ...anxious melancholia, ideas of damnation or possession, suicidal behavior, insensitivity to pain, delusions of nonexistence involving the whole person or parts thereof, and delusions of immortality. (Berrios and Luque, 1995, p.219)[4]

Describing the Cotard delusion as the belief that one is dead or non-existent is thus an over-simplification, which abstracts one way of expressing an altered existential feeling from its context and takes it to be a propositional attitude.

---

[4] The claim that one is immortal might seem incompatible with the claim that one is dead or non-existent but it is not. One could be 'dead' and at the same time endure as a disembodied wraith that has been existentially diminished by death.

There is, however, a fine line between expression of an experience and explanation of it. Perhaps some patients do *infer* from their experience that they are dead (in a sense of 'dead' that differs from 'wholly biologically dead'), rather than using the term 'dead' to *express* their changed experience. If this is so, then 'I am dead' would be a propositional attitude. However, any such attitude would still be symptomatic of the existential orientation. It would be a fair reflection of the altered experience, rather than something that required a huge leap from a slightly strange experience to an outrageous belief by means of anomalous reasoning. Furthermore, the attitude would not be the core feature of the delusion but a symptom of it that might or might not be present. And it would be difficult to distinguish from other utterances that were expressions of the existential predicament rather than inferences from it. It should also be kept in mind that, with such a radically altered sense of existence, the modalities of belief will, of course, be altered. Like Renee, the patient will not *believe* in quite the same manner as someone who does not share her changed experience. So the question of whether or not a patient really does believe that p is not something that can be answered in simple yes/no terms.

Another problem with Young and Leafhead's explanation is that the Capgras and Cotard delusions most likely do differ phenomenologically. Gerrans (2000) observes that, for Cotard subjects, experience of everything rather than just familiar faces is drained of significance. As discussed in Chapter 5, the Capgras delusion is not always restricted to perception of familiar faces either. Even so, it would seem that loss of feeling in the Cotard delusion is more pronounced and widespread than in Capgras. We might think of the difference between the two as a matter of degree. A loss of feeling, which is at first most pronounced in relation to familiar people, intensifies and is experienced as being more widespread. Initially, its impact may only have a conspicuous effect upon those people and objects that used to solicit especially pronounced feelings. Then, as feeling further diminishes, perception of everything is noticeably affected.

Gerrans claims that loss of what he calls 'affect' serves to *explain* the reasoning bias in Cotard subjects. Its progressive loss culminates in feelings of disembodiment and disorientation, which are rationalized in the form of the belief that one is dead:

> I suggest that the difference between the Capgras and Cotard delusions cannot be explained solely in terms of different attributional styles applied to essentially the same affective deficit. The Cotard delusion, in its extreme form, is a rationalization of a feeling of disembodiment based on global suppression of affect resulting from extreme depression. In the Capgras case the affective deficit is more localized,

confined to familiars. [...] Affective processes on which qualitative experiences depend signal, not only changes in body state, but that the experience is occurring *in one's own body*. (Gerrans, 2000, p.111–2)

Hence affect not only structures perceptual recognition but also plays a more general role, amounting to a background bodily orientation within which perception and reasoning operate. This breaks down in the Cotard delusion, and so reasoning impairments and perceptual anomalies have a common source. The experience of disembodiment that he refers to is what I would call a change in existential feeling. However, Gerrans emphasizes *implicit* affect, rather than something that is phenomenologically accessible. The experience, he says, arises due to suppression of 'affective mechanisms by which we monitor and adjust bodily states in response to perceptual and cognitive information processing' (1999, p.591). The mechanisms in question operate at a 'sub-personal' level. In other words, although the 'affects' they generate shape how things are experienced, they are not themselves experienced. As indicated in earlier chapters, I think that what plays the role he describes *is* experienced. When we reflect phenomenologically, what we will not find is a collection of feelings lurking in the background of every experience, all of which have the body as their object. So, if bodily feelings are conceived of as perceptions of internal bodily states, the view that the relevant 'affective processes' are implicit does seem compelling. However, once we reject the assumption of a body-object that experiences its own states in isolation from how it experiences everything else, it is possible to reflect upon the feeling body that is, at the same time, a changeable sense of belonging.

In contrasting the Capgras and Cotard delusions, Gerrans suggests that 'the phenomenology of the Cotard delusion is, at core, disembodiment, whereas the phenomenology of the Capgras delusion is one of estrangement and derealization' (2002, p.49). Such contrasts are misleading. In both conditions, patients complain of 'derealization'. In addition, a feeling of disembodiment is also surely a feeling of estrangement, a sense of detachment from the significant world in which one used to be embedded. And it is important to be careful when talking of a feeling of 'disembodiment'. As discussed in Chapter 4, it is not the release of the self from the body–world relationship. It is a diminishment and transformation of self that is constituted by a changed body–world relationship. Patients may refer to themselves as no longer existing *or* to their being disembodied. In both cases it is clear that the self does not survive intact when the body–world relationship is changed. The self that is disembodied is a diminished self, 'mere fresh air'. The same phenomenon can be described either in terms of disembodiment of self or in terms of extinction of self.

Nevertheless, it does at least seem that the two delusions differ in that one involves paranoia and the other depression. If we acknowledge that these 'moods' participate in the phenomenology of perception, rather than being post-perceptual reasoning biases, then there is a phenomenological difference here. However, this difference may well be explicable in terms of the *extent* to which feeling is diminished, rather than in terms of different *kinds* of feeling. Paranoia involves a general sense of others as menacing, suspicious and not to be trusted.[5] They are a threat to oneself. But the possibility of something being threatening, as Heidegger appreciates, depends upon already finding oneself in the world in a certain way. This way of finding oneself in the world is, I have argued, something that is felt. Now suppose that diminished feeling in the Capgras delusion involves things appearing unpleasantly strange, unfamiliar and threatening. What happens when feeling diminishes still further? It could well be that the possibility of threat is itself lost. A being that no longer feels alive cannot feel its life to be threatened, and so it is at least possible that the paranoia drops out due to intensification of the experience beyond a level where paranoia is an existential possibility. Hence it might be that alternating Capgras and Cotard delusions are symptomatic of a single way of experiencing that varies in intensity, rather than of two different kinds of existential orientation, with a feeling of threat occasionally giving way to a feeling of deadness and vice versa.

So far, I have criticized so-called 'bottom-up' approaches, which claim that the delusion originates in anomalous perception. But this still leaves us with the 'top-down' alternative. This does not have to deal with certain problems faced by bottom-up approaches. For example, if one conceives of experience as an input system that feeds into belief-generating mechanisms, it is not clear how it could possibly motivate the belief 'I do not exist'. As Campbell remarks:

> ...it is very hard to see how vision could be giving you knowledge of your own existence. By the same token, it is hard to see how vision could be giving you knowledge of your own lack of existence. In that case, the Cotard delusion does seem to be a top-down imposition on experience. (2001, p.93)

However, explaining the delusion in terms of anomalous experience is not a problem if it is acknowledged that visual experience includes more than receiving perceptual information about entities in the world. All perception is embedded in a background orientation and it is this that constitutes the sense

---

[5] The points I make here apply to 'paranoia' in both its everyday and it psychiatric senses. The latter is more accommodating, including grandiose delusions in addition to persecutory delusions. In the absence of all self-concern, the possibility of grandiosity would also presumably be absent.

of existence. The relevant visual phenomenology is not just 'visual'. When discussing the Capgras delusion in Chapter 5, I argued that possibilities for activity and for experience through other sensory modalities are incorporated into visual perception. The same applies to the Cotard delusion. Furthermore, the contribution of changed feeling in the Cotard delusion is not restricted to the visual modality. It is an existential alteration that shapes all experience. Closing one's eyes would not make it go away.

Common to both bottom-up and top-down accounts is a tendency to forget that we are in a world at all and to focus instead upon specific contents that are presented to a within-world subject. The question of how the subject finds itself in a world to begin with, a world within which those contents are encountered, is not addressed. The delusional phenomenology cannot be understood if the interpreter presupposes that both she and the patient are already *here* in the same world and then wonders how the patient's experience of things within this shared world differs from her own. When the delusional phenomenology is understood in a within-world way, the patient's experience is abstracted from his reality; the contents of his perceptions are prized free from the place in which he finds himself.

Campbell's (2001) top-down alternative to bottom-up accounts of delusions invokes the concept of a 'framework' or 'hinge' proposition, as employed by Wittgenstein in *On Certainty*. Framework propositions are not propositions that we explicitly doubt or assent to. They are ground-floor commitments that are tacitly accepted and operate as a background to all those propositions the truth or falsehood of which we might explicitly entertain. If delusional beliefs are held as framework propositions, this explains why they are insulated from doubt. In addition, altered framework propositions would surely affect our feelings and thus our perceptions in various ways.

Wittgenstein refers to framework propositions as 'the ground' for discriminations that we make between true and false propositions. They are accepted in a very different way from explicit propositions and it does not make sense to doubt them (1975, p.27). He later states that 'the concept 'proposition' itself is not a sharp one' (1975, p.41). It is therefore arguable that Wittgenstein is not discussing 'propositions' in any familiar sense of the term and that his framework propositions might add up to what I refer to as the sense of reality. However, he emphasizes 'language games' and the distinctive role that some propositions play in these games, propositions that look like empirical propositions but in fact have more 'the character of a rule' (1975, p.65). This is somewhat removed from phenomenological reflection upon the sense of reality. Wittgenstein does succeed in distinguishing different ways in which we might take something to be the case. However, in retaining the term 'proposition' and assuming that the background to explicit conviction and doubt has anything remotely like a propositional form, he fails to make clear the difference between taking something to be the case, regardless of the way in which we do so, and having a sense of what it is to be the case. The sense of reality is not a matter of accepting a proposition of any kind, 'framework' or otherwise. Belonging to the world is a pre-articulate, practical orientation and any attempt to reconstruct it in propositional terms is an over-intellectualisation of something that is presupposed by propositional thought.

Nothingness

The Capgras and Cotard delusions both involve a conspicuous feeling of *absence*. In the Capgras delusion, familiars are perceived as lacking something and thus as replicas or impostors. In addition, there are more generalized feelings of unfamiliarity and unreality, of something being missing. The Cotard delusion involves an even more pronounced and encompassing absence, a loss of the usual sense of existing and being part of the world. It is not just that one no longer feels anything; the loss of feeling is itself something that is felt. What is missing from experience is a real part of the experience; 'nothingness' or 'non-existence' is there. In the case of Capgras, I appealed to Sartre's account of how we can experience absence or 'nothingness' given certain projects, purposes and expectations. However, the all-enveloping absence we find in the Cotard delusion is much closer to something described by Heidegger—an apprehension of the 'nothing'. As discussed in Chapter 2, Heidegger suggests that 'moods' constitute a sense of belonging to the world and that this belonging can break down to varying degrees. Sometimes things 'just don't feel quite right'. The world appears 'uncanny' and we feel disconnected from it. The Cotard delusion involves an extreme variant of the uncanny, where the body through which one ordinarily belongs to the world becomes oddly conspicuous and thing-like, somehow no longer animate or familiar. With this, the feeling of belonging to the world breaks down and is replaced by a sense of utter estrangement.

Heidegger claims that logical negation draws its sense from a more primitive experiential apprehension of 'the nothing':

> Is the nothing given only because the 'not', i.e., negation, is given? Or is it the other way round? Are negation and the 'not' given only because the nothing is given? [...]
> We assert that the nothing is more original than the 'not' and 'negation'. (1978a, p.97)

Appreciating that this is indeed the case is essential to understanding certain modes of existential feeling. The way in which we experience ourselves as existing is quite different from the way in which we accept or infer the existence of a specific entity in the world. A loss of this feeling of existence is not, in any way, akin to the negation of a proposition concerning the existence of an entity. We experience the absence, the non-being. According to Heidegger, it is in the mood of anxiety that we encounter the nothing. Anxiety is the most extreme form of the uncanny, a disintegration of background existential orientation that amounts to the 'complete negation of the totality of beings' (1978a, p.98). The nothing is *experienced* as an absence of ordinary existence-sense, the dissolution of belonging:

> The receding of beings as a whole that closes in on us in anxiety oppresses us. We can get no hold on things. In the slipping away of beings only this 'no hold on things' comes over us and remains. [...] That anxiety reveals the nothing man himself immediately demonstrates when anxiety has dissolved. In the lucid vision sustained by fresh remembrance we must say that that in the face of which and for which we were anxious was 'properly'—nothing. Indeed: the nothing itself—as such—was there. (1978a, p.101)

This is similar in many respects to the kind of experience that Cotard patients report. The patient does not infer that he no longer exists; he has the *experience* of nihilation or effacement. The world loses its reality as the orientation that binds him to it breaks down. The changed body that is implicated in this is experienced as no longer animate. Its phenomenology is one of absence. However, there are differences too. Anxiety, for Heidegger, seems to be a brief episode, whereas the existential orientation that characterizes the Cotard delusion is an enduring way of being that patients inhabit. In addition, there is more to the Cotard experience than the feeling of having no hold on things and of everything falling away. The *possibility* of having a hold on the world, of one's animate body reaching out into the world, even if only in the form of a total loss of practical connectedness and significance, is itself gone. So the Cotard experience is an even greater retreat from everyday belonging than the kind of mood Heidegger describes. 'I am dead' or 'I have ceased to exist' may indeed be the most appropriate description of it.[6]

Up to now, I have consistently referred to the Cotard experience as a 'delusion'. However, I have also claimed that it is the expression of altered existential feeling and that it does not require the adoption of an additional 'belief' on the basis of the anomalous experience. So there is the question of whether this is a 'delusion' at all. I am inclined to continue using the term 'delusion' in this case, whilst accepting, as indicated at the end of Chapter 5, that the term most likely

---

[6] Heidegger claims that anxiety enables an 'authentic' relationship with the world, by breaking down our entrenched self-misinterpretations. Sartre regards it as a consciousness of 'freedom'. This sort of potential is clearly not available to those with the Cotard delusion. They face a debilitating void, rather than the possibility of an authentic existence.

does not identify a homogeneous group of psychological phenomena. There are various other grounds for suspicion regarding the view that 'delusion' refers to a unitary kind of psychological state. For example, Fulford (1994) is critical of the tendency to construe delusions as *factual* beliefs and remarks that *evaluative* delusions have been neglected. He adds that no delusion-specific cognitive impairment has been identified and stresses the dependence of all delusional beliefs upon a 'background structure' (1994, p.227). It is just such a background structure that I have set out to describe here. There is also a fine line between delusional beliefs and other beliefs that are not classified as pathological. As David observes:

> Delusions exist in a world of values, assumptions, prejudices, incorrect inferences, superstitions, wishful-thinking and paranoia (in the non-technical sense). This is what makes delusions possible and also what makes them impossible to pin down. (1999, p.19)

Several other authors have commented on this difficulty in 'pinning down' what delusions are. For example, Broome (2004, p.36) claims that patients and their delusions 'may not have much in common' and Ghaemi (2004, p.50) similarly suggests that 'there simply is no essential feature of delusions'.

Another question that needs to be addressed is whether the Cotard delusion is a 'belief'. I have argued that it is not first and foremost a propositional attitude. However, some authors, in claiming that delusions are beliefs, either tacitly assume or explicitly endorse more permissive conceptions of belief. For example, Bortolotti adopts a fairly liberal conception and then suggests that at least some delusions are beliefs, on the basis that:

> ...according to the best available account of the formation of delusional states, the delusion is an attempt to explain a puzzling experience the subject has or had. Once formed, the delusion is often defended by the subject with tentative arguments. In this respect, delusions do not differ from ordinary beliefs. (2005, p.198)

Even so, this does not accommodate my interpretation of the Cotard delusion. The delusion is, I have suggested, better regarded as an expression than an explanation, even though some element of explanation may also be involved in certain cases. Furthermore, it is not a claim about the contents of the world, which the subject sets out to defend, but an attempt to communicate an altered sense of being. So it does not have a specific 'content' and it is not a 'belief', unless we opt for a conception of belief that is very liberal indeed.

Depersonalization and double-counting

Cotard and Capgras patients often suffer from feelings of depersonalization, in conjunction with feelings of derealization. The term 'depersonalization' refs to something that is found in around eighty per cent of psychiatric in-patients and in a number of different conditions (Medford *et al.*, 2005). More transient episodes can arise in otherwise healthy people during times of trauma, stress, tiredness, illness or bereavement, or as a result of intoxication. Its frequency in the general population is debatable. According to some studies, up to seventy per cent of people experience depersonalization at some point in their lives. But severe depersonalization, which has a serious detrimental effect upon a life, only seems to occur in one to two per cent of people (Baker *et al.*, 2007, p.14).

In this section, I will suggest that depersonalization too can be interpreted in terms of existential feeling and that this serves as a corrective to the double-counting of unitary symptoms. It is difficult to cleanly distinguish the kind of existential feelings found in depersonalization alone from those found in the Capgras and Cotard delusions. It could be that depersonalization always plays a role in these delusions. But it is certainly not restricted to them. Hence the existential feelings constitutive of depersonalization are perhaps necessary but not sufficient for them. Whether the difference consists in a specific kind of depersonalization being present in the delusions or, alternatively, a more pronounced existential feeling of the same kind as that found in the absence of delusions is a question I leave open. It is also debatable whether the term 'depersonalization' refers to a group of very similar experiences or, alternatively, to two or more quite different ways of finding oneself in a world. Stanghellini (2004) suggests the latter, claiming that depersonalization in schizophrenia and in depression differ in their phenomenological character. In Chapter 7, I will caution against drawing too strict a distinction between existential feelings in schizophrenia and depression. However, I do not rule out the possibility that there are different kinds of depersonalization.[7] What I am sceptical about, however, is the view that these differences respect current diagnostic categories, even very broad ones.

Depersonalization, in whatever form, is not classified as a 'delusion', given that patients report feeling 'as if' they are some way but do not claim that they *are* that way, 'dead' for example. But once it is acknowledged that assertions to the effect that one is dead, damned or non-existent are not reports of specific propositional attitudes but expressions of altered existential feeling, the line

---

[7] For example, Baker *et al.* (2007, pp.5–6) note that many patients with depersonalization suffer from anxiety but some do not: 'some sufferers [...] are not visibly anxious or depressed but may be quite introverted or preoccupied. They spend a lot of time dwelling on their thoughts and may appear wrapped up in their own world'. It could well be that 'anxious' and 'non-anxious' variants involve different kinds of existential feeling.

between anomalous experience and full-blown delusion is not so clear. One way of distinguishing delusions from depersonalization is to maintain that people with the latter retain intact reality-testing, whereas those with the former are psychotic and, by implication, do not. In other words, people with depersonalization (at least those without accompanying psychotic symptoms) retain a sense that there is a reality in relation to which their beliefs can be true or false. They also recognize the need to consult that reality in systematic ways so as to test their beliefs. However, given the variability of existential feeling, the line between intact and impaired reality-testing is unclear too. A sense of reality is not something one either has or does not have. It is something changeable, subject to varying degrees and kinds of diminishment and intensification. Any change in the sense of reality will surely have some implications for the practice of reality-testing. The implications are likely to vary, given that 'reality-testing' no doubt includes a range of ways in which we monitor and check our convictions, rather than being a single, unitary ability.

What is depersonalization? According to most accounts, it includes changed experience of both self and world. Medford *et al.* describe it as follows:

> Depersonalisation disorder involves an unpleasant, chronic and disabling alteration in the experience of self and environment. In addition to these classic features of depersonalisation and derealisation, symptoms may also encompass alterations in bodily sensation and a loss of emotional reactivity. (2005, p.92)

They discuss a number of self-reports offered by psychiatric patients with depersonalization (which, as Medford *et al.* note, is closely associated with the phenomenon of 'derealization'). They discuss a number of self-reports offered by psychiatric patients with depersonalization. These patients describe themselves as feeling 'like a robot', 'different from everyone else', 'separate from myself', 'half-asleep', 'as if my head is full of cotton wool'. External reality may appear 'painted, not natural', 'two dimensional' or 'as if everyone is acting out a role on stage, and I am just a spectator' (2005, p.93). Sufferers also complain of a reduction or absence of bodily feelings and diminished feelings of pain, hunger and thirst. Hence there is a consistent association between anomalous bodily experience, estrangement from everything and a sense of the world as no longer real, all of which seem to implicate changed feeling. Other remarks include 'my emotions are gone, nothing affects me' and 'I am unable to have any emotions, everything is detached from me' (2005, p.93).[8] A similar description of depersonalization is offered

---

[8] See also Baker *et al.* (2007, chapters 1 and 2) for a description of depersonalization.

by DSM-IV-TR, according to which 'the individual may feel like an automaton or as if he or she is living in a dream or movie' and suffers from a 'lack of affective response' (2004, p.530).

Something identical to or at least similar to this occurs in a range of different conditions, including some that are not explicitly described in terms of depersonalization. For example, post-traumatic stress disorder can involve a kind of general emotional deadening, in conjunction with heightened anxiety. Frewen *et al.* (2008, p. 177) quote a patient as saying 'I'm living in a tunnel, a fog, no matter what happens it's the same reaction—numbness, nothing. Having a bubble bath and being burned or raped is the same feeling. My brain doesn't feel'.[9] Many patients with post-traumatic stress disorder also have alexithymia (a difficulty in identifying the nature of their own emotional feelings) and Frewen *et al.* hypothesize that this is symptomatic of the emotional numbing.

Descriptions such as 'living in a tunnel' and 'feeling nothing' point to an intimate connection between changed bodily feeling and how the world is experienced. An appreciation of the nature of existential feeling allows us to interpret such complaints in terms of a unitary experiential change. Talk of detachment, things seeming unreal, lack of feeling and an altered sense of body and thus of self all reflect the same existential feeling. As Merleau-Ponty appreciates:

> Depersonalization and disturbance of the body image are immediately translated into an external phantasm, because it is one and the same thing for us to perceive our body and to perceive our situation in a certain physical and human setting, for our body is nothing but that very situation in so far as it is realized and actualized. (1962, pp.339–40)

However, there is a tendency to misinterpret unitary existential feelings in terms of closely related but different psychological symptoms. To illustrate this, I will consider an otherwise rich and informative discussion of the phenomenology of depersonalization offered by Radovic and Radovic (2002).

Radovic and Radovic note that depersonalization is identified solely on the basis of experiential reports, given that no common aetiology has been identified and that no distinctive kinds of behaviours are reliably associated with it. Hence understanding the phenomenology is of central importance when it comes to understanding what depersonalization is. They draw together various autobiographical descriptions, which include feeling detached from body and world, feeling like a spectator, feelings of unreality and strangeness, self-estrangement and loss of feeling. These all indicate that a sense of 'unreality' is

---

[9] Thanks to Paul Frewen for drawing my attention to these remarks.

closely associated with feeling 'cut off' from things, which seem 'remote' or 'detached'. Indeed, Radovic and Radovic (2002, p.274) state that 'the feelings of unreality merge and the patient may not be able to say which aspect of the self or the world it is that feels unreal'. So it seems plausible to suggest that some of the feelings reported in depersonalization are what I call 'existential feelings'; modifications of the self–world relation. In describing them, either side of that relation can be emphasized. The world might be described as looking unreal or the person as feeling strangely different. But although different descriptions have different explicit referents, 'self' and 'world', this need not imply that they are descriptions of different experiences.

Although they do not deny that depersonalization can occur in everyday life, as well as in psychiatric illness, Radovic and Radovic do draw a distinction between the experience of depersonalization and other kinds of everyday experience that might be described in a similar fashion. For example, someone in an apathetic mood might complain that everything is meaningless, and this is a far cry from losing a background sense of familiarity and reality. Or someone might say 'it feels unreal', having just won the lottery (Radovic and Radovic, 2002, p.274). Utterances like this are, I think, quite revealing, in so far as they imply that accepting a proposition such as 'I have won the lottery' is not sufficient for a sense of conviction. One also has to *feel* it. But the relevant sense of 'unreality' can be fairly localized. It is also quite different in nature from the unpleasant and unsettling derealization reported by many psychiatric patients.

However, there are many other kinds of everyday situation where people remark on feeling different, detached, removed from it all and, in conjunction with this, on the world seeming unreal or strangely unfamiliar. For example, someone with jetlag, a bad cold or a hangover might complain of their head feeling as though it were full of cotton wool or of feeling removed from everything, dead to the world or just *not quite right* in some strange and difficult to articulate way. Experiences like this draw attention to the fragility of our sense of belonging to the world. The feelings in question might be sporadic rather than persistent and they might not be as intense as the changes found in psychiatric illness. Even so, given the range of existential feelings that people express, it would be wrong to insist that a sharp boundary be drawn between psychiatric and everyday feelings of unreality and depersonalization. Not all existential feelings of 'unreality' should be identified with 'depersonalization', however. There are many ways in which the horizonal structure of experience can be changed and in which the sense of belonging and reality can be altered. 'Unreality' takes different forms. For example, an intangible world where everything looks strangely distant is not the same as a world devoid of all interpersonal significance. It may be that only some forms of unreality are due to those existential feelings that are also described in terms of depersonalization.

Radovic and Radovic claim that one way in which feelings of depersonalization differ from 'existential reflections' and 'reactions to changes in life' is that people have greater difficulty expressing the former. The difficulty arises partly because patients need to 'assign a precise sense to existential terms like *self*, *world*, and *unreal*' in order to describe their experiences, something that they have not had to do before (2002, pp.274–5). Radovic and Radovic add that some feelings are easier to describe than others because people tend to have similar feelings in certain kinds of familiar situations. Hence one can refer to the feeling of a particularly bad hangover or to the feeling of jetlag. However, it is important to recognize that it is the situation that is described clearly, rather than the feeling. Similarly, although pointing to a life event or a psychological cause might explain *why* one has a particular feeling, it does not convey the nature of that feeling. Some existential feelings have identifiable causes, such as two bottles of poor quality wine or a long haul flight, whereas others do not. In neither case is the phenomenology of the feeling itself clearly articulated.

In attempting to clarify the 'feeling of unreality' that is distinctive of depersonalization, Radovic and Radovic (2002, p.275) propose that the term 'unreal' has three principal uses:

1 Non-existent; merely imagined.

2 Fake; artificial.

3 Not genuine, as in not a 'real friend'; atypical or not optimal.

They go on to suggest that 'feel' has different senses too. It may refer to a belief-like state, where something is taken not to be real. This would relate to (1) and perhaps also (2), above. Alternatively, it may refer to an unusual way of experiencing, where things appear not quite right, thus complementing (3); it is 'a specific kind of quasisensory experience, which is neither simply a belief in the nonexistence of something nor just any atypical feeling' (p. 276). Hence a 'feeling of unreality' can refer to one or the other of the following:

a Changed experience of self or world.

b A belief that something (perhaps self or world) either does not exist or is fake.

They claim that both of these play a role in some cases of depersonalization, given that (b) might be inferred on the basis of (a). Something is judged to be unreal because it is experienced in a strange way.

Although this attempt at phenomenological and conceptual clarification is highly illuminating, it also illustrates the tendency to take too much of the self–world relation for granted when reflecting upon the nature of anomalous experience, resulting in a misleading distinction between 'strange experience' and 'belief in unreality or non-existence'. As I have argued, experience does not *just* present us with specific contents that we then judge to be real or unreal. It also includes a background sense of belonging that determines the manner in which both self and world are experienced. The various phenomenological descriptions offered by Radovic and Radovic and by others all indicate that it is this that is affected in depersonalization. It is neither a matter of having a specific experiential content nor of acquiring a belief on the basis of some such content. An all-pervasive sense of unreality is not the belief that some entity or set of entities is unreal but a shift in existential orientation, a transformation of the modal structure of belief, of the *is* and the *is not*. Those 'quasi-sensory' experiences that encompass the self-world relation as a whole do not merely involve having certain things appear in certain ways, and they cannot be accommodated by any approach that cleanly separates world-experience from belief.

In the absence of a phenomenological appreciation of existential feeling, a feeling that is at the same time a way of finding oneself in the world and a changed sense of reality risks being misinterpreted as a bodily feeling, plus an anomalous experience, plus a belief. Radovic and Radovic's description of depersonalization complements my conception of existential feeling. However, without such a conception, they misinterpret the phenomenology by double-counting existential feeling as changed world-experience plus anomalous belief, when in fact changed experience just *is* the loss of the sense of reality that is referred to as the belief that things are 'unreal'. The same kind of double-counting is evident, I have suggested, in accounts of the Capgras and Cotard delusions. In Chapter 7, I will address the phenomenology of schizophrenia. In the process, I will show how double-counting also occurs in relation to bodily feeling and world experience.

Existential feeling in schizophrenia

This chapter addresses the question of whether and to what extent altered experience and thought in schizophrenia are explicable in terms of existential feeling. The role of existential feeling in schizophrenia is difficult to assess, as the illness is divided into different 'sub-types' and, even within a sub-type, the balance of symptoms changes over time and varies from case to case. Depersonalization and the Capgras and Cotard delusions can all arise in schizophrenia. So an account of existential feeling in schizophrenia must be able to accommodate all three and a lot more besides. In what follows, I argue that many symptoms of schizophrenia are better understood if we abandon conceptions of experience that separate body from world, cognition from feeling and inside from outside. I begin by discussing the close connection between anomalous feeling and changed experience and thought in early descriptions of schizophrenia offered by Emil Kraepelin and Eugen Bleuler. Then, drawing on the more recent work of Louis Sass and others, I suggest that existential feeling is directly responsible for certain delusions and operates as an experiential background that is conducive to the formation of others. In so doing, I reject the distinction between 'positive' and 'negative' symptoms. Following this, I turn to disorganized thought and thought insertion. I propose that both originate in a variant of existential feeling that is characterized by a lack of temporal consistency. The chapter concludes by distinguishing some of the different existential feelings that feature in psychiatric illness more generally and by suggesting that distinctive *kinds* of existential feeling are unlikely to reliably match up with current diagnostic categories.

Early descriptions of schizophrenia

The earliest descriptions of schizophrenia refer to changes in 'affect' or 'feeling', in conjunction with anomalous experience and thought. Kraepelin (1919) emphasizes three central features: absence of affect, an associated loss of volition and a breakdown of psychic unity. Lack of spontaneous action and loss of affect are, he notes, intimately associated: 'nothing matters' and so the world does not solicit activity (p.33, pp.74–5). Bleuler (1950) similarly empha-sizes diminished affect. Some patients, he says, respond to everything with indifference and can sit for years without expressing any feelings. Like Kraepelin, he also refers to a form of mental disorganization that involves a '"splitting" of the different psychic functions' (1950, p.8). To these symptoms he adds 'hallucinations, delusions, confusion, stupor, mania and melancholic affective fluctuations, and catatonic symptoms'. However, he proposes that affective changes and psychic fragmentation are the 'primary symptoms', which are causally responsible for 'accessory symptoms' such as delusions and hallucinations (1950, pp.9–10).

In reflecting on the phenomenology of schizophrenia, it is important to keep in mind that it is not a single, unitary condition that manifests itself in the same way in all cases. Bleuler identifies four variants, which he refers to as paranoid schizophrenia, catatonia, hebephrenia and simple schizophrenia (1950, p.10), and Kraepelin (1919, chapter V) proposes several. Neither author is primarily concerned with phenomenological understanding. What we have instead are lists of inter-related symptoms, many of which take the form of observable changes in behaviour that can be identified and described without any reference to experience. There is no explicit acknowledgement that one need engage with the existential predicament of the patient at all. However, Kraepelin's and Bleuler's emphasis on affective changes is at least consistent with the view that schizophrenia involves anomalous existential feeling. Kraepelin suggests that transient disturbances of occurrent emotion arise due to erosion of a background mood that healthy people take for granted. Emotions are ordinarily regulated by this mood but in schizophrenia there is:

> ...the loss of that permanent colouring of the background of mood which in normal people influences all chance oscillations of the emotions, equalising and checking them and which only then lets them appear in greater strength when an important occasion finds a powerful echo in our being. (1919, p.35)

Bleuler appeals to a breakdown of normal emotional repression, where unpleasant memories are no longer compartmentalized and therefore seep out. But, like Kraepelin, he also mentions certain changeable 'basic moods', amongst which he includes euphoria, sadness and anxiety (1950, pp.41–2). In addition, Bleuler acknowledges a close connection between changed feeling and world experience. This, he says, is especially apparent from the reports of intelligent, articulate patients, who have some awareness of what they have lost. For them, 'reality seems different from what it was before. Things and people are no longer what they are supposed to be. They are changed, strange, no longer have any relationship to the patient' (1950, p.68). Hence, as in the case of Renee (which I discussed in Chapter 2), there is a close connection between diminished feeling, an altered sense of reality and an estrangement from people and things.

When interpreting reports of changed reality, Bleuler presupposes the phenomenological applicability of an internal–external distinction. Reality is construed as something external to the subject, with which she *connects*. In referring to 'the inclination to divorce oneself from reality' (1950, p.14), he fails to appreciate that the everyday *sense* of reality is a phenomenological accomplishment that requires explanation. Instead, he takes for granted the perspective of a subject who is already in the world and assumes that a loss of experienced reality involves *losing contact* with the objects of that world. It is construed in terms of failed access, as a matter of the 'exclusion of the external world' (1950, p.67), of reality being 'blocked off' (1950, p.373). An altered sense of reality and belonging is thus misinterpreted as impaired epistemic access to some external realm.

The assumption of a clear distinction between internal and external is also evident when Bleuler refers to feelings being displaced from subject to object. A feeling is taken to be something with an *internal* phenomenology that can be projected onto something *external*, rather than as something that does not respect such distinctions. According to Bleuler, intelligent patients who reflect upon their predicaments first attempt to attribute the affective changes to themselves and later:

> ...they tend to displace the changes in themselves to the outer world which itself becomes hollow, empty, strange, because of these affective changes. Often the element of strangeness has a touch of the uncanny and hostile. (1950, p.51)

However, the phenomenology of belonging to a world is not one of inner and outer. In taking experience to involve (a) accessing a realm of objects that are out there and comprise *external reality* and (b) feeling one's own bodily states, Bleuler passes over a changed existential background that can be characterized in terms of both bodily and worldly changes. He does acknowledge that disturbed affect contributes to aberrant thought processes but describes altered experience of, and thought about, reality in terms of inferences concerning the nature of reality, rather than in terms of changes to a sense of reality that all such inferences presuppose (1950, pp.381–4). Even so, some of Bleuler's observations are suggestive of a changed sense of reality and a shift in the modalities of conviction. For example, he notes that patients are often indifferent to their delusions. One patient commented 'perhaps they are pathological, perhaps they are real' and did not care either way (1950, p.41). Such indifference indicates a kind of conviction that differs in character from *everyday believing*.

Hence, although Bleuler and Kraepelin are more preoccupied with observable symptoms than with phenomenology, the symptoms they describe are quite compatible with altered existential feeling, given the intimate association that is acknowledged between changed feeling, detachment from the world and an altered sense of reality. However, as illustrated by Bleuler's misconstrual of the sense of reality, unless the interpreter *brackets* or *suspends* a sense of belonging that she ordinarily takes for granted and appreciates that it is changeable, a unitary existential feeling will be misinterpreted as a range of symptoms had by a subject who shares the interpreter's world. This kind of mistake is something that Laing (1960, p.15) comments on: 'the mad things said and done by the schizophrenic will remain essentially a closed book if one does not understand their existential context'. He is equally critical of the associated tendency to split unitary experiential structures into distinct psychological and bodily components, into 'mind and body, psyche and soma, psychological and physical' (1960, p.17).

The tendency to interpret existential feeling in terms of distinct symptoms persists in more recent descriptions of schizophrenia. For example, it is commonplace to distinguish between 'positive' and 'negative' symptoms, where the former involve something being added to experience or thought and the latter involve something being taken away. For example, DSM-IV-TR (2004, p.299) identifies the following positive and negative symptoms of schizophrenia:

- Positive: delusions, hallucinations, disorganized speech, self-monitoring of behaviour. (This category is then subdivided into psychotic and disorganized symptoms.)
- Negative: lessened range and intensity of emotional expression, decrease in fluency and production of thought and speech, loss of volition.

According to classifications like this, diminished feeling is distinct from anomalies in experience and thought, such as delusions and cognitive disorganization. Even though it is recognized that these symptoms interact in various ways, it is taken for granted that they are not to be identified with each other. If this is correct, then many symptoms of schizophrenia, including all the so-called 'positive' ones, will not be interpretable in terms of 'negative' existential feeling, even though they might cause or be caused by existential feeling.

Thinking of our mental life in this way, as something that can be added to or subtracted from, is dubious to say the least. Our phenomenology is not a cooking pot that can contain varying amounts of several distinct ingredients. And it is not at all clear that phenomenological changes are ever simply *additions* or *subtractions* (see Sass, 2003). A description of changed existential feeling might emphasize something *lost* or something *added* but the same existential feeling could be described in both ways. We saw this with the Capgras and Cotard delusions, where the negative absence of feeling is, at the same time, the positive experience of others as impostors or of oneself as non-existent. Both delusions can occur in schizophrenia and so some schizophrenic delusions just *are* changes in existential feeling. Hence, in some cases at least, it is a mistake to double-count *negative* loss of *internal* feelings and *positive* changes to the *external* world.

Phenomenological accounts of schizophrenia

Several authors have drawn on insights from phenomenology to argue that feeling and altered existential orientation in schizophrenia are intimately con-nected. The phenomenological changes that they refer to are quite compatible with what I call 'existential feeling'. However, what they lack is a detailed phenomenological account of how it is that something can be both a feeling and a background sense of belonging. So, although much work has already been done on phenomenological changes in schizophrenia, my conception of existential feeling still has a role to play in clarifying, supporting and supple-menting claims that others have made regarding 'affect', 'emotion', 'mood' and 'existential orientation'. In addition, an appreciation of (a) the variety of exis-tential feelings and (b) the fact that the same existential feeling can be described in a number of different ways together serve to challenge some of the phenomenological claims that have been offered.

One of the most detailed phenomenological descriptions of schizophrenia offered in recent years is that of Sass.[1] Central to Sass's account is what he calls 'hyperreflexivity' (e.g. 2003, p.153). This is a kind of 'exaggerated self-con-sciousness' whereby a medium of activity, something that is ordinarily inhabited, becomes an object of experience and/or thought (Sass and Parnas, 2007, p.68). When catching a ball, one is not usually aware of one's arm in an object-like way but one does sometimes attend to it as such. This self-aware-ness might be an outcome of voluntary reflection but it often takes the form of an involuntary and uncomfortable 'self-consciousness', which is sometimes inextricable from a sense of being watched by others. When this occurs, what was a seamless, purposive activity becomes clumsy and effortful. The practical connectedness that previously characterized one's relationship with the ball is lost. Now consider what would happen if a non-localized background feeling of belonging changed in a comparable way. It would cease to be a way of relating to things and become instead an experience of one's own body as object-like.

---

[1] Some of the relevant work is co-authored with Josef Parnas (see Parnas and Sass, 2001; Sass and Parnas, 2007).

Sass proposes that something like this is involved in schizophrenia. What was taken for granted, presupposed by experience and thought, becomes an explicit object of awareness. The change encompasses bodily feeling, action, perception and thought. We do not usually experience our thoughts as objects that appear before our awareness, just as we do not experience our hands as objects of awareness when we type. But schizophrenia, Sass suggests, involves globally heightened reflexivity and with it an alienation from the world, from our bodies, and from our experiences and our thoughts. Experience without normal affect is no longer 'lived'; it is 'more like a mechanical, purely receptive sensory process'. And inner speech 'becomes transformed from a *medium of thinking* into an object-like entity with quasi-perceptual characteristics' (Parnas and Sass, 2001, pp.105–7).[2]

There is a significant difference between voluntary hyper-reflection and the involuntary hyper-reflexivity that occurs in schizophrenia (Sass and Parnas, 2007, p.69). I could make an effort to reflect upon my activities, feelings, experiences and thoughts, scrutinizing them from a perspective of self-imposed detachment. However, schizophrenia does not arise through an act of will and it is more extreme than anything that deliberate reflection alone could accomplish. It is also more intense and encompassing than more everyday experiences of 'feeling self-conscious'. The object-like conspicuousness of bodily feelings, thoughts and the like is a change in the patient's existential orientation as a whole, rather than in the way she attends to particular things. It is a way of being in the world rather than something that she does within a pre-given world.

Sass (e.g. 2003) is dismissive of distinctions between positive, negative and disorganized symptoms of schizophrenia, which he thinks originate in misleading mechanistic conceptions of experience and thought. Changed feeling is inextricable from hyper-reflexivity, and it is hyper-reflexivity that sets the scene for the various positive and disorganized symptoms. What we have here is not causal, mechanistic association but phenomenological inextricability. Sass notes that 'flat affect' might seem like an absence but adds that it is also accompanied by the presence of something 'abnormal and anomalous: mask-like faces or incongruous facial expression' (2003, p.158). The relevant 'affect' has a phenomenology that does not respect distinctions between inside and outside; the same existential change is both the feeling and the strange experience. This view is wholly compatible with the account of the nature and role of existential feeling that I developed in Chapters 2 to 4. Hence my account

2 Laing (1960, p.71) suggests something similar, claiming that in schizophrenia '*the body is felt more as one object among other objects in the world than as the core of the individual's own being*' and that this involves becoming 'hyper-conscious'.

can be applied so as to further clarify the phenomenological structure of the relevant 'affects' and thus lend additional support to such views.

Sass documents some of the bodily changes reported by schizophrenic people, indicating that a diverse range of feelings, which would ordinarily operate as an inconspicuous background to experience and activity, become salient objects of experience. People report:

> ...sensations of movement or of pulling or pressure inside the body or on its surfaces; electric or migrating sensations; awareness of kinaesthetic, vestibular, or thermic sensations; and sensations of diminution or enlargement, of heaviness or lightness, of sinking or emptiness, or of numbness or stiffness of the body or its parts. (2003, p.163)

He focuses more specifically on the importance of changes in those feelings or 'affects' that are associated with characteristically *emotional* experience:

> It could be argued [...] that affective abnormalities are among the most *central* features of the schizophrenic condition, for they seem closely bound up with the alterations of personhood or self-experience, and of the sense of reality, that are so distinctive of this psychiatric illness. (2004b, p.127)

The role of feeling is similarly stressed by Stanghellini (2004), who claims that changes in feeling, resulting in an experience of disembodiment, are primarily responsible for altered experience. The background through which oneself, other people and the world as a whole are ordinarily experienced breaks down. Stanghellini's discussion includes several remarks offered by schizophrenic patients that refer to changes in felt belonging, such as 'I cannot feel my *being* anymore' and 'I feel disconnected from myself' (2004, pp.123–6).

Feeling is not simply *diminished* in schizophrenia. Like Kraepelin, Sass observes that there are also situationally inappropriate and sometimes overly intense affective reactions:

> ...many schizophrenic patients seem neither to feel nor to evoke a natural sense of emotional rapport. Both the affective response and the affective expression of these patients frequently seem odd, incongruent, inadequate, or otherwise off-the-mark. (2004b, p.128)

With changed feeling and hyper-reflexivity, there is disengagement from activity and a loss of the familiar, significant world that once offered up a range of possibilities for activity. The patient can undergo what Sass, drawing on Heidegger, calls 'unworlding', an absence of felt, purposive connectedness that is, at the same time, a loss of the experienced functionality of things. Things seem strange, detached, unfamiliar and insignificant. Closely associated with unworlding is an objectification of the lived body that Sass refers to as 'bodily alienation'. Also present is 'subjectivization', where the patient comes to inhabit a somewhat solipsistic experiential realm that is stripped of the usual sense of public reality (Sass, 2004*b*). This diminished or absent sense of public reality is at the same time a change in the modalities of belief. The *shared* world against which convictions are ordinarily checked has been eroded and so the patient does not *believe* in quite the same way anymore.

Sass also adds 'disengagement' to the list of phenomenological changes, to refer to the feeling of detachment involved in schizophrenic experience. This is the 'plate-glass feeling' that some uses of the term 'derealization' also refer to (2007, p.371), where an ordinarily taken-for-granted connectedness to the world is interrupted as if by a haze, veil, film or wall of tainted glass.

Parnas and Sass (2001) recommend that delusions and other so-called 'positive symptoms' be interpreted against the backdrop of this existential shift, which usually precedes their onset. Hence the prodromal or pre-psychotic stage of the illness is not only a causal precursor for full-blown schizophrenia but a phenomenological precondition too. Disorders of self, they suggest, are later 'thematized' as delusions or hallucinations (2001, p.111). They thus reject the kind of approach advocated by Young and others, on the grounds that changed experience and thought are not 'a matter of cognitive principles or intellectual rules so much as of what might be termed *general existential orientations*' (2001, p.114). To have a delusion is not just to have a false belief about the world; delusions are embedded in existential changes.

In both the Capgras and Cotard delusions, I argued that the relevant 'belief' is a fairly accurate expression of the changed phenomenology. I added that the modalities of belief will also have shifted. With an altered sense of reality, patients cannot *take things to be the case* in the usual way, as the sense of 'is' and 'is not' has changed. However, this account will not apply in the same way to all those delusions that occur in schizophrenia. The association between an altered existential orientation and the delusion that one plays for Chelsea football club is contingent, in a way that the impostor claim is not. Due to an existential change, the spouse is experienced as an impostor, a fake. But assertions about being a Chelsea player, having a mouth full of dead birds, being chased by the CIA and the like do not reflect existential feelings in such a direct fashion. Altered existential feeling alone does not dispose the patient to have a thought with the specific content that he is a Chelsea player.[3] Nevertheless, 'beliefs' like these still arise in the *context* of a changed existential orientation. The erosion of a public reality and of the usual

---

[3] The 'Chelsea player' claim was persistently made by one of Matthew Broome's patients (personal correspondence).

distinction between reality and unreality may dispose the patient towards all manner of strange assertions, associations and narratives. Many of these will reflect, in an indirect way, the nature of her existential feeling. For example, *being chased* by some person or organization might be symptomatic of paranoia.

Although these delusions do not relate to changed existential feeling in quite the same way as the Cotard and Capgras delusions, they too differ from everyday kinds of belief.[4] This is because the sense of reality that is presupposed by such beliefs has been lost. The patient inhabits a different realm, with a different kind of conviction. The public world is no longer there and she cannot have concrete beliefs about entities in the world (at least not in any of the ways in which healthy people hold beliefs) if the sense of 'an object independent of me that is also available to others' has been removed from the space of experiential possibilities. The practical possibilities that ordinarily structure experience are also gone and so the patient's utterances and thoughts about the world no longer relate to a realm of potential activities. Experience is dreamlike in some respects; 'the patient does not feel being fully existing or alive, *fully awake* or *conscious*, or fully *present and affected*' (Parnas and Sass, 2001, p.105).[5]

Sass maintains that subjectivization, unworlding, bodily alienation and disengagement are different phenomena, rather than being different ways of describing a single, unitary existential orientation, given that they occur to different degrees in different cases. However, he is not suggesting that they are wholly separate from each other. One could not experience what Sass calls unworlding without at least some change in the feeling body. Such changes would in turn involve a level of disengagement from the public world and thus some degree of subjectivization, which would in turn be closely related to bodily conspicuousness. Hence, although these changes might differ in their relative salience from case to case, they remain essentially interconnected. All, I suggest, can be understood as inextricable aspects of unitary existential feelings. A particular aspect might be more or less prominent in a particular case, and such differences are symptomatic of differences in the *kinds* of existential feeling involved. It may also be that some apparent differences between cases reflect different emphases in patients' reports, more so than contrasting experiential structures.

---

[4] See Hamilton (2007) for a defence of the view that there is no simple fact of the matter as to whether certain delusions are beliefs.

[5] See also Sass (1992, chapter 9) for a discussion of schizophrenic experience and the loss of a sense of public reality.

Inconsistency

Existential feelings have a temporal structure, and differences between kinds of existential feeling do not consist solely of differences in the structure of a static possibility space. For example, an existential feeling might be distinctive in its recalcitrance to change. In describing herself as stuck in a bell jar 'stewing' in her own 'sour air', Sylvia Plath's protagonist communicates a fixed, enduring transformation of the possibility space; it is unbearable partly because of its imperviousness to everything (Plath, 1966, p.178). In contrast to this, non-pathological existential feelings change subtly in response to experienced events and occasionally in a way that is more pronounced and noticeable. An existential orientation that did not change following the death of a close friend or family member would be an orientation that was lacking somehow, impervious to the world. Existential feelings can also be anomalous in being excessively changeable or prone to sudden, violent shifts. In addition, they might change in unstructured, disorganized ways.

Consider again the concept of a horizon. Experience unfolds in a structured, harmonious fashion, as possibilities offered up by the world are actualized through our activities, in accordance with certain expectations, and reveal further possibilities in the process. This flow would be disrupted if the possibilities offered up lacked structure and shifted in such a way as to break up patterns of salience and expectation. Something like this seems to happen in schizophrenia, which is not simply a fixed, frozen existential orientation, involving quasi-solipsistic detachment and alienation of the lived body. The structure of experience is fragmented by changeable feelings that do not relate to each other in stable ways and therefore do not facilitate the unfolding of an organized possibility space, a world structured by consistent patterns of significance. This is something that Binswanger (1975) draws attention to, in claiming that schizophrenia includes both an 'inconsistency of experience' and a feeling of being overwhelmed by the world. Presumably the two are closely connected. A world of unstructured and ever-changing possibilities would be a world over which one had no reliable practical hold. There would be an all-pervasive feeling of lacking control, of there being an endless realm of unpredictable happenings that one might be passively subjected to. As Binswanger says, 'natural experience is that in which our existence moves not only unreflectively, but also unproblematically and unobtrusively, as smoothly as a natural chain of events'. When this breaks down, a person can no longer live 'serenely' in relation to things. The 'revolutionary spirit' he says, is not the person whose world is turbulent. The world must first be structured in order for it to be challenged. In schizophrenia, it is the presupposed world that is afflicted. It cannot be challenged by the patient, as she does not find herself in it to begin with; the consistent grounding required to embark upon any project is lacking (Binswanger, 1975, pp.251–2). A chaotic world over which one has no hold is not a place in which one can establish order and so, Binswanger suggests, patients retreat from it and try to find order elsewhere:

> What makes the lives of our patients such a torment is that they are not able to come to terms with the inconsistency and disorder of their experience, but, rather, constantly seek for a *way out* so that order can be re-established. (1975, p.253)

It is arguable that this inconsistency is at the same time a distinctive kind of anxiety, a sense that nothing is secure, nowhere is safe. Indeed, Sass and Parnas suggest that:

> At times, schizophrenia patients appear to experience something closely akin to Heideggerian *Angst*: the anxiety born of registering the arbitrariness of any particular way of looking at life and the vertigo that this can engender. (2007, p.79)[6]

However, if Binswanger is right, then the two existential feelings are not quite the same. A lack of consistency and consequent absence of tranquil belonging differs from the total loss of a cohesive sense of belonging. In the former case, it is not that all possibilities fall away and the world offers nothing. The world does still offer something but the possibilities that it offers all take the form of impositions before which one is helpless, passive. They are potential happenings, rather than potential activities.

DSM-IV-TR (2004, p.300) describes symptoms such as conversations slipping off track, tangential responses to questions and, in extreme cases, speech being reduced to 'word salad'. If inconsistency in schizophrenia is interpreted as I have suggested, then these so-called 'disorganized' symptoms also turn out to originate in changed existential feeling. Without the structured unfolding of possibilities, experience would be jumbled and the same surely goes for thought and talk, which would be embedded in an existential background without rhythm, flow or coherent patterns of anticipation. We think and speak in the context of a presupposed world. Our thought is surely not immune from its fragmentation. Thus, in addition to involving a consistent loss of practical significance, it is arguable that schizophrenic experience also involves an unstable, disorganized possibility space, a world that is both diminished and fragmented.[7]

---

[6] Sass and Parnas (2007, p.79) add that other patients experience a more 'nihilistic anxiety', comparable to Sartrean Nausea.

[7] My concern here is with phenomenology rather than with neurobiology. However, it is worth noting that the existential changes I describe are compatible with at least some recent versions of the dopamine hypothesis. For example, Broome *et al.* (2005) discuss the view that mesolimbic dopamine plays a role in determining patterns of significance

Binswanger's emphasis on the inconsistency of experience is compatible with Sass's view. The 'unworlding' that Sass refers to could be construed in terms of a *fading away* of the significant world or, alternatively, in terms of its *fragmentation*. Sass (2004b, p.136) emphasizes the latter. But, in both cases, the world would no longer offer up the usual possibilities. And either could lead to the endpoint that Sass describes, a somewhat solipsistic delusional realm. Even so, the two kinds of experience are importantly different. The fading of possibilities and happenings need not amount to an experience of losing control. *All* possibilities for relating to things could disappear, including those that constitute a sense of powerlessness. However, a chaotic world remains a world of happenings, which no longer offers up coherent patterns of activity, and there is thus a feeling of having no control over things. This feeling need not be unpleasant; a person could well be indifferent to it. But it might well take the form of an unpleasant sense of helplessness, vulnerability and anxiety. And the latter fits better with descriptions such as Renee's, which refer to anxiety, dread, all-embracing fear and objects 'defying me' with their 'presence' (Sechehaye, 1970, p.56). As Binswanger puts it, the patient cannot 'freely allow the world to be' and is 'increasingly surrendered over to one particular world-design, possessed by it, overwhelmed by it' (1975, p.284). What he surrenders to, I suggest, is not a fixed possibility space but an unstructured realm that no longer offers up coherent patterns of activity. This surrender before chaos is not quite the same thing as an unworlding that takes the form of an erosion of all practical possibility. A diminished horizon need not be a chaotic horizon.[8] Different cases of 'schizophrenia' will differ to some extent in their phenomenological character, and different phenomenological changes will occur at different stages of the illness. Hence it might be that 'fading' better describes some experiences that occur in schizophrenia and 'fragmentation' others. Furthermore, fading and fragmentation are not incompatible. The possibility space as a whole could be diminished and at the same time fragmented.

Thought insertion

I have proposed that existential changes in schizophrenia incorporate both diminished feeling and unruly feeling. Some of the so-called 'positive

----

and salience in the experienced world. They suggest that anomalous increases or decreases in dopamine levels could result in mundane things seeming significant and vice versa. Such changes are stimulus-independent and so previously organized patterns of salience are replaced by disorder.

[8] See also Wiggins and Schwartz (2007) for a Husserlian interpretation of schizophrenia that appeals to a breakdown of passive synthesis.

symptoms' of schizophrenia are actually expressions of changed existential feelings and others need to be understood as arising against a backdrop of changed existential feeling. In this section, I will focus specifically on the symptom of 'thought insertion'. Many patients with schizophrenia report having thoughts that are not their own. These thoughts belong to other people, often specific individuals, and are somehow projected into the patient. Such claims are not easy to make sense of, partly because it is difficult to understand how a person could have a thought and at the same time think that it belongs to someone else. As with the Capgras and Cotard delusions, I want to suggest that assertions regarding inserted thoughts communicate something that is *experienced*; they are not reports of beliefs that the patient has arrived at by means of an inference from experience. An experience of thought insertion has a specific content and so is not itself an existential feeling. Nevertheless, such experiences are embedded in a background of anomalous existential feeling and are largely symptomatic of it.

As discussed in Chapters 5 and 6, there is a tendency to treat delusions as states with specific contents and to neglect the existential context in which they arise. The same neglect is evident in the case of thought insertion. To illustrate this, I will focus on the influential account offered by Frith (1992). Frith advocates a neuropsychological, symptom-based approach. The idea is that, rather than trying to understand kinds of 'mental disorder', such as 'schizophrenia', we focus upon specific symptoms and attempt to explain them in terms of breakdowns in underlying psychological mechanisms. Closely related to this project is that of associating the postulated mechanisms with particular brain areas. This approach has the advantage of bypassing debates over what schizophrenia is and whether it even exists. Even if the category 'schizophrenia' were to be abandoned, the symptoms would remain. Hence neuropsychological explanations of those symptoms would not be undermined.

Frith's account of schizophrenia does not acknowledge the kinds of existential changes that I have discussed here. He appreciates that the positive symptoms have a phenomenology, and accepts that thought insertion is a matter of experience rather than of holding a propositional attitude. However, when it comes to the negative symptoms, there is a curious refusal to engage in any way with the phenomenology. Frith draws a distinction between 'symptoms' and 'signs'. The former are revealed by first-person reports whereas the latter consist of behaviours that are observed by a third party (1992, p.12). So 'I hear voices' would be a symptom, whereas a lack of facial expression that is not remarked upon by the patient would be a sign. Hallucinations, delusions and other positive symptoms feature in self-descriptions of experience, whereas negative symptoms such as 'flattening of affect' are observed by others.

Frith therefore suggests that we adopt the categories of 'positive symptoms' and 'negative signs'. He treats the latter as behavioural in nature. Flattening of affect, for example, amounts to much the same thing as 'poverty of gesture' (1992, p.51). According to Frith, these negative signs are usually more debilitating in the long-term than the positive symptoms. Unlike positive symptoms, which come and go, they are an ever-present feature of the condition. Even so, he restricts himself to a purely behavioural conception of them, devoid of any reference to the relevant phenomenology. The outcome is an account of positive symptoms that fails to acknowledge the changed experiential context in which they arise.

Turning specifically to thought insertion, Frith begins by considering the view that what patients misattribute to another agency is their own inner speech. This is supported by the observation that some patients visibly move their mouths and tongues or whisper when they report hearing voices or being subjected to alien thoughts. Even when there are no observable movements, enhanced muscle activity can often be detected in the area of the mouth (Frith, 1992, p.71). However, this hypothesis does not seem to accommodate all cases and, as Frith notes, inner speech in non-pathological cases need not involve any muscular activity. The same will most likely apply to schizophrenia.

Frith also recognizes that not all thought is inner speech. It is often 'much more abstract than hearing voices'. What patients experience in at least some cases might be better described as 'experience of receiving a communication without any sensory component', which they then describe to others in auditory terms (1992, p.73). So the term 'thought insertion' refers to an experience that can involve differing degrees of abstraction from the spoken word. There is, presumably, a continuum between those thoughts that are experienced as being speech-like and those that are not.

Frith's explanation of thought insertion is based on the premise that thought and speech are *actions* or at least like action in important respects. He considers the example of eye movement and notes that, when we move our eyes, the visual world does not shift with them. The reason for this, he explains, is that there is a 'corollary discharge' as an eye movement is initiated (1992, p.74). A signal is sent out at the same time as the instruction to the eye muscles, allowing the outcome of the eye movement to be anticipated. This signal is picked up by a comparator, which matches the anticipated outcome with the actual outcome. When they match up, we have a sense of agency. When they fail to do so, the sense of agency is absent. In the case of an eye movement, there are two ways in which a match might fail to occur. When you move your eyeball with your finger, there is no corollary discharge and so it is perceived as a happening. And when the eye fails to move after the corollary discharge, perhaps due to paralysis of the relevant musculature, there is also no sense of agency, as intentions are not matched up with predicted effects. Frith suggests that the same kind of mechanism is at work in limb movements and also in speech. The phenomenological correlate of the corollary discharge is an intention to act, which precedes all our actions. Central to Frith's account of thought insertion is the claim that an analogous mechanism is involved in thought; there is an intention to think just as there is an intention to speak or act. The experience of thought insertion arises due to a monitoring defect, an absence of this intention. The result is an experience of unbidden thoughts being imposed from elsewhere, rather than arising through one's own agency.[9]

There are several problems with this account, the most obvious being its phenomenological implausibility. Frith claims that 'thinking, like all our actions, is normally accompanied by a sense of effort and deliberate choice as we move from one thought to the next' (1992, p.81). But this is not true. In many instances of thought, perhaps the majority, the thought occurs to us without any intention, effort or prior context. Sometimes we do *try* to think about something or actively intend to think through something but on many occasions our thoughts arise unbidden. Seemingly random memories and ideas 'pop up out of nowhere' and the irritating song that keeps playing 'in the back of one's mind' is not something that is knowingly solicited. But such thoughts are not experienced as inserted. Much the same applies to our actions, many of which are habitual and effortless. This is readily apparent from Frith's own example; we unthinkingly move our eyes all the time and it is only occasionally that an eye movement is preceded by an intention.

---

[9] Frith goes on to claim that the self-monitoring of thought is a 'special case' of 'a more general mechanism' called 'metarepresentation', which gives us the ability to reflect upon our own and others' experiences and thoughts (1992, pp.115–6). He suggests that all the symptoms of schizophrenia are explicable in terms of a breakdown of this mechanism and categorizes its effects as 'disorders of willed action', 'disorders of self-monitoring' and 'disorders in monitoring the intentions of others' (1992, pp.113–5). As already pointed out, Frith does not describe the phenomenology of affective changes and instead construes them as changes in observed behaviour. However, when the relevant phenomenology is described, it becomes apparent that it includes an altered sense of reality and of belonging to the world. This cannot be understood in terms of a cognitive mechanism that scrutinizes 'mental representations'. Metarepresentation of experiences and thoughts cannot mysteriously inject a sense of reality into them. Like them, it presupposes the sense of reality. So changed existential feelings cannot be explained in terms of a faulty metarepresentation mechanism. Existential changes can, however, explain the symptoms that the concept of 'metarepresentation' is invoked to explain.

In addition to this objection, there is the concern that a thought-monitoring mechanism is redundant. Our ability to interact with the world requires that we be able to distinguish our own activities from things that happen to us. However, as there is no way our thoughts could possibly belong to somebody else, there is no point in having a mechanism that monitors the genesis of thoughts in the same way.

These two objections are addressed by Campbell (1999), who offers a modified version of Frith's account. Like Frith, he takes thought to be a 'motor process' and also considers thought insertion in isolation from any changes in the structure of experience as a whole. But, unlike Frith, he acknowledges that the corollary discharge or, as he calls it, the 'efference copy' is not associated with an *experience* of intention or effort. The processes that facilitate a sense of thought ownership are not themselves experienced. Campbell also suggests that a thought-monitoring mechanism of this kind could have a function. It might be concerned with 'keeping thoughts on track' and with keeping patterns of thought coherent (1999, p.616). As inappropriate or incongruous thoughts arise, they can be blocked or modified.

This kind of approach indicates that thought insertion owes little, if anything, to changed existential feeling. However, an alternative model proposed by Gallagher (2005, chapter 8) suggests otherwise. Gallagher distinguishes between the sense of ownership and the sense of agency. In thought insertion, a person experiences a thought as something that belongs to her but, at the same time, as something that she has not produced. So the task is to explain why there is a sense of ownership but no sense of agency.[10] He cites a number of experimental results, all of which point to the conclusion that the distinction between ownership and agency corresponds to the distinction between 'ecological, sensory-feedback control' and 'pre-action, forward control' (2005, p.178). So, contrary to Frith and Campbell, it is disturbance of anticipation that is responsible for thought insertion, rather than breakdown of a process that matches an anticipated action with perceptual feedback.

Gallagher raises several other concerns regarding the role of the corollary discharge or efference copy in Frith's account. Some of these are placated by Campbell's amendments but others remain. For example there is the regress problem. In Frith's account, the problem is that an intention to think is itself a

---

[10] See also Stephens and Graham (2000) for a distinction between the 'subjectivity' and 'agency' of thoughts. As they observe, 'the subject regards the thoughts as alien not because she supposes that they occur outside her, but in spite of her awareness that they occur within her' (2000, pp.126–7).

thought and so requires a prior intention to think it and so on. Even if the *intention to act* is not something that one is aware of, a variant of this problem still arises in those cases where the intended action is a thought. Intending to perform action p does not require actually performing p, whereas intending to think p is itself a thought with the content p. Even if the anticipation of a thought about p is unconscious, it is still an anticipation of a thought with content p and, by implication, a mental state with some content approximating p. This would surely need to be monitored too, for the same reasons that thought p needs to be monitored. Without the monitor, intentions to think—conscious or otherwise—would not remain on track, and if intentions to think became incoherent, surely conscious thoughts would become incoherent too. So a regress of monitoring is required. And if intentions to think do not need to be monitored, it is not clear why thoughts need to be monitored either. What requires monitoring is overt speech and activity, not thought.

Perhaps this objection can be countered by maintaining that intending to think p does not embody the full content of p but something vaguer or less specific. Indeed, it might be that, on some occasions, it is enough to have an intention 'to think something' without knowing anything at all about the content. However, the danger of a regress remains. Intending to think a thought with some content is still a thought content, regardless of how vague the anticipated content is. Hence it too needs to be monitored.

Even if this objection can be countered, there is still what Gallagher calls the problem of *specificity*. If a monitoring process is no longer functional, surely all thoughts would be bereft of the sense of agency. However, this is not what happens in schizophrenia. A simple response is to maintain that the process breaks down only on some occasions. But then there is the problem that inserted thoughts reported by patients are not random. They often have a consistent thematic content and are even claimed to be the thoughts of a particular person. The selectiveness of the breakdown therefore requires explanation.

Gallagher also complains that Frith-type models are too static. A sense of agency is not a matter of tacitly producing 'I did it' tags in conjunction with discrete, synchronic, decontextualized, mental entities called thoughts. Thinking is a temporal process, with thoughts arising from other thoughts and flowing harmoniously into further thoughts. In order to explain the content-specificity of inserted thoughts, he turns to affective states and notes that the temporal structure of experience and thought is affected by mood. For example, when you are extremely bored, everything seems to slow down and, when you are enjoying something, time seems to pass more quickly.[11] He adds that some experience and thought contents are associated with heightened emotions. So it could be that the usual harmonious flow of experience and thought is only disrupted when specific themes arise, those that are associated with certain unruly emotions, such as sudden feelings of intense anxiety.

How might this generate an experience of thought insertion? In emphasizing the temporal structure of thought, Gallagher appeals to Husserl. For Husserl, thoughts do not just come one after the other, each occupying a different time slice. Thought has a protentional–retentional structure, by which Husserl means that a thought is experienced as anchored in the thoughts that precede it (retention) and also has an anticipatory element (protention). In thinking a thought, what is to come next is not already present in the form of a tacit efference copy. Rather, we apprehend the thought as a salient but not wholly determinate possibility; we experience its coming.

Hence the structure of thought is like the horizonal structure of world experience. When we look at a chair, its hidden sides are not part of what is actually perceived. However, the *possibility* of accessing them is part of the experience and, as one moves around the chair, experience unfolds in line with tacit, bodily expectations. We do not anticipate the exact perceptual content of what is to come next. Nevertheless, the possibility space is still constrained in a structured way. Bodily expectation provides a sense of what might come next and a directive for how to actualize it. The horizonal structures of thought and world-experience are inseparable. As argued in Chapter 4, the 'universal horizon', the possibility space that determines the shape of all experience, is not exclusively directed at what is *outside*. It is a way of finding oneself in the world that encompasses both self and world. The 'I' that thinks already finds itself *there*, and so thoughts too are shaped by this background horizon.

Gallagher claims that affective disturbances of protention generate the experience of thought insertion. One still experiences a thought as one's own, given that it retains its retentional structure. But the protentional structure is absent. There is no background feeling of anticipation, no scene from which the thought emerges. It just suddenly appears and seems alien, surprising,

----

[11] Heidegger (1983, 2001) discusses the temporal phenomenology of boredom. He states that, in a mood of all-encompassing boredom 'there is no longer a sense of future, past, or present' (2001, pp.208–9). So it is not just a case of time 'speeding up' or 'slowing down'. There is also a change in the *structure* of temporal experience. Experienced distortions in the duration and structure of time are frequently reported in psychiatric illness. See Schreber (2000) for autobiographical descriptions of changed temporal experience in schizophrenia. See Jaspers (1962, pp.79–88) for a discussion of several different ways in which the experience of time can be altered in psychiatric illness.

as though it came from elsewhere. The experience is restricted to those thoughts that arise in conjunction with certain pronounced feelings. Hence there is a degree of content-specificity.

Of course, most people do not experience thought insertion when they feel anxious or have some other heightened emotion. This, I suggest, is where existential feeling comes in. The unruly occurrent emotions are accompanied by diminished background feeling. Given this, the schizophrenic person would be particularly susceptible to thought insertion. As discussed earlier, changed existential feeling in schizophrenia can affect thought in at least two ways. Thoughts in general can seem strangely object-like and thought can also be fragmented, due to the effect of erratic episodic feelings upon its horizon structure. So the patient's existential predicament renders her especially vulnerable, given that the protentional–retentional structure is already diminished and disrupted. In certain instances, the breakdown of this structure is sufficiently severe to constitute the experience of thought insertion.[12] Specific occurrences of thought insertion are thus symptomatic of an existential change, involving diminished and disorganized feeling. The sense that a thought has come from elsewhere is part of the experience, rather than a belief that is formed via inference from an anomalous experience, and the relevant experience depends upon an altered existential orientation.

Diagnoses and existential feelings

So far, I have claimed that existential changes are largely responsible for at least some psychiatric conditions. I have also warned against (a) misconstruing an existential change as the adoption of a propositional attitude and (b) double- or triple-counting unitary symptoms by interpreting them in terms of bodily feelings, experiences and beliefs. However, I have not addressed, in any depth, the questions of how many different kinds of existential change are involved in psychiatric illness and whether different kinds of existential feeling are associated with different kinds of illness. These issues are complicated by two factors. First of all, the same existential feelings can be described in different ways. For example, Cotard patients might describe themselves as being detached from their bodies or as being non-existent. Conversely, different existential feelings can be described in similar ways.

---

[12] Gallagher (personal communication) thinks that schizophrenia involves a process whereby affective anomalies disrupt the affective background as a whole, rendering it more susceptible to such anomalies, which disrupt it further, and so on. See also Sheets-Johnstone (forthcoming) for a discussion of how the flow of experience and thought is disrupted in schizophrenia.

For example, I have suggested that a 'feeling of unreality' does not always take the same form. A second problem is that diagnostic categories in psychiatry are themselves questionable. Take schizophrenia for example. As noted earlier, Bleuler and Kraepelin both identify different subtypes. The current DSM-IV-TR classification refers to five: paranoid, disorganized, catatonic, undifferentiated and residual (2004, p.298). Opinions differ as to whether these should be thought of as closely related diseases, as distinctive symptom clusters or as wholly uninformative taxonomic impositions. Kraepelin, who first described the condition, is non-committal as to whether or not a common aetiology is involved and observes that, even if it is, the course of the illness varies from case to case. 'Dementia praecox', he says, encompasses a number of 'morbid pictures' and it is 'an open question whether the same morbid process is not after all the cause of the divergent forms, though differing in point of attack and taking a varying course' (1919, p.1). Bleuler (1950, pp.3–5) is more confident in claiming that a genuine 'disease' is at work.

Since then, many researchers, working in a range of fields, have questioned the existence of schizophrenia and/or the utility of the concept 'schizophrenia'. Some have claimed that the diagnosis and treatment of schizophrenia are founded upon a range of dubious ideological and political motivations and assumptions. Others have appealed primarily to scientific findings. For example, Poland offers a scientifically based case for the view that 'schizophrenia' does not pick out a real phenomenon and that the concept is not even a useful one:

> The research programme spawned by the concept [of schizophrenia] has not proven to be productive, and it is becoming increasingly clear that diagnostic categories like schizophrenia (and, especially schizophrenia) do not play a useful role in either clinical assessment or the design and implementation of effective treatment plans for people with severe and disabling mental illness….(2007, p.183) [13]

Despite controversy regarding the utility of diagnostic categories and the reality of mental disorders, some have suggested that schizophrenia is characterized by a distinctive kind of existential change. Fuchs (2005), for example, draws a contrast between existential changes in schizophrenia and in depression, claiming that the former involves detachment from the lived body and the latter objectification of it. Like Sass, he emphasizes that the body as a whole is not ordinarily experienced in an object-like way but as a medium of experience and activity. Both schizophrenia and depression, he suggests,

---

[13] See also Bentall (2003), who suggests that categories such as 'schizophrenia' be dropped altogether, in favour of symptom-based diagnoses. See Cooper (2005) for a more general discussion of philosophical issues regarding the classification of psychiatric illnesses.

involve anomalous bodily experience. In depression, there is 'corporealization'; one identifies oneself with an object-like body:

> The melancholic patient experiences a local or general oppression, anxiety, and rigid-
> ity (e.g., a feeling of an armor vest or tire around the chest, lump in the throat, or
> pressure in the head). Sense perception and movement are weakened and finally
> walled in by this rigidity, which is visible in the patient's gaze, face, or gestures. (2005,
> p.99)

What is lacking, Fuchs goes on to say, is the 'seeking and striving' dimension of
experience. The world is no longer a space of significant possibilities; it
does not solicit activities. This is something that patients are all too aware
of, complaining of an unpleasant 'feeling of not feeling', rather than the
absence of feeling that is found in schizophrenia (2005, pp.99–100). Fuchs
claims that the Cotard delusion is the most extreme form of this existential
predicament, where 'the environment looks dead; persons and objects
seem hollow and unreal, the whole world is emptied' (2005, p.100).[14]

According to Fuchs, in schizophrenia the body is also objectified but
one feels disconnected from it, like a 'disembodied mind' (p.96). The depressed
person is no longer motivated to act, whereas the schizophrenic person
is detached from her actions, which are object-like rather than inhabited.
So both conditions include alienation from the world but this alienation
takes different forms. Stanghellini argues for much the same phenomenological contrast:

> In schizophrenic states the body, and the self in general, is experienced as a sort of
> object that is disconnected from one's own life. [....] The melancholic person's aguish
> is due to her impossibility to transcend her own inanimate body. (2004, p.157)

Fuchs and Stanghellini both refer to 'melancholia', rather than to
'depression' but I take the difference to be a largely terminological one, which
does not have any implications for the phenomenological contrasts they
draw. Fuchs (2005, p.105) states that his 'melancholia' is a variant of depression that corresponds roughly with what has also gone by the name
'endogenous depression'. He adds that it is not clearly distinct from other
kinds of depression. And I assume that neither author is using the
term 'melancholia' in its historical sense, given that the category was
very broad and also incorporated the symptoms of what is now called schizophrenia. Hence it could not be meaningfully contrasted with schizophrenia
(Radden, 2003, pp.39–40).

---

[14] DSM-IV-TR (2004, p.301) similarly contrasts the painful affect that is common in
depression with the loss of affect in schizophrenia.

In both accounts, the dualistic terminology, although rhetorical rather than metaphysical, is misleading.[15] For example, Fuchs states that the role of the body is to connect the subject to the world and then to hide itself away, so that it does not appear as an object to the subject. But talk of a pre-existent subject that then connects to the world through its body or of a self that is disembodied is suggestive of an entity that can exist independently of its existential orientation and be separated from its relationship with body and world. However, the self that is estranged to some degree from the body is also a changed, diminished self. As pointed out in Chapter 4, it does not exist *outside of* the relationship between body and world. Rather, the anomalous mode of self-experience is itself constituted by a changed relationship between body and world. The feeling of estrangement from body and world is at the same time a bodily feeling.

Leaving aside concerns about dualistic metaphors, does the contrast between a corporealized self and a disembodied self capture a genuine distinction between the kinds of existential feeling typical of depression and schizophrenia? To some extent perhaps but the boundaries between the two are not at all clear. And it is likely that metaphorical language contrasting disembodied and corporealized selves serves to exaggerate the differences between existential predicaments that are quite similar. One problem with the contrast is that most people diagnosed with schizophrenia for the first time will have suffered from depression in the previous year (Broome *et al.*, 2005). The diagnoses are therefore closely linked and not mutually exclusive. There is also a more general concern regarding the association of types of existential change with diagnostic categories. It is curious that Fuchs, Stanghellini and others take broad psychiatric categories for granted when interpreting and distinguishing existential changes. Such categories are based upon symptoms that a clinician can read off a patient's behaviour without ever contemplating what it is to have a changed sense of belonging or a changed feeling of reality. Given that the diagnostic categories are not informed by an appreciation of existential feelings, it is unlikely that they will reflect distinctive kinds of existential change. Indeed, an appreciation of existential feeling might well serve to challenge descriptions of symptoms and, consequently, certain symptom-based classifications. For instance, I have argued that it serves as a corrective to the double- or triple-counting of symptoms. Existential feelings are therefore unlikely to track diagnostic categories in any reliable fashion. Diagnoses do refer to altered existential feelings, under descriptions such as 'diminished

---

[15] Leder (2005) raises this concern in relation to Fuchs' discussion.

affect', but they do not incorporate an adequate phenomenological apprecia-tion of the changes that they refer to. So they are not sufficiently sensitive to the ways in which these changes might differ phenomenologically.

The lack of a clear phenomenological boundary between depression and schizophrenia is further evident when we consider the Cotard delusion. This is associated with cases of extreme depression but can also occur in schizophre-nia. It is arguable that the Cotard delusion is an expression of a particularly pronounced form of depersonalization (e.g. Weinstein, 1996, p.20), a view that seems all the more plausible once it is acknowledged that the delusion is not a propositional attitude but an existential orientation. Depersonalization likewise occurs in depression and in schizophrenia (Phillips et al., 2001). If the same kind of existential orientation can feature in both depression and schizophrenia, it is unlikely that these conditions have such divergent bodily phenomenologies.

Stanghellini (2004, pp.156–9) claims that there are two very different kinds of depersonalization at play in schizophrenia and depression, which map onto the contrast between disembodied spirits and their corporealized opposites, the Cotard delusion being a case of the latter. However, as noted in Chapter 6, a Cotard patient might describe herself as being dead or as being disembodied. Hence, in this case at least, the different descriptions express what is acknowledged to be much the same predicament. It is arguable that this point has more general application and that the contrast between corpo-realization and disembodiment reflects differences in the language used by patients to describe their experiences, more so than it does different existential feelings. In fact, some self-descriptions include references to both. For example, Jaspers (1962, p.122) quotes a patient who says 'I am only an automaton, a machine; it is not I who senses, speaks, eats, suffers, sleeps; I exist no longer; I do not exist, I am dead; I feel absolutely nothing'. This patient is first identified with an altered, machine-like entity but then distances herself/himself from the body that is so different from the being he/she once was. To add to this, the self that is estranged from bodily goings on is a self that has ceased to exist.

A lack of clear boundaries is also apparent with respect to the contrast between an 'absence of feeling' and the 'feeling of not feeling'. Granted, some cases do seem to fall into one or the other category. But it is not clear that absence of feeling in schizophrenia is always quite so different in character from a painful feeling of not feeling that occurs in depression. Jaspers quotes another schizophrenic patient who says 'There is nothing left; I am cold as a block of ice and as stiff; I am frozen hard' (1962, p.111). This person is evidently aware that something is missing from her experience, that she has lost something and that her sense of self is impoverished as a result. Regardless of whether or not this existential orientation involves a *painful absence*, it certainly involves a sense of *absence*. And, in this case too, the person identifies himself/herself with the deanimated body, rather than emphasizing a detachment from it.

It is interesting to note that Styron, in describing his depression, reports at one point a curious sense of there being a neutral, detached observer, watching his torment from elsewhere:

> A phenomenon that a number of people have noted while in deep depression is the sense of being accompanied by a second self—a wraithlike observer who, not sharing the dementia of his double, is able to watch with dispassionate curiosity as his companion struggles against the oncoming disaster, or decides to embrace it. (2001, p.64)

I certainly do not wish to suggest that this experience is exactly the same as that reported by certain schizophrenic patients. Indeed, there is most likely a range of existential feelings involved in depression and schizophrenia. Even so, perhaps the difference here is not a difference in kind. It could well be that one comes to further identify oneself with this 'wraith', as a sense of one's animate, feeling body increasingly fades.

That said, I do concede that there is a phenomenological distinction to be drawn between detachment from one's deeds and a bodily conspicuousness that hinders activity. For example, in talking to somebody, I might find myself struggling to come up with the words, straining to voice one and then the next with unusual effort and awkwardness. In contrast, I might find a narrative pouring effortlessly from me, without my having to think through what I'm saying. After a while of this, there is sometimes the odd feeling of being removed from my words, of no longer inhabiting them even though they continue to flow. The same goes for my typing, which can be either laboured and awkward or quite effortless. In certain instances of the latter, I feel strangely detached from it, as though it is going on without me. Nevertheless, when this kind of experience occurs, the activity eventually breaks down. So long as I am oblivious to my typing, which goes on in the background of my experience, it carries on quite happily. However, once I remove myself from my habitual activity and gaze upon it, that activity is not sustained for long. My hands eventually become clumsy and my typing ceases to proceed harmoniously. The disruption ensures that the divorce is never complete. The same goes for schizophrenia, where practical activities are of course not unaffected by existential changes.

So there is something to be said for the contrast between a detached, hyper-reflexive experiencing, which changes a practical orientation into an experienced object, and the inhabiting of an orientation that becomes increasingly object-like. However, it is not clear why these two modes of experience should be mutually exclusive. One could feel more object-like and, at the same time, detach oneself from certain activities, which one no longer struggles to inhabit but instead views from elsewhere. The patient might emphasize the aspect of experience that is most salient or troubling, rather than articulating one of two wholly distinct ways of experiencing.[16]

As well as failing to respect distinctions between types of illness, many of the existential feelings involved in psychiatric illness will not be exclusive to psychiatric illness. People experience similar feelings in less pronounced ways in everyday life and it might be that some existential feelings occur in much the same form and with the same intensity in both psychiatric and non-psychiatric contexts. For example, it could be that two people share a similar existential orientation but that one is better able to deal with it or even to regulate it. To further complicate matters, the way in which one understands one's predicament and the way in which one deals with it can serve to change the predicament in question.[17]

Kinds of existential feeling

Existential feelings will not fall neatly into separate taxonomic boxes; they form a continuum. Shifts from one feeling to another can be sudden but are often gradual. Existential feelings cannot be classified along one dimension, with opposing extremes at either end. They change in a number of different *ways*, and current diagnostic categories are unlikely to be a reliable guide for distinguishing different variants. However, the variety of existential feeling cannot be charted through armchair reflection alone either. Without descriptions of anomalous experience supplied by patients and clinicians,

---

[16] In appealing to hyper-reflexivity, Sass, unlike Fuchs and Stanghellini, does not subscribe to a contrast between corporealization in depression and disembodiment in schizophrenia. He remarks that schizophrenic people 'can sometimes feel very much like they are nothing but a body, even though at other times they may feel totally devoid of a body' and that schizophrenia involves 'opposites' that are somehow 'complementary' (personal communication). In addition, he emphasizes that 'persons with schizophrenia are surely heterogeneous with respect to many aspects of affective experience and expression' (2007, p.352), this heterogeneity applying to different patients and also to different stages of the illness. The aim of his phenomenological account is to describe some of the most conspicuous and commonplace phenomenological changes, rather than to describe them all.

[17] The fact that an understanding of one's existential feeling can, to some extent, reshape the feeling suggests that there may be a difference between the existential feelings of intelligent, articulate schizophrenic people, who have some insight into the nature of their condition, and others who do not. So we should not be too quick to generalize from cases like Renee's to the experiences of other patients. Thanks to Matthew Broome for this point.

we would be oblivious to the possibility of certain existential changes. For example, the possibility of an existential orientation involving the experience of thought insertion is not something that we would most likely contemplate in the absence of such descriptions. But kinds of existential feeling cannot simply be *read off* the reports offered by psychiatrists and patients, given that these reports do not themselves interpret patients' symptoms in terms of existential changes. An understanding that someone has a particular illness that is likely to affect her in predictable ways does not amount to an understanding of her existential orientation. Interpretations of utterances, expressions, gestures, feelings and actions that begin with an appreciation of existential feeling will differ from those that do not. What is therefore required is a hermeneutic approach, where phenomenology and psychiatry work together: patients' experiences are interpreted in terms of existential feeling, and interaction with patients then facilitates a better phenomenological understanding of the feelings in question.

I will not attempt to offer a comprehensive classification of existential feelings in psychiatric illness here. It is a project that would demand extensive collaborative work between phenomenologists, clinical practitioners and patients. My emphasis in this book has been on interaction between phenomenologists and psychiatrists, more so than between phenomenologists and patients. However, further study will require ongoing interaction between the three groups, whereby clinicians interpret patients in terms of existential feeling (often aided by patients' own remarks and self-interpretations) and their descriptions are refined, elaborated and criticized by phenomenologists. Of course, direct interaction between phenomenologists and patients will also have a role to play. But the interpretive skills of the phenomenologist are different from, and no substitute for, the skills of the clinician. As a phenomenologist lacking in clinical experience, I can only offer part of the story. Even so, by drawing on what I have discussed so far, it is possible to indicate at least some of the ways in which kinds of existential feeling differ from each other.

One important distinction is that between consistent and changeable existential feeling. A central difference that sets apart many of those diagnosed with depression from others with schizophrenia is that the former inhabit an enduring existential orientation that is recalcitrant to change. Experience retains its consistency. But what is consistent is a diminished possibility space, an unpleasant feeling of loss, isolation, imprisonment and hopelessness that shapes all experiences. Descriptions of schizophrenic experience generally suggest a possibility space that unfolds in a disorganized way. This may or may not be blended with the kind of diminishment that characterizes depression.

So a major difference between kinds of existential feeling is diachronic in nature, rather than being a structural difference between two kinds of fixed, enduring orientation.

It is also important to recognize that some existential feelings are neither rigid nor disorganized orientations but *processes* that unfold over time. How one reacts to an existential feeling can enhance, diminish or reshape it. For example, Medford *et al.* observe that:

> In some patients, symptoms of depersonalisation and anxiety occur together, apparently feeding each other—the strangeness and sense of isolation occasioned by depersonalisation fuels the anxiety and the depersonalisation then intensifies as a defence against this anxiety. (2005, p.95)

And Sass (2003, p.173) claims that unworlding and other existential changes arouse further feelings, ranging from anxiety to wonder and awe. These, I suggest, are not simply additions to a pre-existent orientation, which itself remains constant throughout, but changes to it. A world bereft of all practical significance could be experienced through an all-encompassing sense of panic, lack of control, suffocation, utter indifference or mystery. So the falling away of practical significance does not always have the same character. Neither does bodily conspicuousness. As discussed in Chapter 4, this too can take a number of different forms. There is not a simple, linear gradient between harmoniously belonging to the world and a bodily conspicuousness that estranges one from the world. There are many different kinds of bodily conspicuousness and inconspicuousness, and of worldly belonging and detachment. Some of these are not recalcitrant to change but shift over time in structured and often complicated ways.

All kinds of existential change can be described in terms of changes in the possibility space that shapes our experiences. For example, all possibilities for activities and happenings might be heightened or diminished. Alternatively, the space might be overly constrained, offering less than it once did. Or it might be excessively open, offering a bewildering array of possibilities, none more enticing than others, and a consequent lack of practical focus. Excessive, diminished and constrained possibilities all seem to feature in schizophrenia and may be associated with different stages of the illness. At one point, Renee complains of things being 'limitless'. She later refers to a 'boundless Fear' and a 'sense of vastness, infinity', suggesting a possibility space that is no longer restricted in the usual way. It is completely open and yet also strangely bereft of ordinary enticements (Sechehaye, 1970, pp.25–37). Sass (1992, chapter 9; 1994) suggests that, in some cases at least, the later stages of schizophrenia are characterized by a mode of experiencing that is akin to solipsism, incorporating a *loss* of the possibilities integral to interpersonal and social reality.

Some changes that occur in psychiatric illness involve particular *kinds* of possibility being heightened and others diminished. For example, the balance between possible activities and happenings might shift one way or the other. The world could appear as something to be acted upon in all manner of ways or, in contrast, as a series of potential happenings before which one is passive. A sense of potential activities and happenings is not simply *neutral* in tone. The activities that the world offers take different forms. They can appear as effortless, easy, pleasurable, difficult, intimidating, daunting, painful, safe or dangerous. Things can also make impossible demands, appearing as 'to be done but not possible to do' or as 'to be done by others but impossible for me'. Experience of happenings before which we are passive also has many different forms. Happenings can be irrelevant to the self, in which case they can still appear in a range of ways—as fascinating, mysterious, horrifying, irrelevant or meaningless, for example. Alternatively, they can be experienced as potentialities relating to the self, perhaps as overwhelming, threatening, oppressive or sinister. In certain existential changes, the *variety* of ways in which activities and happenings are experienced is lost, replaced by one all-encompassing experiential tone. One finds oneself in the world in such a way that everything is oppressive, threatening, painfully irrelevant or mysteriously detached. The universal horizon undergoes an enduring change in structure. A contingent kind of possibility becomes a way in which everything is encountered. For example, one can feel vulnerable before the world as a whole, which takes on an overall shape of existential threat. Laing uses the term 'implosion' to describe:

> …the full terror of the experience of the world as liable at any moment to crash in and obliterate all identity, as a gas will rush in and obliterate a vacuum. The individual feels that, like the vacuum, he is empty. But this emptiness is him. (1960, p.47)

Things before which one is passive or helpless can still appear as potential loci of activity for everyone else. A change that seems to characterize some instances of depression is that the possibilities still appear but not as opportunities to be taken up by oneself. The possibility of anything being self-involving or enticing is eradicated from experience and this lack takes on the form of a painful sense of absence and isolation. In some cases at least, the possibilities are still perceived as enticing for others, as possibilities that move people and ought to move people but that, in one's own case, do not. This amounts to a feeling of estrangement, isolation and imprisonment, Plath's 'bell jar'.

The diminishment, loss or alteration of *interpersonal* possibilities is central to many existential changes. For example, in Chapter 5, I argued that the Capgras delusion arises due to a diminished or absent sense of the personal. Another change in interpersonal possibilities is when other people all appear as sources of possible activities that might be inflicted upon one, rather than as potential partners in dialogue. For example, Lysaker *et al.* (2005) suggest that interpersonal experience in schizophrenia is often structured by a consistent feeling of threat. There is a sense of others as invasive, as potential destroyers of a fragile self. Laing similarly talks of people with schizophrenia feeling 'exposed', 'vulnerable' and 'isolated'. A schizophrenic person, he observes, 'may say that he is made of glass, of such transparency and fragility that a look directed at him splinters him to bits and penetrates straight through him' (1960, p.38).

In contrast to this somewhat Sartrean phenomenology is an existential orientation where one is untouched by others, incapable of being moved by them in any way, and thus feels a profound sense of estrangement and isolation. A sense of others could also be diminished or absent without that loss being felt. As discussed in Chapters 2, 5 and 6, there is an important distinction to be drawn between absent or changed possibilities and an experience of possibilities as absent or changed. Things can be missing but things can also appear *as* lacking, missing or out of reach. The loss of possibilities can be a conspicuous part of the experience and this loss is not always felt in the same way; it can involve anxiety, mystery, paranoia and a host of other feelings. Another case where a sense of loss or absence is a conspicuous part of the experience is the feeling of intangibility, which I discussed in Chapter 4, where things appear as lacking in a way that renders them strangely inaccessible, out of reach, not quite there.

Some existential changes are alterations in the structure of anticipation. As discussed in Chapter 4, we experience some things as certain, others as uncertain and others as doubtful. For example, I might take for granted that, when I turn my coffee cup round, the side that I cannot currently see will be the same colour. However, the possibilities could be less determinate than this, thus taking on the shape of uncertainty. Or they could take the form of doubt; a feeling that further manipulation of the object will reveal it to be other than what it seems to be. Any one of these modalities might be heightened, diminished or extinguished. For example, the emphasis on erosion of practical commonsense in schizophrenia (e.g. Blankenburg, 2001; Stanghellini, 2004) suggests a loss of habitual, practical certainty from the horizonal structure and an existential feeling where doubt and uncertainty surround everything.

All these variants of existential feeling can also be described in terms of (a) various kinds of belonging and estrangement, (b) kinds and degrees of bodily conspicuousness or (c) some or all objects of experience appearing a certain way, such as unreal, unfamiliar, contingent and so on. Existential feelings are also describable in terms of different modes of concern, directed at either self or world. The world can be significant, insignificant, meaningful or meaningless.

It can matter or not matter. And the self can be something that is oppressed, suffocated, threatened, safe or unsafe.

Hence there are many different kinds of existential feeling and these can all be described in different ways too, with reference to self, body, world, the relationship between them or to *everything*. Many if not all existential changes are also subtle or pronounced changes in the sense of reality. This, I have suggested, consists of a background feeling of practical belonging. The possibility of something being *the case*, *real* or *there* is not something that is primitive to all experience and thought, about which no more can be said. It is a changeable and fragile modality, the variants of which are amenable to phenomenological description.

Part III

Existential feeling and philosophical thought

Chapter 8

What William James really said

Up to now, existential feelings have been my *object* of enquiry. However, as I indicated in the introduction, they are also integral to my phenomenological method. Changes in existential feeling, which are experienced by the phenomenologist or described by others, serve to make explicit the contribution made by existential feelings to experience. What we ordinarily take for granted becomes salient in its diminution, absence or change. Emphasis upon a single kind of existential shift, such as 'anxiety', is not methodologically sufficient. There are many kinds of existential feeling to be explored, rather than a single, normal, consistent way of belonging to the world that can be disturbed by only one or two unusual and extreme kinds of existential change. In addition, some existential changes are quite subtle, rather than being sudden, world-estranging events. In this part of the book, I offer a more general account of the role played by existential feelings in philosophical enquiry, showing how they contribute to philosophical commitment, conviction, doubt and disagreement. Although my emphasis throughout is specifically upon philosophy, much of what I say will apply more generally.

The philosophy of William James features as a central theme throughout these last three chapters. It merits this level of attention for several reasons. First of all, James's theory of emotion is the starting point for many recent philosophical discussions of emotion and feeling. We saw in Chapter 1 that it is usually portrayed as a view that can be summarily dismissed, illustrating in the process the need for an alternative approach that places more emphasis on the cognitive dimensions of emotion. However, as this chapter will show, such portrayals rest upon a serious misinterpretation of James's position. In identifying emotions with feelings of bodily changes, James does not divorce them from world-experience or from thought. Rather, he rejects the cognition–affect distinction altogether. The account he actually offers is similar to my view of existential feeling in (a) recognizing that feelings structure all experience and thought, and (b) emphasizing those feelings that have existential import. James uses the term 'emotion' to refer to a wide range of feelings.

Hence I begin by using this term, rather than by referring to existential feelings, and I use 'emotion' interchangeably with 'feeling', given that James takes emotions to be bodily feelings. As the discussion progresses, it will become clear that he is not just interested in 'standard emotions'. He also recognizes that there are numerous feelings that do not have established names and that some of these operate as existential backgrounds.

James's relevance is not exhausted by his offering a view that is in many respects complementary to my own. The interpretation of his position offered in this chapter sets the scene for Chapter 9, where I explore the roles of existential feelings in philosophical enquiry, and for Chapter 10, where I address the question of when an existential feeling is rightly regarded as 'pathological'. James emphasizes that philosophy is done by the whole person; those feelings that are so central to our lives are central to our philosophy too. He adds that differing existential orientations influence philosophical thought in a number of ways. He also emphasizes the close connection between psychiatric illness, and metaphysical and religious dispositions, claiming that medical pathologies can at the same time be ways of experiencing the world that give the sufferer genuine and profound insights. His work is therefore unique in offering a theory of feeling that is at the same time employed to reflect upon the role of feeling in philosophical enquiry and upon the relationship between philosophical dispositions and pathologies of experience. In addition, James discusses how a background of feeling fuels his own explicit philosophical position.

Physiology and philosophy

As discussed in Chapter 1, James's account of emotion is often seen as an easy target, to be dismissed for rendering emotions epiphenomenal, trivializing them, failing to recognize that they play a role in world-experience, separating them from cognitive evaluations and so on. Where such criticisms have gone wrong is in failing to recognize that *feelings* for James are not the *mere feelings* that they are so often presumed to be. Criticisms almost always refer only to his 1884/1890 account, which emphasizes the physiological processes involved in emotion. However, it is important to appreciate that James's concern with emotion is first and foremost philosophical. His view of the nature and role of emotion is not exhausted by an account of the relevant physiology, accompanied by a dubious thought experiment that invites us to imagine stripping all the feelings away from an emotion and to realise in the process that no emotion would remain. James stresses that his physiological account is influenced by an independently formulated philosophical theory. His philosophical conception of emotion serves as a background framework that shapes his physiological theorizing:

> ...although [a theory of brain physiology] seems to be the chief result of the arguments I am to urge, I should say that they were not originally framed for the sake of any such result. They grew out of fragmentary introspective observations, and it was only when these had already combined into a theory that the thought of the simplification the theory might bring to cerebral physiology occurred to me, and made it seem more important than before. (1884, p.189)

Not all of this framework is explicit in the 1884 and 1890 discussions, and critics tend to neglect the broader philosophical context. As we saw in Chapter 1, a common complaint against James is that he fails to assign a cognitive role to the emotions, identifying them with feelings of bodily changes and trivializing them in the process. I will now turn to several of James's other philosophical works in order to piece together a theory of the *role* played by emotions that complements his account of what emotions *are*. Interpreting James (1884, 1890) in the light of these works suggests that many criticisms of his view are misguided, in taking for granted conceptions of affect, cognition and the distinction between them that James himself rejects.[1]

One potential problem with the approach I take here is that James's later philosophical works might put forward views that are distinct from or even opposed to those ventured in the 1884 and 1890 account. However, I think that there is a great deal of continuity between these writings, at least so far as emotion is concerned. Indeed, any tensions are largely due to the later James putting forward stronger or more explicit statements of views he was already leaning towards in his earlier writings on emotion. Some of these views were even put forward before his physiological account of emotion and are retained as central themes in later works. For example, there is the 'The Sentiment of Rationality' (in James, 1897). This is made up of material from an article of the same title, which appeared in *Mind* in 1879 and from an address that James presented to the Harvard Philosophical Club in 1880. Its content coheres well with many of the themes in the later *Varieties of Religious Experience* (1902) and *Pragmatism* (1981). Furthermore, the identification of emotions with feelings of bodily changes is explicitly retained by James (1894)

---

[1] My complaints are directed at philosophers working on the emotions, more so than James scholars, who are often more charitable towards his account. To offer two examples of the latter, Gerald Myers (1986, p.242) acknowledges that James does not always distinguish cognition from affect and Wesley Cooper (2002, p.74) rejects the oft held view that emotions, on James's account, are trivial by-products of behaviour, whilst also emphasizing the unity and coherence of James's philosophy.

and he still endorses the James–Lange theory, with its emphasis on 'affections of the body', in an essay that was first published in 1905 (see James, 1912, p.142).[2]

Hence the overall position that emerges is, I will suggest, fairly cohesive. It is also quite different from, and far richer than, the view that many critics of James take him to hold. For James, feelings or affects are not *mere* accompaniments to distinct cognitive states and processes but inextricable from them. By 'cognitive', I mean both intentional states and deliberative processes. Rather than taking a conception of intentionality for granted and identifying emotions with bodily feelings that are distinct from intentional states, James reconceptualizes intentionality so as to include bodily feeling in its structure. Emotions are thus essential to the structure of world-experience. In this role, they also shape our decision-making and behaviour.

The charge that James (1884, 1890) renders emotions epiphenomenal is perhaps understandable, given that he neglects in these discussions to formulate an explicit account of the cognitive role played by emotions. However, he does at least indicate that they have a role to play in *behaviour*. Adopting a broadly Darwinian approach, James claims that organisms' nervous systems are evolutionarily pre-tuned to ecological niches, responding perceptually only to those features of the environment that are salient in relation to potential behaviours. He remarks that 'peculiarly conformed pieces of the world's furniture will fatally call forth most particular mental and bodily reactions' (1884, p.190) and that 'each creature brings the signature of its special relations stamped on its nervous system with it upon the scene' (1884, p.191). Bodily feelings are integral to an organism's physiological tuning to the environment. Certain features of the world automatically summon good or bad feelings, independent of explicit reasoning processes, and these feelings play a role in regulating behaviour, in steering an organism away from those things that feel bad and towards those things that feel good. Because bodily feelings are innately pre-tuned to certain kinds of environmental cues, they are able to systematically structure behaviour in a manner that generally conforms to the organism's evolved needs and capabilities.[3]

---

[2] The essay, entitled 'The place of affectional facts in a world of pure experience' also appeared in 1912 as Chapter 5 of James's *Essays in Radical Empiricism*. I will quote from the latter here.

[3] James's view of the organism–environment relation does not conform to a traditional lock and key conception of organisms and niches, and bears greater similarity to an account offered by Lewontin (1978, 1982). According to Lewontin, organisms *construct* rather than *fit into* their environments. Their evolved needs and capacities bind together salient environmental features into a niche, which is created as much as it is discovered.

James adds that the relevant physiological changes are not hard-wired to respond only to a rigid, inflexible set of perceptual cues. Changes can be associated with novel stimuli through learning, constituting a dynamic framework of dispositions that renders only certain features of the environment behaviourally salient: 'a nervous tendency to discharge being once there, all sorts of unforeseen things may pull the trigger and let loose the effects' (1884, p.195). Feelings are automatically generated during perception, as a result of innate or learned associations, and structure behaviour by making some activities salient and deterring an organism from others. For example, the sight of a cliff edge, coupled with a bad feeling, serves to partially specify the behaviour 'back off'.

There are many similarities between James's position and that of Damasio. For example, Damasio claims that:

> Preorganized mechanisms are important not just for basic biological regulation. They also help the organism classify things or events as 'good' or 'bad' because of their possible impact on survival. In other words, the organism has a basic set of preferences—or criteria, biases, or values. Under their influence and the agency of experience, the repertoire of things categorized as good or bad grows rapidly, and the ability to detect new good and bad things grows exponentially. (1995, p.117)

Damasio also distinguishes between primary and secondary emotions, the former of which are hard-wired (e.g. fear of heights), whilst the latter involve learned associations between perceptions and feelings (e.g. a distaste for ice cream). However, a significant difference between the two accounts, which I mentioned in Chapter 1, is that Damasio chooses to regard the physiological changes, rather than feelings of those changes, as the 'emotions'. And, unlike James, he does not situate his account in the context of a broader philosophical theory.

As I will now show, the emphasis on how a felt, bodily orientation regulates our activities is also there in many of James's philosophical works (1897, 1902, 1912, 1970, 1981).[4] In addition, he claims that this orientation is inseparable from the way in which features of the world are experienced and from how we relate to the world as a whole in our experience. Hence his philosophical work offers a phenomenological analogue of his Darwinian account of the physiology of emotion.

....

For James too, the perceived environment is an indissociable amalgam of organism-independent features and organismic concerns. The set of things to which an organism is responsive does not comprise a disinterested representation of *things outside*. It is a construct that reflects both the way the world is and what the organism brings to it.

[4] *The Meaning of Truth* (James, 1970) was originally published in 1909 and *Pragmatism* (James, 1981) in 1907.

The role of emotion in experience and thought

The claim that emotions structure world-experience might look like a substantial departure from the 1884 and 1890 account, where James says that emotions follow perceptions rather than contributing to them. However, this apparent tension is, I think, due to a terminological ambiguity rather than a genuine conflict. James sometimes fails to distinguish clearly between 'perception' as a physiological process and 'a perception' as the phenomenological product of that process. Similarly, whether the 'object of perception' is the 'external cause of the perception' or the 'experienced outcome of perception' is not always clear. Taking such distinctions into account, the early James seems to be saying that it is not 'an object as perceived' but 'sensory stimulation of our perceptual systems by an object' that automatically triggers bodily changes, as one would expect from a reflex-like process. Consider his statement that 'the emotion is nothing but the reflex bodily effects of what we call its "object", effects due to the connate adaptation of the nervous system to that object' (1884, p.194). He is not talking about the *object as perceived* but of the *object that is perceived*. References to neural adaptations concern what causes the experience rather than the object as it is experienced.

Given this interpretation, James's account of what emotions *are* can be supplemented by his account of their *role*, to arrive at the view that emotions are feelings of bodily changes, which are triggered during perception and contribute to the phenomenological structure of perception. Jamesian 'feeling' is not distinct from cognition but a constituent of cognition; it plays a role in structuring the experiential world that forms the backdrop to our various deliberations.

James alludes to this sort of reconceptualization in his earlier writings on emotion, when he remarks that 'if our hypothesis is true, it makes us realize more deeply than ever how much of our mental life is knit up with our corporeal frame, in the strictest sense of the term' (1890, p.467).[5] Although he does not explicitly challenge the philosophical distinction between cognition and feeling (as is understandable given that his explicit concern is with physiology), he certainly entertains the possibility:

> Cognition and emotion are parted even in this last retreat [science],—who shall say that their antagonism may not just be one phase of the world-old struggle known as that between the spirit and the flesh?—a struggle in which it seems pretty certain that neither party will definitively drive the other off the field. (1884, p. 203)

---

5 Like James, Damasio claims that 'contrary to traditional scientific opinion, feelings are just as cognitive as other percepts' (1995, xv).

However, in other writings, there are more decisive statements of the view that emotion and cognition are indissociable aspects of world experience, rather than distinct categories. In *The Will to Believe*, James explicitly assigns a cognitive role to emotions, in aiding decision-making and belief-formation when other factors fail to provide grounds for preferring one option over another:

> Our passional nature not only lawfully may, but must, decide an option between propositions, whenever it is a genuine option that cannot by its nature be decided on intellectual grounds; for to say, under such circumstances, 'Do not decide, but leave the question open,' is itself a passional decision,—just like deciding yes or no,—and is attended with the same risk of losing the truth. (1897, p. 11)

There are some situations where, having weighed up all the evidence and run through all the reasons, we still have no grounds for favouring one option over another. In such cases, our feelings guide us because we have no other source of preference. Without the influence of our passions, we would be deliberatively paralysed. Emotions provide a kind of pre-deliberative, evaluative backdrop. Some options simply *feel* better than others and when we have exhausted all other grounds for choice and are still presented with more than one option, our only alternative is to fall back on these pleasant or unpleasant feelings of body states to guide our choices.[6]

Of course, one could recommend abstaining from choice in such cases until there is sufficient evidence to arbitrate between rival opinions. However, James makes the point that abstention is not always the rational or neutral choice when it comes to our practical affairs. In many scenarios, not acting at all will serve to ensure the worst possible outcome. Consider the example of a goalkeeper facing a penalty kick. He can dive one way or the other and only one of them will be right. But not committing himself would be the worst strategy. James adds that abstention is itself an emotional choice, rather than a neutral strategy that is adopted in the absence of feeling. For instance, a reluctance to commit oneself or to accept something can originate in a *feeling* of caution.

James also makes the point that being non-committal is not always a wise strategy, even in our intellectual affairs. Even if we are concerned with belief, rather than with those practical decisions where deciding not to act is as significant a choice as any other, refraining from judgement can still be the wrong way to go. There are some truths, he says, that can only be revealed to someone who has already adopted certain prior commitments. Take the

---

[6] See Stocker and Hegeman (1996) for a more recent discussion of the evaluative roles played by emotions.

example of whether or not to believe that B is one's friend. An agnostic stance regarding the matter may be the best way to ensure that B is not one's friend, by culturing a shared attitude of distrust. Commitment to a friendship can itself serve to make it the case that someone is a friend. As James puts it:

> There are, then, cases where a fact cannot come at all unless a preliminary faith exists in its coming. *And where faith in a fact can help create the fact*, that would be an insane logic which should say that faith running ahead of scientific evidence is the 'lowest kind of immorality' into which a thinking being can fall. Yet such is the logic by which our scientific absolutists pretend to regulate our lives! (1897, p. 25)

He is not saying that, in managing our beliefs, we should just choose what to believe on the basis of what feels best. The point is not that we can or should simply *go with our emotions* and choose what to believe or how to act *in spite of the evidence*. The relevant feelings come into play only in relation to what James calls 'live options'. In other words, feelings arbitrate between beliefs and actions that are already judged to be intellectually respectable, to which one is already disposed. So they are not the sole basis for choice. Many of the feelings that regulate beliefs and activities do not feature in the usual lists of emotions. For example, James (1897, p.77) refers to the feeling of familiarity, which, he claims, is also a feeling of rationality. The felt familiarity of something can add up to a sense of its rightness. (Presumably this does not apply to all feelings of familiarity though; there is often some kind of 'feeling of familiarity' when we witness a familiar mistake.) As will become clear in Chapter 9, it is not only focused feelings that have an epistemic role to play. James also acknowledges the role of background feelings, which make us receptive to certain kinds of evidence and doctrinal commitment.

A similar role for emotions in choice-making has been suggested more recently by a number of authors, including de Sousa (1980, 1990), Johnson-Laird and Oatley (1992) and Damasio (1995, 2000). Johnson-Laird and Oatley, for example, claim that 'emotions help to specify which goals will be actively pursued, and which abandoned, or assigned to a subsidiary or dormant status' (1992, p.208), and de Sousa suggests that:

> When faced with two competing arguments, between which neither reason nor determinism can relevantly decide, emotion can endow one set of supporting considerations with more salience that the other. We need emotion [...] to break a tie when reason is stuck. (1990, p.16)

However, these authors do not credit James with offering a sophisticated version of the same view a century earlier.

That emotions function as arbiters in some instances of choice is only the beginning of the Jamesian story. Emotions, according to James, do not merely intervene in deliberative processes. They partially constitute the experiential world, the contents of which form the material for our deliberations. We do not just have feelings about aspects of a pre-given reality, which in turn influence our decision-making. Rather, bodily feelings shape the manner in which things appear to us and structure our reasoning as a consequence. So feeling regulates decision-making by first setting up the experienced world in which decisions are made and only then, where uncertainty remains, by disposing us towards one or another live option.

It might at first seem that James (1884, 1890) explicitly retains the distinction between feeling and cognition, referring to both cognition and affect as though they were separate phenomena: 'Without the bodily states following on the perception, the latter would be purely cognitive in form, pale, colourless, destitute of emotional warmth' (1884, p.190). He goes on to ask that we imagine abstracting all our various feelings of bodily changes from an emotional state and claims that 'a cold and neutral state of intellectual perception is all that remains' (1884, p.193), suggesting that cognition is distinct from bodily feelings. However, in commenting on 'the dryness of it, the paleness, the absence of all glow' (1884, p.202), he seems to indicate that experience is somehow deficient when feeling is diminished, rather than being cognitively complete but cleansed of affect.[7] The same sentiment is conveyed more decisively in *The Varieties of Religious Experience*, where James echoes his earlier thought experiment and contemplates what experience would be like in the absence of emotions:

> Conceive yourself, if possible, suddenly stripped of all the emotion with which your world now inspires you, and try to imagine it *as it exists*, purely by itself, without your favorable or unfavorable, hopeful or apprehensive comment. It will be almost impossible for you to realize such a condition of negativity and deadness. No one portion of the universe would then have importance beyond another; and the whole collection of its things and series of its events would be without significance, character, expression, or perspective. Whatever of value, interest, or meaning our respective worlds may appear endued with are thus pure gifts of the spectator's mind. (1902, p.150)

So absence of emotion amounts to 'deadness', a state of cognitive and behavioural paralysis rather than fully functional cognition stripped of *mere* feeling. A phenomenology without emotional feeling is a phenomenology that guts

---

[7] Vallelonga (1992, pp.236–7) accuses James of explicitly enforcing an artificial Cartesian schism between affect and cognition. However, Viney, in the same volume, suggests that 'a careful reading of the *Principles* and the later philosophical work shows that James recognized the artificiality of sharp distinctions between emotion and thinking' (1992, pp.246–7).

the world of all its significance. The experienced world is ordinarily enriched by the feelings that are sewn into it, that imbue it with value and light it up as an arena of cognitive and behavioural possibilities. So cognition without feeling is not, according to James, in any sense complete. It is an extreme phenomenological privation that strips the world of all meaning, akin to extreme depression or 'melancholia'. He discusses Tolstoy's autobiographical account of depression in *A Confession*, which emphasizes its existential aspect, and observes how:

> In Tolstoy's case the sense that life had any meaning whatever was for a time wholly withdrawn. The result was a transformation in the whole expression of reality. [....] Things were meaningless whose meaning had always been self-evident. (1902, pp.151–3)

Diminution or loss of feeling is not a refinement of cognition but a mark of what James calls the 'sick soul'. His discussion indicates that our most basic familiarity with the world, our sense of belonging, is structured by emotional feeling. Feeling is not peripheral or epiphenomenal but gives the world a kind of meaning that we ordinarily take for granted. In fact, James claims that the sense of reality itself is not a product of thought but something that is composed of feeling; 'the feeling of reality may be something more like a sensation than an intellectual operation properly so-called' (1902, p.64). He is critical of overly intellectualized conceptions of conviction more generally and argues that the beliefs that drive us are not the unfeeling states philosophers now call propositional attitudes. Rather, our *beliefs* are felt convictions. This is evident in his 1890 description of changed existential orientation in depression, which he attributes to a loss of certain emotional feelings:

> In certain forms of melancholic perversion of the sensibilities and reactive powers, nothing touches us intimately, rouses us, or wakens natural feeling. The consequence is the complaint so often heard from melancholic patients, that nothing is believed in by them as it used to be, and that all sense of reality is fled from life. They are sheathed in india-rubber; nothing penetrates to the quick or draws blood, as it were. (1890, p. 298)

In this quotation, James indicates that our convictions are comprised of feeling and also that the sense of reality presupposed by them is similarly a matter of feeling. Diminished feeling is a change in the modalities of belief, which affects all beliefs. Nothing, as James says, is believed in 'as it used to be'. With this there is an alteration in the sense of belonging. The melancholic is 'sheathed in india-rubber', stuck in an unchangeable existential orientation that offers no hope of escape.

If world-experience is construed in terms of detached, unconcerned representation of an external reality by a subject, then ascribing such a significant role to feeling makes little sense. But James, like Heidegger and Merleau-Ponty, is critical of approaches that cast our experience as first and foremost a matter of detached contemplation, to be construed in terms of a contrast between internal and external. As already noted, he emphasizes a practical orientation towards things. Perception of the environment is shaped by needs, capacities and potential behaviours, and feeling plays a role in this shaping. The body, for James, is an invariably active 'sounding-board' that 'reverberates' with varying degrees and qualities to all sensations (1890, pp.470–1). When those 'reverberations' that tune an organism to the world are distorted or diminished, cognition is incomplete. As a phenomenological correlate of this biological claim, he maintains that feeling binds us to things, making them relevant. Without the world-structuring orientation that they provide, we would be disorientated, cut-off from a world that no longer solicited actions or thoughts and was consequently devoid of all value and relevance.

It could be objected that James (1884, 1890) conceives of emotions as occasional events, rather than an ever-present, experience-structuring field, and that they are therefore unlike my 'existential feelings'. However, although James focuses on strong occurrent emotions, he explicitly intends his claim that emotions are feelings of bodily changes to apply more generally. It might seem that subtle intellectual or aesthetic emotions are very different from feelings of body states. As James notes:

> These are the moral, intellectual, and aesthetic feelings. Concords of sounds, of colors, of lines, logical consistencies, teleological fitnesses, affect us with a pleasure that seems ingrained in the very form of the representation itself, and to borrow nothing from any reverberation surging up from the parts below the brain. (1890, p.468)

But he goes on to suggest that:

> In all cases of intellectual or moral rapture we find that, unless there be coupled a bodily reverberation of some kind with the mere thought of the object and cognition of its quality; unless we actually laugh at the neatness of the demonstration or witticism; unless we thrill at the case of justice, or tingle at the act of magnanimity; our state of mind can hardly be called emotional at all. (1890, pp.470–1)

Hence he claims that 'the bodily sounding board is at work, as careful introspection will show, far more than we usually suppose' (1890, p.471). Indeed, given his depiction of depression as a crippling absence of world-orienting feeling, it is clear that some such feelings provide a constant background to our activities, the absence or diminution of which amounts to a significant change in the structure of world-experience. Feelings are integral to the structure of all experience, rather than being an occasional ingredient in the perception of certain objects or situations. It is background feelings that play the most important role in our lives, comprising our existential background, rather than just those occurrent preferences that we have within a taken-for-granted world.

However, James does not draw a clear distinction between occurrent emotions and the existential background. Instead he emphasizes the extent to which emotions in general serve to *construct* the world of everyday experience. For James, any experienced situation is an amalgam of the way the world is and what we add to it through the emotions. Our relationship with the world is one of practical 'commerce' rather than detached, theoretical 'correspondence' between mental states and the way things are. Emotions are indeed reports of bodily states but, as the structure of experience is always a reflection of our needs, concerns and bodily capabilities, such feelings are not wholly 'internal' to the subject:

> ...the practically real world for each one of us, the effective world of the individual, is the compound world, the physical facts and emotional values in indistinguishable combination. Withdraw or pervert either factor of this complex resultant, and the kind of experience we call pathological ensues. (1902, p.151)

This conception of emotion as part of a world-constituting practical orientation is an important aspect of James's pragmatism and I will now draw on his formulation of pragmatism in order to further elaborate his account of emotion and locate it in the context of his broader philosophy.

Pragmatism

James's pragmatism treats all *conceptualized worlds* or *realities* as structures that enable our various practices. Whether we are referring to abstract scientific formulations or to the conceptual structure that is integral to everyday experience, conceptualized worlds are essentially maps, implicit or explicit tools that we use to guide our activities. Hence, if there is a genuine difference between two rival conceptualizations, there must be some difference in their practical consequences:

> There can *be* no difference anywhere that doesn't *make* a difference elsewhere—no difference in abstract truth that doesn't express itself in a difference in concrete fact and in conduct consequent upon that fact, imposed on somebody, somehow, somewhere, and somewhen. The whole function of philosophy ought to be to find out what definite difference it will make to you and me, at definite instants of our life, if this world-formula or that world-formula be the true one. (1981, p.27)

The connection that James proposes between worlds, construed as conceptual frameworks or patterns, and practices is not a contingent one. Worlds are inevitably tied to practices, given that they are partially made up of a background of values, concerns, interests and preferences that are themselves indissociable from our practical dispositions. James places the emphasis on world-construction rather than on world-revelation, as he thinks that a multitude of different, equally coherent conceptualizations could conceivably originate in the range of different capacities, concerns and preferences that regulate our activities. Many different conceptual worlds could be made that hold together, providing guiding frameworks for a host of different practices. This pluralism is especially apparent when we reflect upon other species and the very different ways in which they are attuned to things:

> Were we lobsters, or bees, it might be that our organization would have led to our using quite different modes from these of apprehending our experiences. It *might* be too (we can not dogmatically deny this) that such categories, unimaginable to us today, would have proved on the whole as serviceable for handling our experiences mentally as those which we actually use. (1981, p.79)[8]

James also claims that divergent sets of human concerns serve to *make* different conceptual universes. Reality is flexible enough to be shaped into all sorts of different patterns: 'in many familiar objects every one will recognize the human element. We conceive a given reality in this way or in that, to suit our purpose, and the reality passively submits to the conception' (1981, p.113). The predominance of some conceptual patterns over others is, according to James, not primarily a mark of their superior rationality or better fit with the world, but a symptom of historically entrenched, practical common sense and of the feeling of coherence that accompanies familiar categories (1981, chapter V). World-experience is never simply the outcome of our perceptual representations *conforming* to things outside. All objects of experience, whether encountered through everyday perception or from a theoretical standpoint, have our own contributions sewn into their structure and are thus partially *made* by us:

> ...even in the field of sensation, our minds exert a certain arbitrary choice. By our inclusions and omissions we trace the field's extent; by our emphasis we mark its foreground and its background; by our order we read it in this direction or in that. We receive in short the block of marble, but we carve the statue ourselves. (1981, pp.111–2)

Intentionality is conceptualized in practical terms, as a structure that does not merely reveal but also differently configures the experienced world. Given this, one can see why feeling, for James, is not something distinct from intentionality, peripheral to cognition, trivial or epiphenomenal. The experienced world is shaped by a habitual practical orientation from which feeling is inextricable.

----

[8] Damasio again echoes James, in claiming that 'if our organisms were designed differently, the constructions we make of the world around us would be different as well. We do not know, and it is improbable that we will ever know, what 'absolute' reality is like' (1995, p.97).

An account of emotion and 'world-making' offered more recently by Goodman (1978, 1984) is very close to that of James. Goodman claims that there is a plurality of made worlds, meaning conceptual systems that are taken for granted in experience, activity and thought. He suggests that emotion and feeling 'function cognitively in aesthetic and in much other experience' (1984, pp.7–8). Playing on Kant, he goes on to remark that 'feeling without understanding is blind, and understanding without feeling is empty' (1984, p.8). However, the role that James ascribes to emotions need not be couched in terms of Goodmanesque world-making and can also be extricated, to some extent, from the specifics of James's own formulation of pragmatism. Several philosophers have more recently said similar things about the everyday world being emotionally configured and about objects being experienced and conceptualized through our emotions. For example, de Sousa (1990) claims that emotions 'give us frameworks in terms of which we perceive, desire, act and explain' (p.24) and that they circumvent cognitive paralysis by '*controlling the salience of features of perception and reasoning*' (p.172). James's view also has some similarity to the proposal put forward by Roberts (1988, pp.191–2) that emotions are 'concern-based construals', which are not interpretations laid on top of already experienced objects but involve 'a *characterization of the object*, a way the object presents itself'.

In emphasizing the experiential role of emotion and also the fact that we encounter the world as feeling organisms that are entangled with it, rather than as detached onlookers that passively and unfeelingly gaze upon it from afar, James's account also has considerable affinity with my view of existential feeling. However, his pragmatism suggests a construal of experience whereby we are presented with the world-in-itself, which we carve up into conceptual patterns in accordance with our emotional dispositions. This differs from the view that emotions constitute existential backgrounds, as Jamesian emotions determine *how* we experience and conceive of what *is* rather than the sense we have *that* there is a world at all. The view that we impose patterns upon a pre-given world or 'carve the marble into a statue' is a partial return to the subjective–objective or internal–external perspective that James himself tries to escape from when he emphasizes the world of the feeling organism over that of the disembodied theorist. However, as noted earlier, James also acknowledges that states such as depression drain away the sense of reality, rather than just disrupting the conceptual patterns that we impose upon the world in our experience and thought. And this distinctive role for emotions is something that another of his doctrines, *radical empiricism*, might well accommodate.

Radical empiricism

When offering his biological account and when reflecting upon the phenomenological role of emotion, James stays methodologically rooted within the natural attitude, describing the role that emotions play in carving up a world the existence of which remains presupposed. He does not conceive of anything akin to the Husserlian *epoché* and so does not enquire as to how a sense of there being a reality that can be carved up by conceptual patterns is constituted in the first place. However, his doctrine of radical empiricism does attempt something like this. Pragmatism and radical empiricism are offered by James as complementary doctrines but there is some debate as to how they fit together. Wesley Cooper (2002, pp.69–70) suggests that James is a pragmatist at the empirical level and a radical empiricist when it comes to metaphysics. I think something like this is right. The radical empiricist is concerned with something that all within-world experience, thought and activity presuppose. James's project is now more like that of the phenomenologist. His aim is to uncover something that world-experience in the natural attitude takes for granted, whereas his pragmatism assumes the natural attitude and offers an account of how we experience, conceptualize and act upon a world that we are already in.

What makes this doctrine a form of 'empiricism'? James maintains, as empiricists do, that all his philosophical conclusions are susceptible to revision in the light of experience. His brand of empiricism is 'radical' because it does not adopt the kinds of tacit metaphysical presuppositions that so-called empiricists often do when making judgements as to what experience tells us. The radical empiricist does not start by quietly taking a particular, contingent conception of our relationship with the world for granted. So radical empiricism is not a 'half-way' empiricism like 'scientific naturalism', which 'dogmatically' affirms a form of monism, rather than looking to experience itself for guidance (James, 1897, vii–viii). James does champion a monistic position of sorts but he come to this view through reflection upon experience, rather than by presupposing some entrenched dogma. So the radical empiricist attempts to reflect upon the deliverances of experience in a way that is not constrained by a priori assumptions regarding how the world is and how we find ourselves in it; she tries to let experience speak for itself.

This method is somewhat like the Husserlian *epoché*, in that it advocates the putting out of play of all presupposed conceptions of our relationship with the world in order to reflect upon the deliverances of experience. One of its outcomes is the conclusion that there is a level of experience that does not incorporate a distinction between subject and object. What James calls 'pure experience' does not distinguish self from world. He adds that feelings should be understood at this level. They are neither subjective nor objective and do not ultimately respect the subject–object distinction. James claims that both 'common sense and popular philosophy are as dualistic as it is possible to be', with respect to distinctions such as that between subject and object (1912, p.137). Contrary to popular views, he suggests that contrasts between the subjective and objective aspects of experience or between the internal and external are symptomatic of different emphases in the descriptions we offer, rather than genuinely different categories of experience:

> There is no thought-stuff different from thing-stuff, I said; but the same identical piece of 'pure experience' (which was the name I gave to the *materia prima* of everything) can stand alternately for a 'fact of consciousness' or for a physical reality, according as it is taken in one context or in another. (1912, pp.137–8)

James goes on to say that the example of emotion 'illustrates beautifully my central thesis that subjectivity and objectivity are affairs not of what an experience is aboriginally made of, but of its classification' (1912, p.141). Emotions can be described as states of the subject or as ways in which their objects appear. For example, we can talk of a ''state' of pain' or of a 'painful place' (1912, p.142). According to James, the subjective feeling of an emotion and how its object appears are not different features of the emotion but different ways in which a single, unitary phenomenon is referred to. A subjective feeling is at the same time a way in which its object appears:

> The man is really hateful; the action really mean; the situation really tragic—all in themselves and quite apart from our opinion. We even go so far as to talk of a weary road, a giddy height, a jocund morning or a sullen sky. ... (1912, p.144)

For James, emotions are feelings and these feelings are neither subjective nor objective. He does not distinguish those feelings that constitute existential orientations from others that do not. Nevertheless, as the contrast between his earlier remarks regarding melancholic changes in the sense of reality and the above reference to perceiving an action as 'really mean' might suggest, he is at least sensitive to the fact that some feelings, but surely not all feelings, amount to existential orientations. What James calls 'pure experience' does, I think, serve to accommodate what I call existential feeling, given that it involves a level of experience that is prior to subject and object, and prior to any sense of a subject-independent reality. It is a ground that we take for granted when we experience or think about anything. Existential feelings might be construed as different shapes that pure experience can take on.

Perhaps one of the reasons James fails to draw a distinction between certain rather mundane feelings and what I call existential feelings is that he is sceptical of the exercise of classification more generally. His pragmatism implies that emotions will be classifiable in a range of equally legitimate ways, and he thinks that scientific conceptualizations are not in any way privileged over the conceptual frameworks that comprise the commonsense backdrop for everyday behaviours. The difference between them is just that they are tailored to different purposes and concerns:

> Every way of classifying a thing is but a way of handling it for some particular purpose. Conceptions, 'kinds', are teleological instruments. No abstract concept will be a valid substitute for a concrete reality except with reference to a particular interest in the conceiver. The interest of theoretic rationality, the relief of identification, is but one of a thousand human purposes. (1897, p.70)

It follows that any scientific account, including James's own physiological account of emotion, is but one of a plurality of different formulas, gelling only with some concerns. James (1890) explicitly endorses pluralism in the case of emotion, claiming that attempts to classify the emotions get us nowhere, contingent as they are on different purposes, none of which are objectively more legitimate than others:

> If then we should seek to break the emotions, thus enumerated, into groups, according to their affinities, it is again plain that all sorts of groupings would be possible, according as we chose this character or that as a basis, and that all groupings would be equally real and true. The only question would be, does this grouping or that suit our purpose best? (1890, p.485)

However, his account also implies that what he calls 'emotions' are not just conceptualized ingredients of a particular world-formula. They are the glue that binds worlds together into coherent conceptual patterns and imbues them with a significance that motivates us to act.[9] So 'emotion' refers to something that is not a feature of some contingently conceptualized world but a *precondition* for the meaningfulness of all the variously constituted conceptual worlds that form the backdrop for deliberation and action. Emotions can be categorized in any number of different ways but are themselves pre-conceptual enabling conditions for all acts of conceptualization; they operate

---

[9] Several recent authors have claimed that the emotions are not a 'natural kind'. For example, Rorty remarks that they are a 'heterogeneous group' (1980, p.1) and Griffiths proposes a 'three-way fracturing of the emotion category into socially sustained pretences, affect program responses and higher cognitive states' (1997, p.17). James's pluralism is more radical, as he rejects the idea of 'natural kinds' altogether.

at a level of experience that underlies all conceptual thought. Hence James's philosophical account is more fundamental to his view of emotion than the physiological account that he also offers. It addresses the constitution of an experienced world that physiological studies take for granted and it also supplies a coherent interpretive backdrop for his physiological claims.

To draw everything together, interpreting James's 1884/1890 account in the light of his other writings reveals a theory according to which:

1 Emotions are feelings of bodily changes, which are triggered reflexively during perception.
2 These feelings are partly constitutive of a practical orientation towards things.
3 This practical orientation structures all experience and conceptualization.
4 Emotions are thus a constituent of intentionality, which is construed in practical terms rather than as the disinterested representation of things external to us.
5 Emotions are neither subjective nor objective but feature in experience in a way that is prior to such distinctions.
6 Emotions structure how we experience, think and act within a world, and some of them also constitute a sense of reality and belonging that operates as a background to all world-experience.

There are some problems with this view. For example, premise (1) suggests that all emotions arise during perception, but it is clear that emotions can also be solicited by our thoughts and beliefs about the world, and by what we imagine. Hence the account needs to be broadened to acknowledge that emotions can be induced by more than just perception. Nevertheless, regardless of how emotions are *elicited*, the other aspect of (1), that emotions are feelings of bodily changes, can be retained, as can points (2) to (6). Another problem with the view is that many of the states we refer to as emotions do seem to have more to them than James admits. Emotions can be complex states with a narrative structure (Goldie, 2000). Now James could retort that any additional features of emotion that are posited are symptomatic of how emotions are conceptualized and classified, and that he doesn't care much for classification. However, if most of those states that we refer to as emotions are indeed *feelings as conceptualized in certain ways*, then refusing to admit this and focusing on feelings instead would amount to surreptitiously changing the subject and ignoring at least some emotions. For current purposes, I am happy to accept this criticism. I am interested in feelings and I think that most of what James says can be fruitfully regarded as relating to feelings, rather than to emotions. Indeed, many of the feelings he discusses, such as those that structure decision-making and give things their significance, do not have established names and do not appear in lists of standard emotions. As we will see in Chapter 9, the same goes for those feelings that guide philosophical enquiry.

What James says about *feeling*, even though it does not amount to a comprehensive account of *emotion*, is not vulnerable to the usual list of criticisms that are offered. James emphasizes the extent to which world-experience implicates the feeling body and he does not construe bodily feelings as ways of perceiving one particular object—the body. Feelings are not merely feelings of bodily changes; they do not have the body alone as an object; and they need not have the body as a primary object. James also recognizes that some feelings are constitutive of the sense of reality and significance, of the way in which we find ourselves in a world. Hence we arrive at the conclusion that for James, as for Solomon, certain emotions are the *meaning of life*. Solomon claims that they cannot play this role if they are mere feelings, whereas James claims that they play this role and that they are feelings. Hence Solomon's (1993) criticisms of James, which I mentioned in Chapter 1, are misplaced. James cannot be criticized for trivializing states that constitute a meaningful experiential world by maintaining that they are feelings, when what he actually says is that feelings are what constitute a meaningful experiential world. Furthermore, in claiming that the relevant feelings have a phenomenology that is pre-subjective and pre-objective, his account coheres with Solomon's view that emotions are not states of the subject or perceptions of a distant, external world but constitutive of the world that we inhabit; they are 'not occurrences but activities; they are not 'inside' our minds but rather the structures we place *in our world*' (Solomon, 1993, p.108). Solomon's account is frequently criticized both for its marginalization of bodily feelings and for its phenomenologically implausible emphasis on the extent to which we choose our emotions. By bringing feeling into the structure of world-experience and by emphasizing that the world is experienced by animate, feeling organisms rather than by disembodied, unfeeling minds, James avoids the neglect of bodily feelings.

One might raise the concern that attributing so much to feeling leads to a construal of how we find ourselves in the world that is overly passive. According to James, we do not control our feelings; they happen to us. Hence his position departs from Solomon's view that emotions are choices we make but it slides into the equally implausible opposite extreme of maintaining that they are passive events that wash over us:

> [Emotions are] almost always non-logical and beyond our control. How can the moribund old man reason back to himself the romance, the mystery, the imminence of great things with which our old earth tingled for him in the days when he was young and well? (1902, p.151)

This aspect of his position surely applies to what I call 'existential feelings' too. I argued in Chapter 6 that it is indeed sometimes impossible to see beyond one's current existential predicament. This is most likely so with the depression that James describes as feeling as though one were sheathed in india-rubber. Nothing gets through; nothing affects you. But many existential feelings, I have suggested, incorporate openness to other existential possibilities, a sense of their own contingency, the possibility of change. However, James (1884, p.197) does claim that we can, to an extent, control our bodily states (and presumably our environment) and, in so doing, supply the conditions under which particular emotions are or are not experienced. Implied by this is the view that we can, to a degree, regulate our emotions. In some cases at least, we can seek out the conditions that bring forth certain feelings and thus sustain, enhance or reshape the ways in which we find ourselves in the world. So we are not, after all, wholly passive before our feelings. In addition, some of the feelings that James discusses are not *passive* in a way that is to be contrasted with rational deliberation and choice, as they are important participants in decision-making processes.

It is also worth noting the similarity between James's view of emotion and Heidegger's account of mood, which I discussed in Chapter 2. Like James, Heidegger construes intentionality in terms of purposes and practical concerns. He also recognizes that, in addition to being directed towards things *in* a world, intentionality includes a background structure that constitutes how we find ourselves in the world. Moods, according to Heidegger, are an inextricable aspect of this structure; they are a background that gives sense to all our practical and theoretical dealings with things. For Heidegger, as for James, we do not *represent* the world in some abstract, detached manner but are in commerce with it, teleologically entwined and inseparable from it, with moods playing an essential role in constituting our everyday familiarity with things.

There are also more specific parallels. Like Heidegger, James draws a contrast between feelings of homeliness and unhomeliness, claiming that the latter can arise due to an uncomfortable sense of expectancy that lacks a specific object. Feeling at home in a place is, according to James, a matter of reducing felt uncertainty, of gaining a practical appreciation of the space of possibilities that comprises a situation; 'when after a few days we have learned the range of all these possibilities, the feeling of strangeness disappears' (1897, p.78). He adds that the same goes for people, when we gain a feeling of their character. James even refers to a certain feeling of pointlessness, insignificance and lack of motivation as a 'nameless *unheimlichkeit*' (1897, p.83).

To summarize, in this chapter I have (a) attempted to correct a persistent misinterpretation of a historical figure, (b) suggested that James, like Husserl,

Heidegger and Merleau-Ponty, says various things that complement my account of existential feeling and (c) further emphasized that feelings need not respect distinctions between internal and external or subjective and objective. However, another aim of the chapter is to set the scene for a discussion of the role of feelings in philosophical enquiry. As we will see in Chapter 9, James has a lot to say about this. Amongst other things, he indicates that some feelings take the form of existential backgrounds that dispose us to a range of philosophical positions, in addition to regulating our convictions and doubts.

Chapter 9

Stance, feeling and belief

This chapter explores the role of existential feelings in philosophical enquiry. In the process, it considers whether the kinds of anomalous feeling found in psychiatric illness might also underlie certain philosophical concerns. I introduce the topic by briefly discussing a case study offered by Louis Sass. Then I return to the writings of William James. In the last chapter, I offered an interpretation of James's account of emotion, according to which emotions are feelings of bodily changes, which structure all experience and thought. As I show in this chapter, James also claims that some feelings operate as existential orientations, and he makes numerous remarks to the effect that these orientations can motivate and also partly constitute philosophical positions. Following that, I turn to the writings of some more recent philosophers in order to further explore the role of existential feeling in philosophy, focusing on a book by Bas van Fraassen. I propose that some existential feelings amount to broad philosophical dispositions, which motivate the explicit positions that philosophers defend. These feelings also play a role in regulating episodic doubts and convictions that are indispensable to philosophical thought. I go on to discuss how discrepancies can arise between explicit philosophical claims or implicit presuppositions regarding how we find ourselves in a world and how we *actually* find ourselves in the world. In so doing, I consider what it means to really *believe* the claims that one makes. The chapter concludes by suggesting that acknowledgement of the role played by existential feeling in philosophy need not threaten the rationality of philosophical enquiry. Existential feelings can contribute to non-rational dogmatic commitments but they can also play a role in critical reflection, as can an explicit understanding of their role.

Feelings and philosophical positions

Sass (1994) compares the world of the schizophrenic person, as conveyed by Daniel Paul Schreber in his *Memoirs of my Nervous Illness*, to the predicament of the philosopher, as described by Wittgenstein. According to Sass, the two have much in common. Wittgenstein's work is preoccupied with the diagnosis and cure of problems that originate in philosophers' artificial detachment from everyday social experience, a detachment that involves both alienation and a disposition towards excessive reflection on what is ordinarily taken as given. In these respects, the philosopher's situation is not unlike that of the schizophrenic. They are both alienated from what most of us are rooted in. What troubles the philosopher is often symptomatic of this alienation and lack of homeliness:

> ... Wittgenstein's characterization [of philosophy as a sickness] can almost be taken literally: the sicknesses of the understanding he examined in his later work, sicknesses bound up with the philosopher's predilection for abstraction and alienation—for detachment from body, world, and community—have a great deal in common with the symptoms displayed by Schreber and many other mental patients with schizophrenia or related forms of illness. (Sass, 1994, x)

Of course, the two are not wholly similar and Sass acknowledges that, whereas madness engulfs a whole life, a philosophy is a more circumscribed intellectual position (1994, p.15). Nevertheless, it seems likely that a philosophical position is at least symptomatic of an existential orientation that does structure a life, and this is a view I will explore here. The diagnosis that Sass offers, according to which philosophy is associated with detachment and alienation, coupled with an excess of abstract reflection, does not apply to all philosophical thought. His aim is to offer a comparison between Wittgenstein's portrayal of confused thinking in philosophy and Schreber's way of being, rather than a comprehensive account of a universal philosophical predicament. Not every philosopher or philosophy will be driven by the same concerns or the same existential feelings.

In what follows, I will take a more general look at the role of feelings in philosophical enquiry. I will suggest that different ways of finding oneself in a world operate as pre-articulate dispositions that motivate explicit philosophical positions. Although I admit that some philosophers and philosophies are most likely influenced by the kind of predicament that Sass describes, I also emphasize the converse, where a tendency towards abstractions that are divorced from everyday experience is symptomatic of the philosopher feeling *too* at home in the world, so at home in fact that she becomes largely oblivious to it.

The view that different philosophies have their source in different existential backgrounds is advocated by James in several of his works. He applies his philosophical position concerning the nature and role of feeling to the activity of philosophizing, making clear throughout that his philosophy is first and foremost an articulate expression of his own feelings. According to James, broad philosophical claims concerning how the world is and how we gain epistemic access to it are not and cannot be evaluated by means of rational argument alone. He ascribes a more significant role to feelings, claiming that the experienced plausibility of a view is primarily a matter of how it is felt: a philosopher judges a conception of the world 'by certain subjective marks with which it affects him' (1897, p.63).

A weak version of this view would be that the 'subjective marks' steer a philosopher towards one already formulated world-view rather than another. But James makes the stronger claim that it is only through certain feelings that philosophical positions coalesce and make sense to a person. It is feelings that hold a philosophy together as an harmonious whole. A 'strong feeling of ease, peace, rest' and 'relief' constitutes both a sense of the position's coherence and a disposition towards endorsing it (1897, p.63). He states that:

> Nothing could be more absurd than to hope for the definitive triumph of any philosophy which should refuse to legitimate, and to legitimate in an emphatic manner, the more powerful of our emotional and practical tendencies. (1897, p.88)

Use of the term 'absurd' implies something stronger than just 'inadvisable' or 'mistaken', and this is no accident. James is suggesting that these tendencies contribute to the experienced meaningfulness of the philosophies that we explicitly formulate. So any philosophy that did not satisfy some such tendency would indeed be an incoherent enterprise. Philosophizing does not consist of abstract thought decoupled from the feeling person:

> Pretend what we may, the whole man within us is at work when we form our philosophical opinions. Intellect, will, taste, and passion co-operate just as they do in practical affairs. (1897, p.92)

As the word 'pretend' indicates, this is something that is seldom explicitly acknowledged. James remarks elsewhere that 'there arises [...] a certain insincerity in our philosophic discussions: the potentest of all our premises is never mentioned' (1981, p.9). Our most fundamental philosophical commitments are partly comprised of feeling but these commitments remain inarticulate, implicit.

The view that feelings contribute to the perceived meaningfulness of philosophical positions is implausible when applied to specific claims and arguments. The meaning of an assertion or the cogency of an argument surely does not depend upon a particular kind of feeling. However, the kinds of position to which James refers are much more general in scope. They are broad philosophical doctrines, such as rationalism, empiricism, naturalism or antinaturalism. These doctrines, he suggests, are partly made up of kinds of inarticulate sentiment and so cannot be exhaustively described in terms of propositional commitments. They operate as backgrounds to explicit theorizing, determining the kinds of debate that are deemed worthy of engaging with, the kinds of argumentative strategy that are favoured, which arguments are taken seriously and which are dismissed altogether as somehow wrong-headed in their premises or general strategy.

Hence explicit philosophical claims, theories and systems elicit feelings and these feelings are symptomatic of underlying dispositions. James refers to these dispositions as 'temperaments'. The philosopher, we are told:

> ...*trusts* his temperament. Wanting a universe that suits it, he believes in any represen-tation of the universe that does suit it. He feels men of opposite temper to be out of key with the world's character, and in his heart considers them incompetent and 'not in it,' in the philosophical business, even though they may far excel him in dialectical ability. (1981, p.8)

Temperaments are already in place before reasoned argument gets to work. Where they diverge, philosophers do not connect and arguments ventured by both sides fail to convince. Each participant takes for granted her own way of belonging to the world and does not explicitly contemplate the contribution that different modes of belonging to the world might make to the disagree-ment. Philosophy is not just a matter of trading arguments or of formulating positions on the basis of reason and evidence. A substantial element of a philosophical position comes ready-made in the way that one finds oneself in a world:

> ...the philosophy which is so important in each of us is not a technical matter; it is our more or less dumb sense of what life honestly and deeply means. It is only partly got from books; it is our individual way of just seeing and feeling the total push and pressure of the cosmos. (James, 1981, p.7)
>
> ...in the metaphysical and religious sphere, articulate reasons are cogent for us only when our inarticulate feelings of reality have already been impressed in favor of the same conclusion. (James, 1902, p.74)

By 'feelings of reality', I think James means something very similar to what I have described using the term 'existential feeling'. Philosophers, like everyone else, vary in the manner and extent to which they find themselves at home in the world. Associated with inter- and intra-personal variations in the feeling of belonging are variations in the sense of reality. Some people consistently belong to the world in such a way that they are never troubled by existential worries. For others, the feeling of reality is diminished, fragile or changeable. These different ways of belonging dispose people towards different explicit philosophies.

James is not advocating a form of *psychologism* here, according to which an understanding of why philosophical positions are adopted or dismissed consists in an account of the motivating psychology involved, rather than an appeal to the rationale of those positions. The kind of feeling he refers to is not something that could ever be comprehensively understood in terms of an empirical psychology. Existential feelings, I have argued, constitute the sense of reality and so cannot be fully accommodated by any enquiry that presupposes the sense of reality and takes, as its starting point, a being that is already in a world. James similarly acknowledges that feelings play a role which is presupposed by any account of what the world contains.

James construes the history of philosophy as a 'clash of temperaments' (1981, p.8) and, in several of his works, he claims that disagreements between rationalists and empiricists ultimately come down to this. For example, he contrasts the 'tender-minded' empiricist with the 'tough-minded' rationalist (1981, p.10). James does not restrict his remarks to *kinds* of temperament that are shared by large groups of philosophers. He also offers diagnoses of how the feelings of particular *individuals* shape their metaphysical commitments. For instance, in the case of McTaggart:

> When Mr. McTaggart himself believes that the universe is run by the dialectical energy of the absolute idea, his insistent desire to have a world of that sort is felt by him to be no chance example of desire in general, but an altogether peculiar insight-giving passion to which, in this if no other instance, he would be *stupid* not to yield. (1970, pp.260–1).

A philosopher's *belief* in the nature of the universe is inextricable from his *desire* for it to be that way. The universe, as conceived of in that way, solicits conviction in the form of a feeling of truth, coherence, rightness. The pull of this is irresistible. Feeling opens up a space of philosophical possibilities and at the same time renders some of them enticing. However, it is important to recognize that feelings of conviction are not always *positive* in tone. A feeling of dread or horror can also be a feeling of revelation.

Although James concedes that rational debate is ineffective when underlying existential orientations differ, I do not think he is advocating a form of relativism or irrationalism with regard to philosophical enquiry, where we have a wide range of temperaments and no possibility of rational comparison or debate. The first thing we can do is articulate the kinds of existential feeling that underlie our explicit doctrines. James is quite happy to voice his own and encourages others to do the same:

> ...since we are in the main not sceptics, we might go on and frankly confess to each other the motives of our several faiths. I frankly confess mine—I can not but think that at bottom they are of an aesthetic and not of a logical sort. The 'through-and-through' universe seems to suffocate me with its infallible impeccable all-pervasiveness. Its necessity, with no possibilities; its relations, with no subjects, make me feel as if I had entered into a contract with no reserved rights, or rather as if I had to live in a large seaside boarding-house with no private bed-room in which I

might take refuge from the society of the place. [....] It seems too buttoned-up and white-chokered and clean-shaven a thing to speak for the vast slow-breathing unconscious Kosmos with its dread abysses and its unknown tides. (1912, pp.276–8)

He adds:

I show my feelings; why *will* they not show theirs? I know they *have* a personal feeling about the through-and-through universe, which is entirely different from mine, and which I should very likely be much the better for gaining if they would only show me how. (1912, p.278)

Understanding the phenomenology of existential feeling and describing the differences between existential feelings are not easy tasks. Complaining that the rationalist universe is comparable to the alienating anonymity of a shared seaside boarding-house is, I suppose, a start. Nevertheless, a clearer and more detailed description of how one finds oneself in a world and how that orientation attunes one to an explicit philosophical position is surely possible. The 'confessing' of existential feelings that contribute to our philosophical commitments is itself a philosophical project, which involves careful phenomenological reflection rather than a few minutes of simple and honest soul-searching.

Where would this project get us? At the very least, it could help to distinguish those instances of philosophical disagreement that are due to differing existential orientations from those that are due to other factors, such as whether or not a particular argument is accepted as watertight. However, James does not stop here. He also indicates that some feelings are *better* guides to truth than others:

That we all of us have feelings, [...] that they may be as prophetic and anticipatory of truth as anything else we have, and some of them more so than others, can not possibly be denied. (1912, p.279)

Under the assumption that this is so, the question arises as to how existential feelings that are conducive to fruitful philosophical enquiry might be distinguished from those that are not. In the remainder of the chapter, I will offer a partial answer.

As I will discuss in Chapter 10, James suggests that some philosophical and religious thought arises from the kinds of feelings that occur in psychiatric illness. For example, a philosophy might originate in feelings of insecurity regarding the self–world relation, perhaps in the sense that the world might not be real and that nothing is dependable. But that a view crystallizes out of anomalous or even psychotic experience need not, he says, count against it. However, he does suggest another criterion for drawing a distinction, by contrasting philosophies that genuinely engage with our predicament with others that just pretend to. Some philosophies, he says, immerse themselves in abstractions that have no bearing on how the world is actually encountered. They have, he suggests, become disconnected from a feeling of belonging to the world that they continue to quietly presuppose. The philosopher who explicitly doubts the existence of the world or wonders how it is that we manage to connect up with it could well be quite happily at home in it. Thus, although the existential predicament of the schizophrenic person might have genuine similarities to that of some philosophers, it has only superficial linguistic similarities to that of others. In fact, the schizophrenic who has lost the sense of reality and the philosopher who doubts the existence of the world are sometimes polar opposites. The former has an all-encompassing sense of homelessness, whilst the latter is so at home in the world that she does not even know it.

Many of James's criticisms are directed at the rationalist, who he charges with retreating into a realm of cosy abstractions and with becoming disconnected from how she and most of the rest of us find ourselves in the world. The rationalist universe, he says:

> …is far less an account of this actual world than a clear addition built upon it, a classic sanctuary in which the rationalist fancy may take refuge from the intolerably confused and gothic character which mere facts present. It is no *explanation* of our concrete universe, it is another thing altogether, a substitute for it, a remedy, a way of escape. (1981, p.14)

When it comes to philosophies that have become disconnected from the realities of experience, it is helpful to distinguish two different kinds of detachment. One is where the proponent feels a strong sense of conviction with respect to an explicit claim, without recognizing the content of that claim to be wholly removed from how she actually finds herself in the world. Take the claim 'I doubt that the world exists'. A philosopher cannot really doubt the world's existence so long as her experience and thought continue to take for granted a sense of reality and belonging. But, all the same, she might well have a genuine feeling of conviction regarding her assertions, having failed to appreciate their discordance with the reality that she continues to obliviously presuppose. So there is a kind of double-think going on here and this, I suggest, is the kind of failing that James wants to charge the rationalist with. Another kind of detachment is where the philospher has no feelings at all in relation to the proposition that he accepts or rejects. For example, he might simply put the word 'not' in front of 'the world exists' and claim to have doubted the world's existence in the process. Hence there are at least three different kinds of explicit 'belief' that could be communicated by the claim 'I doubt that the world exists':

1 One undergoes an existential shift involving an erosion of the feeling of reality and comes to genuinely believe that the world's existence is doubtful.

2 One is oblivious to what one takes for granted but has a genuine feeling of conviction towards the proposition 'the world might not exist'.

3 One takes the proposition 'the world exists', puts the word 'not' in front of it and claims to have doubted that the world exists.

Claiming that the assertion 'I doubt that the world exists' communicates a 'propositional attitude' does nothing whatsoever to distinguish between these alternatives. However, we can see that (1) is a genuine kind of doubt, where the sense of reality is no longer taken for granted; (2) is also a genuine kind of doubt but it is a confused doubt, which can be exposed as such by reflecting upon the existential background that it continues to take for granted; (3) is not a genuine doubt at all but a linguistic exercise, which consists solely of adding the word 'not' to something. But still the philosopher might not explicitly *know* this; she might think that she doubts something even though she is not really doing so. Perhaps she mistakenly assumes that, for philosophical purposes at least, this is what *doubt* consists of.

So an appreciation of the role of existential feelings and of feelings more generally can, I suggest, serve to clarify the differences between kinds of philosophical conviction and thus play a methodological role in philosophical enquiry. In the remainder of this chapter, I will further discuss how existential feelings and also reflection upon these feelings can contribute both to doctrinal commitments and to philosophical critique. To do so, I will turn to some more recent philosophical discussions that address the nature of philosophical commitment.

Philosophical stances

A simple objection to the view that existential feelings are integral to broad philosophical doctrines is that such doctrines can be comprehensively described in terms of the acceptance of a series of inter-related propositions. All of these propositions are perfectly intelligible, regardless of how someone feels. So feelings might well dispose a person towards a particular view but they are dissociable from the content of that view. In response, it should be noted that some philosophical doctrines, such as empiricism and naturalism for example, have proved very difficult to characterize in this way. Indeed, it is arguable that the attempt to do so is either ill-conceived or even, in some cases at least, self-refuting. Van Fraassen (2002) argues that the latter applies to empiricism. It cannot, he says, be a metaphysical position adopted on the basis of something other than experience, as its acceptance would then be contrary to the empiricist's reliance upon experience. It cannot consist in the dogmatic and unwavering acceptance of an empirical proposition either. That too would be contrary to empiricism, a doctrine that takes all empirical claims to be contestable. In order to characterize empiricism without falling into one trap or the other, van Fraassen offers an alternative account of it as a *stance*, rather than a set of propositions that are taken to be true:

> A philosophical position can consist in a stance (attitude, commitment, approach, a cluster of such—possibly including some propositional attitudes such as beliefs as well). Such a stance may of course be expressed, and may involve or presuppose some beliefs as well, but cannot be simply equated with having beliefs or making assertions about what there is. (2002, pp.47–8)

Van Fraassen calls this the *empirical stance* rather than the *empiricist stance* but takes the empiricist to be someone who adopts this empirical stance as a basis for enquiry. I suggest that we distinguish between the *strong* and the *weak* empiricist, where the former is committed to thinking about science and pursuing philosophy *exclusively* through the empirical stance, whilst the latter adopts it only for certain purposes. Van Fraassen's insistence that empiricism be free of all metaphysical presuppositions that are not based on experience suggests that he is a strong empiricist (sometimes, at least). A proponent of the weak view would not be troubled by the thought that empiricism is not all-encompassing or self-supporting. In what follows, I will reject strong stance empiricism but I will not challenge the legitimacy and utility of adopting an empirical stance for at least some purposes.

We might think of a stance as an attitude or group of inter-related attitudes that someone explicitly adopts towards a subject matter. The proposal by Teller (2004) that stances be construed as 'epistemic policies' suggests such a view; policies are usually knowingly adopted on the basis of deliberation. However, Teller also notes that it is important to distinguish between implicit and explicit stances. One can unreflectively inhabit a stance, rather than taking it as an object of cognition or explicitly assenting to it. It is not always clear whether van Fraassen's 'empirical stance' is something that he takes to be knowingly adopted or implicitly inhabited. In any case, the two kinds of stance will be intimately related, given that an implicit orientation will dispose one towards the adoption of certain explicit attitudes and beliefs. Thus we might think of implicit and explicit stances as *aspects* of a more encompassing philosophical stance, rather than as wholly distinct. It is the implicit aspect that I will focus on here.

At various points, it does seem that van Fraassen conceives of a stance as an implicit, pre-articulate background, rather than as a conceptual framework that is explicitly adopted by a subject who already finds herself in a world. For example, he compares his conception of a 'stance' to Husserl's conception of the 'natural attitude' and also suggests that stances are 'existential orientations' (van Fraassen, 1994). As I discussed in Parts I and II, the natural attitude is not akin to the propositional attitude of believing that some entity exists. It is something that is already in place before any such attitude is adopted, a sense of belonging to a world that operates as a backdrop to all experiences and thoughts. So an implicit stance, construed in this way, is not something adopted within a pre-conceived world. Earlier in the book, I also argued that what Husserl calls the 'natural attitude' varies in structure, from person to person and time to time, with some people having more consistent orientations than others. Different variants might well dispose people towards different questions, lines of enquiry, commitments and degrees of commitment.

In addition to construing stances as existential orientations, van Fraassen acknowledges that they incorporate feeling and approvingly draws on the work of James, to argue for the view that a shift in stance requires a kind of felt transformation of the world (van Fraassen, 2002, lecture 3).[1] Given these references to existential orientations and feelings, I suggest that the implicit stance or the implicit aspect of a stance can be characterized, at least in part, in terms of existential feeling.

Van Fraassen (2002, p.155) appreciates that there are many different kinds of stance and contrasts two very broad existential orientations: a secular contentment with the scientific world-view, and an 'abiding wonder' at the being of the world that is more typical of the religious life. The former is incorporated into a range of doctrines that go by the name 'naturalism' or closely associated labels such as 'physicalism' and 'materialism'. Van Fraassen argues that naturalism, like empiricism, involves a distinctive kind of stance. So it too cannot be adequately described in terms of a set of explicit propositions that the naturalist assents to. The attempt to do so risks attributing metaphysical commitments to the naturalist that are in tension with naturalism.

One way of characterizing naturalism is to maintain that it is synonymous with physicalism, the doctrine that everything is physical. But, van Fraassen asks, what does it mean to say that everything is physical? It cannot be a metaphysical claim, accepted in advance of scientific enquiry, given that physicalism is scientifically motivated. And it is surely not the unwavering acceptance of everything that current physics tells us about the world. It is not at all clear what current physics does tell us and, even if it were, a doctrine that placed so much weight on current scientific theories would be unjustifiable, given that most of these theories are very likely to be incomplete or false. Perhaps physicalism is committed to the view that reality consists only of what some future physics will include, presumably a complete physics. However, even under the assumption

---

[1] Van Fraassen (2002, p.104) also appeals to Sartre's account of emotion as something that 'magically' transforms the world and thus facilitates a shift in philosophical, scientific or everyday orientation (see Sartre, 1994).

that such an accomplishment is possible, we do not know what a complete physics would look like or whether it would be a science of *physics* in a sense to be contrasted with other scientific domains. So it is not clear what is meant by 'physical' and neither is it clear what it is for something to be 'non-physical' in such a way as to contradict physicalism (van Fraassen, 2002, pp.51–3).[2]

Hence doctrines such as physicalism and naturalism are presumably not committed to specific metaphysical claims. Their faith in the deliverances of science requires that they neither rest on metaphysical presuppositions regarding the nature of the universe nor dogmatically insist on the truth of certain contingent scientific claims. Van Fraassen concludes that, although such doctrines might superficially look like theories, they are actually stances, evaluative attitudes rather than assortments of propositional beliefs. Central to a naturalistic stance is a feeling or desire that philosophy be guided by science:

> ...materialists may take themselves to be maintaining a theory while they are in reality merely expressing attitudes, in ways that lend themselves to such expression only under conditions of confusion and unclarity. (2002, p.50)
>
> If the 'physicalist' or 'naturalist' part of this philosophical position is mainly the desire or commitment to have metaphysics guided by physics, then it is something that cannot be captured in any thesis or factual belief. (2002, p.59)

Van Fraassen is not alone in thinking that, contrary to appearances, naturalism is not a factual doctrine. For example, Rea (2002) argues that, despite being the 'academic orthodoxy', naturalism has no 'rational foundation' (2002, p.1). It is not, first and foremost, an explicit position but a non-rational, ordinarily pre-articulate sense of which sources of evidence and methods of evidence-collection we ought to trust:

> In order to even begin an inquiry, we must already have various dispositions to trust at least some of our cognitive faculties as sources of evidence and to take certain kinds of experiences and arguments to be evidence. (2002, p.2)

Rea refers to these as our 'methodological dispositions' and claims that they together comprise a largely implicit 'research program', which determines the scope of acceptable evidence (2002, p.4). The terms 'methodological' and 'research programme' are slightly misleading, as many of the relevant dispositions are not explicitly recognized by the naturalist. Nevertheless, these terminological concerns do not detract from his conclusion that 'what unifies those who call themselves naturalists is not a particular philosophical thesis but

---

[2] Several others have argued that physicalism, if treated as a metaphysical thesis, is empty. For example, Crane and Mellor (1990, p.206) claim that 'in no non-vacuous sense is physicalism true'.

rather a set of methodological dispositions, a commonly shared approach to philosophical inquiry' (2002, p.22). If naturalism is advocated as an ontological thesis, it is, Rea says, 'vacuous, obviously false, or incompatible with possible developments in the natural sciences' (2002, p.59). His view therefore complements, for the most part, van Fraassen's claim that naturalism is a stance.

The assertions of certain naturalistically inclined philosophers lend support to this diagnosis. For example, Searle (2000, p.90) remarks that 'a sane philosophy *starts* with atomic theory and evolutionary biology and with the fact that we are identical with our living bodies, and goes on from there'. He offers no argument for this and instead takes it to be an uncontroversial premise. It seems to be a commitment that he *inhabits*, something he just takes to be immediately obvious on the basis of a conviction that he neglects to describe, rather than a debatable doctrine that is amenable to rational debate.

Dennett likewise adopts a naturalistic attitude as the starting point for philosophical enquiry. He describes this as a 'tactical choice' (1987, p.5). Why make such a choice? The final court of appeal again seems to be a very general and rather vague sense of what the world is like, what the important philosophical questions are and how they are best approached. Dennett contrasts his naturalism with Nagel's (1986) assertions to the effect that an objective, scientific view will never be able to accommodate everything, and he proceeds to charge Nagel with mysticism. The disagreement between them, as both acknowledge, stems from contrasting ground-floor intuitions concerning the nature of the world, the scope of our epistemic abilities and the goals to which philosophy should aspire. For Dennett, whether a 'starting point' ultimately bears fruit adds a pragmatic criterion for assessing its success. However, whether or not one regards a doctrine as having 'borne fruit' will, I assume, depend to some extent upon the stance that one has already adopted.

Some of Dennett's comments suggest that the difference between his philosophical orientation and that of Nagel comes down to different feelings. For example, he states that 'our tastes are different' and that 'Nagel is oppressed by the desire to develop an evolutionary explanation of the human intellect' whilst he, in contrast, is 'exhilarated'. He adds that Nagel recommends embracing what to him looks like a '*reductio ad absurdum*' (1987, p.5). This appraisal of the situation implies that it will not be resolvable via rational argument. As Dennett acknowledges, 'the feeling then is mutual; we beg the question against each other' (1987, p.6). Nagel goes so far as to say that the difference between them 'will presumably end only in the grave, if then' (1995, p.86). So, if these two philosophers are anything to go by, it does indeed look as though disagreements between naturalists and their critics are partly a matter of philosophical dispositions that are in place before explicit reasoning gets to work.

A similar assessment is offered by Baker, with reference to the choice between a physicalist philosophy and her own version of pragmatism:

> Both the physicalist and the pragmatist are rational, but neither is moved by the other's arguments. To the methodological physicalist, the pragmatist looks shallow and unprincipled; to the methodological pragmatist, the physicalist looks rigid and out of touch with reality. Hence, the impasse. (2001, p.37)

Sounding rather Jamesian, she adds that 'the sublime elegance of physicalism is seductive, but the rough-and-tumble of pragmatism seems closer to reality, as we all know it' (p.38).

Hence there is plenty of evidence, in the form of both arguments and 'confessions', to support the view that differences between philosophies owe at least something to background existential orientations that are not themselves the products of enquiry. Pre-reflective, felt commitments shape philosophical thought and make some explicit positions appear more enticing than others.

Stance, commitment and critique

A phenomenological approach incorporates reflection upon the structure of existential orientations that are more usually *implicit*, meaning that they operate as backgrounds to experience and thought rather than being objects of experience and thought. The kind of philosophical enquiry I have pursued here does not itself rely upon the implicit assumption of a single, constant existential background. Rather, it is made possible by the changeability of existential feeling. A shift in existential feeling reveals something of what was previously implicit, and different kinds of shift cast light on different ways of belonging to the world. Once a way of belonging to the world is revealed to be contingent, it need not be taken for granted by one's enquiries in the way it previously was.

Existential phenomenology is a background theme throughout van Fraassen's discussion of stances. In addition to describing stances as 'existential' he suggests that philosophical work should be an 'authentic, engaged project in the world', a project that is 'self-conscious and conscious of what sort of enterprise it is' (2002, p.195). To unthinkingly inhabit a stance is a rather unphilosophical thing to do and van Fraassen does not do this. Instead, he attempts to make his own existential orientation explicit. However, this exercise does not ultimately sway his faith in empiricism. Having made the empirical stance explicit, he then affirms his commitment to it. He also claims that a stance view of empiricism serves to insulate it from certain justificatory demands. One can legitimately be called upon to justify explicit premises but not, in the same way, to justify a stance. He defends a form of voluntarism, according to which a person is rationally *permitted*, rather than rationally *obliged*, to adopt a particular stance. This alleged immunity from rational critique has itself been subject to criticism. For example, Ladyman (2000, p.845) states that it is unclear 'why adopting an unjustifiable stance or attitude is any more respectable than simply accepting a proposition [...] which cannot be justified by its own lights'.

In defence of van Fraassen, whenever an implicit stance is *operating*, it cannot itself be an object of criticism or indeed an object of description. Whilst one is busy *being* an empiricist, one cannot justify one's stance and the same goes for stances more generally. The empiricist cannot begin to describe, let alone justify, her stance unless she *disengages* to some extent from the empiricist project, unless she *brackets* that project and reflects upon its structure.

It might be objected that the same stance can be adopted either implicitly or explicitly and that making an implicit stance explicit does not therefore require any change in one's commitment to it, any disengagement or reorientation of stance. However, whereas implicitly inhabiting a stance implies unthinking *acceptance* of it, explicit contemplation of that same stance accommodates a range of different attitudes towards it, including rejection, doubt or acceptance. Hence, the project of describing a stance involves suspending commitments that are ordinarily unthinkingly accepted, facilitating in the process the possibility of explicit attitudes towards them other than that of acceptance.

Consider Husserl's procedure with respect to the natural attitude. In order to describe this everyday stance, he suspends it through the *epoché* and comes to inhabit a different existential orientation, a *phenomenological stance* if you like. Whilst accepting the world, one might ask what exists or what grounds there are for believing that certain things exist. But, having withdrawn from the natural attitude and suspended a commitment to the existence of things, one can now study the structure of that attitude and of the commitment that it incorporates. Suspending the natural attitude in this way is not an easy thing to do and, as stated in the Introduction, I do not advocate as part of my own method a complete *epoché*, through which the structure of everyday experience is bracketed in its entirety. However, regardless of whether or not such a radical and complete perspectival shift is actually possible, the point remains that one has to suspend commitment to a stance—at least to some extent—in order to describe that stance. This applies to the empirical stance too. Rather than committing to evaluative judgements that are typical of empiricism, such as 'to get knowledge, we should look to experience', one brackets them by bracketing the stance that they are embedded in. One studies them, rather than simply adopting them. Husserl makes the same point with reference to what he calls the naturalistic stance, the attitude of scientific naturalism:

> As long as we live in the naturalistic attitude, it itself is not given in our field of research; what is grasped there is only what is experienced in it, what is thought in it, etc. (1989, p.183)

Through a phenomenological stance, we can attempt to make explicit the structure of the empirical stance. And this is pretty much what van Fraassen does. He brackets his commitment and attempts to describe its structure, rather than thinking and living *through* that commitment. However, characterization of a stance need not be followed by re-affirmation of that stance. It can result in an appreciation of the stance's contingency, its inability to encompass all that is. The shift in existential feeling that facilitates contemplation of an existential orientation that one used to take for granted is, at the same time, a sense of there being other possibilities. It has to be, given that the changed existential orientation which phenomenological enquiry itself involves is one such possibility.

In addition to revealing the contingency of stances that were previously inhabited and describing them, this kind of phenomenological enquiry also has the potential to criticize and undermine certain stances, by exposing their pretensions and confusions. For example, the *naturalistic stance* is taken by Husserl (1989, p.29) to be a theoretical attitude that involves a spectatorial 'disengaging' from practical dealings.[3] He claims that this stance continues to tacitly presuppose a practical appreciation of the existence of things that is integral to the natural attitude, whilst at the same time explicitly denying that there is anything more to the world than what can be revealed to a naturalistic stance. Naturalism of the kind that Husserl takes issue with is partly comprised of the felt conviction that certain epistemic practices are adequate to the task of understanding absolutely everything. But the existential background that these practices themselves presuppose cannot be examined by means of them. The way in which the naturalist finds himself in the world is at the same time his obliviousness to how he finds herself in a world and, consequently, a disposition to misinterpret his relationship with the world. In Parts I and II, I similarly criticized popular philosophical approaches to experience and belief for being oblivious to a sense of belonging that they themselves quietly assume.

---

[3] See Heidegger (1962, Division One: III) for a similar characterization of naturalism.

Hence the project of describing stances can incorporate critique, and the very *possibility* of such a critical project itself amounts to a criticism of the view that philosophy is to be done by *committing* to a particular stance. Van Fraassen describes becoming an empiricist as 'similar or analogous to conversion to a cause, a religion, an ideology, to capitalism or to socialism, to a worldview' (2002, p.61). The empirical stance, although initially implicit, can be made explicit and then knowingly and legitimately adopted. However, once a stance that facilitates description of pre-reflective empiricist commitment has been adopted, one is not then in a *philosophical* position to authentically commit to the empirical stance, given that a realm of enquiry has been discovered that is not encompassed by the empirical stance. The philosopher can, at this point, either knowingly commit to something partial and restrictive or adopt a more open, critical attitude towards stances and a broader conception of philosophical enquiry. One could authentically adopt an empirical stance as an *aspect* of philosophical enquiry but wholesale commitment to it in the form of strong empiricism is unwarranted. Philosophy as conversion to a cause should be contrasted with philosophy as ideological critique.[4] Given that van Fraassen's view of stances accommodates the possibility of the latter, the former amounts to a rather unphilosophical stance.

Phenomenology, I have suggested, can include a form of critical reflection upon the structure of stances that does not itself require the dogmatic adoption of a particular existential orientation.[5] However, the rejection of philosophy as dogmatic commitment should not be contrasted with a philosophy that involves no commitment at all. One can commit oneself for certain purposes and also adopt an overall philosophical approach that is fairly consistent in its orientation, whilst at the same time remaining open to other possibilities. A significant difference between kinds of philosophical stance, as with existential orientations in general, is that between stances which are open to other possibilities and others which are closed off. There is also a difference between openness and lack of rootedness though. A philosopher can be open to possibilities without drifting along in an unstructured fashion from one view to another.

---

4 Rowbottom (2005, p.221) likewise objects to aspects of van Fraassen's account on the basis that philosophical enquiry is characterized by a 'critical attitude', rather than by inflexible commitment.

5 A phenomenological approach incorporates an attitude of critical reflection towards what is ordinarily taken for granted but is certainly not the only possible critical attitude. Hence I do not seek to endorse an exclusively phenomenological approach to philosophy. However, neither do I want to be excessively permissive and maintain that any old critical stance is legitimate.

Feeling and epistemic disposition

I have claimed that an appreciation of the role of existential feeling in philosophical enquiry, and also the practice of reflecting upon one's own and others' existential feelings, can both be integrated into philosophical enquiry. In addition, I have stressed that this need not amount to the endorsement of dogmatic commitment. Indeed, a failure to acknowledge the role of background commitment is more likely to result in dogma and confusion. However, existential feelings and feelings more generally play other important roles in philosophical enquiry too, which do not depend upon their being explicitly acknowledged and reflected upon. We have already seen that they play a role in commitment. But not all feelings take the form of stable, enduring background orientations. Existential feelings change and can thus play a role in the revision or abandonment of commitments. In addition, enquiry is regulated by episodic feelings.

James observes that, before any enquiry can even get off the ground, its scope must be limited. The enquirer must already have a sense of what is significant and worth pursuing.[6] He also recognizes that, once a course of investigation has been embarked upon, feelings play the further role of managing both doubt and conviction. This latter role has been discussed more recently by Hookway (2002, 2003), who argues that feelings play an indispensable role in all intellectual activity. For example, they tell us when to stop asking questions, searching for evidence, testing a hypothesis or vacillating over whether or not to accept some claim or finding. Our subject matter does not tell us when to stop and, in most cases, there is no rational calculus that can be employed in order to determine that we have now done enough. It is our doubts that keep us asking questions and prevent us from settling with what we've got. The kind of doubt involved has, Hookway recognizes, a *felt quality*—a phenomenology—analogous to some other strong emotions. There is a "gut reaction"—a "felt doubt"' (2002, p.256). Even in those scenarios where it is possible to gather all the relevant data, do the calculations and make an informed assessment of whether or not the data are adequate, felt doubt can still be a useful strategy. It is much faster than systematic, unfeeling assessment of all the evidence and therefore offers a cognitive shortcut.

Felt doubts are not the abstract doubts of sceptics but real doubts that embody a feeling of dissatisfaction, tension, unsettledness or unease with the point that one has reached. Many of our evaluations have a pre-articulate,

---

[6] See also de Sousa (1990) for the complementary claim that emotions shape experience, thought and activity by configuring the experienced world in terms of 'patterns of salience'.

habitual and felt character. Skilful judgement is ordinarily a matter of being attuned to a situation type in a bodily, pre-reflective way, rather than of being able to mechanically weigh up the evidence and perform complex inferences:

> When properly trained in the mastery of concepts and techniques of inquiry, when properly educated in the exercise of judgment, our habitual evaluations enable us to inquire well without excessive reflection. (Hookway, 2003, p.88)

However, successful enquiry cannot be regulated by doubt alone. Enquiry must end somewhere. So we need to have the right balance of feelings. In addition to the feelings that sustain consistent, long-term doctrinal commitments, there are also episodic feelings of *conviction*. Some feelings constitute a sense of satisfaction with a conclusion or result, the sense that one has done enough. As Hookway puts it:

> ...the end of inquiry must be regulated by an emotional change. This certainly involves the elimination of anxiety about one's epistemic position, and it may also involve an emotional acknowledgement that one's position renders further inquiries inappropriate. (2002, p.258)

He adds that people differ in their epistemic dispositions and suggests that distinctions between good and bad epistemic dispositions should not be drawn exclusively at the level of the individual. It would not benefit enquiry if everyone had exactly the same dispositions, however virtuous those dispositions might be. A degree of variation between people may contribute to the good of an intellectual community, even if many of their epistemic leanings appear suboptimal when viewed from an individualistic standpoint: 'what could be seen as mismanagement of individual epistemic performance can contribute to the success of a community of inquirers' (Hookway, 2002, p.262).

What does all this have to do with *existential* feelings? The relevant feelings are not existential feelings; they are more focused episodic responses to things and are experienced by people who already find themselves in a world. However, they are at least symptomatic of existential feelings. Some people commit more readily than others; some are riddled with doubts and some have inappropriate doubts; others don't have sufficient doubt and are prone to incautious acceptance; and others are erratic. These differences reflect existential feelings. For example, the way in which one finds oneself in the world might be shaped by an all-enveloping sense of uncertainty or doubt. Alternatively, the world might be a cosy place, characterized by a feeling of trust.

Hookway refers to the feelings that regulate enquiry as 'emotions'. However, many different kinds of feelings are implicated in philosophical and scientific thought, as in our intellectual and practical affairs more generally. Most of the relevant feelings are not ordinarily referred to as 'emotions' and many of them do not even have fixed, established names.[7] There are feelings of strangeness, insight, tranquillity, unsettledness, completeness, limitation, novelty, contingency, coherence, anxiety, satisfaction, frustration, mystery, meaninglessness, significance, homeliness, completeness, peace, satisfaction and many others. These can take the form of specific episodes or they can be consistent existential backgrounds that shape all experience and thought, regulating the kinds of episodic feelings that one undergoes.

Authentic and inauthentic philosophies

Explicit philosophical positions can relate to existential orientations in a number of different ways. James contrasts a rationalist system that is alienated from how its proponent actually belongs to the world with philosophies that remain attached to the realities of our experience. Like James, van Fraassen claims that there is sometimes an estrangement between what a philosopher claims and how we actually find ourselves in the world. He appeals to a distinction between *authentic* and *inauthentic* philosophical positions, and is especially hard on contemporary analytic metaphysics. This, he argues, is disconnected from the world we live in and instead plays around with abstract constructs that are produced via obfuscatory re-description of already familiar phenomena: 'its mighty labours address simulacra of no importance at all' (2002, p.4). I think he is right to distinguish philosophies that grapple with our predicament from those that are obliviously cut-off from it. However, it is also important to recognize that there is no *necessary* connection between the kind of conviction involved and the explicit content of the view that is adopted.

Existential feelings do at least comprise *dispositions* towards certain kinds of questions, arguments and positions. Nevertheless, a range of different feelings could conceivably come into play when different people explicitly respond to the same philosophical issue in the same way, and quite different responses could arise from the same kind of existential feeling. Hence an explicit philosophy does not require a specific kind of existential feeling and an account of contrasting existential feelings will not serve to distinguish inauthentic and authentic philosophies at the level of explicit methods, claims, styles and positions. Putting all analytic metaphysicians in the 'inauthentic philosophers' camp is therefore unwarranted. The same applies to empiricists. Empiricism,

---

[7] Van Fraassen recognizes this, remarking that 'none of the familiar emotions that anyone would list as feelings or passions may be involved' (2002, p.107).

construed as an existential orientation, is neither necessary nor sufficient for adherence to a body of explicit philosophical claims. One could assent to those claims typically made by 'empiricists' without knowingly or unknowingly adopting what van Fraassen refers to as an empirical stance.

Furthermore, as suggested by the three different kinds of doubt that I listed earlier in this chapter, the distinction between authentic and inauthentic philosophies needs to be further refined. A philosophy could be inauthentic in so far as it reduces to a purely linguistic exercise that is indifferent to the world it claims to address. Alternatively, the philosopher might have a genuine feeling of conviction regarding an explicit position but fail to appreciate the estrangement of that position from a world that she tacitly takes for granted. A third possibility is an authentic philosophy, one that does manage to engage, to some extent at least, with the way in which we find ourselves in the world.

Philosophies of all three kinds might be aggressively defended by their proponents. Even if a series of doubts amounts to no more than selective use of the word 'not', with no associated feelings of conviction, the philosopher may still care passionately for the position he has assembled and defend it resourcefully. The concern and defensiveness involved is analogous to the way in which someone might care for and protect a model ship that she has assembled perfectly, having paid scrupulous attention to every detail. The finished product has no bearing on how the world is but it is a cherished achievement nonetheless and is not to be surrendered without a fight.

In contrast to this, James's rationalist and van Fraassen's analytic metaphysician might both be quite authentic, in the sense that they have a genuine feeling of conviction towards a doctrine; they *feel* its rightness. In other words, they at least hold a philosophical position, rather than forgetting altogether what it is to hold a position and playing with word games instead (games whose proponents still care very deeply about winning). Even so, if James and van Fraassen are right, the relevant philosophies are themselves inauthentic, in being abstract simulacra that do not engage with the predicament that they claim to. The philosophers themselves are not inauthentic though; they do not know that their conceptual systems have lost touch with the way in which they belong to the world.

It is an open question as to which philosophies have and have not become disconnected from the realities of experience in this way. So, given the assumption that a particular philosophy is the product of sincere conviction rather than word play, the question of whether it is authentic or inauthentic becomes a matter for philosophical debate over whether or not it succeeds in engaging with how we belong to the world, rather than of hurling the label 'inauthentic' around once rational argument has broken down. Philosophical critique can likewise be employed to expose the inadequacies of inauthentic positions that consist of technical, linguistic exercises wholly divorced from their alleged subject matter. However, we are not simply back with the somewhat uncontroversial conclusion that philosophy involves debate. In addition to this, I am suggesting that an appreciation of the nature and role of existential feeling (and of feelings more generally) in enquiry can itself contribute to philosophical debate, in a number of ways.

The mere *acknowledgement* that there is an existential background to experience itself serves to expose some of the confusions involved in certain philosophical approaches. For example, the scientific naturalist presupposes a way of being in the world that her naturalism denies. In Part II, I raised a similar concern about accounts of perception and thought that conceive of our relationship with the world in terms of specific contents and the subsequent formation of propositional attitudes. Such accounts are confused, in their failure to recognize that experience also incorporates a way of finding oneself in a world, within which all specific thoughts and experiences are situated. There are plenty of other candidates for guilty status. For example, most statements of the so-called 'problem of consciousness' construe consciousness exclusively in terms of how things are experienced by a being that is already situated in a shared world. The fact that experience also sets up a world, *within* which one experiences oneself as having a particular contingent, subjective perspective, is generally ignored. Aspects of experience are thus abstracted from an existential context in which they are embedded, a context that is equally part of experience. In assuming 'consciousness' to consist of these aspects alone, an account of the nature of consciousness is doomed from the start. It passes over structures of world experience that are presupposed by all within-world experiences, lifting objects of experience from the space of possibilities through which they appear and misconstruing the feelings through which things are revealed as object-like *internal* states with qualitative feels. Much the same concerns apply to conceptions of intentionality that conceive of it as the achievement whereby a subject's internal mental representation somehow manages to hook up with something in the external world in such a way as to be *about* that thing. Before we hook up with any object in experience or thought, we already belong to a world and this sense of belonging participates in the structure of all intentional states.

Hence, in discussions of consciousness and intentionality, there is a general tendency to misconstrue being in the world as a within-world phenomenon. No account of a within-world 'consciousness' can do justice to the question of how it is that experience opens up a world in the first place and no 'mental representation' can float free from the existential context that talk of 'representations' and the like fails to acknowledge. Phenomenological enquiry can, I suggest, help to expose such confusions.

The kind of confusion that some philosophies fall into, consisting of a sincere affirmation of what is said which is at the same time detached from how one finds oneself in the world, is not dissimilar to the mode of understanding that Heidegger calls *Gerede*, often translated as 'idle talk'. This is a kind of habitual banter that is not necessarily *thoughtless* but is, however, estranged from a world that it obliviously takes for granted. There is a sense in which we sincerely understand what is said by others and sincerely affirm what we ourselves say. But we lose sight of what is talked about by becoming absorbed in the routine of the talk:

> We do not so much understand the entities which are talked about; we already are listening only to what is said-in-the-talk as such. What is said-in-the-talk gets understood; but what the talk is about is understood only approximately and superficially. (1962, p.212)

We come to interpret things in established ways and to skilfully discuss them in an habitual, comfortable, effortless fashion. In so doing, we also lose sight of the background that our established patterns of interaction rest upon:

> ...the obviousness and self-assurance of the average ways in which things have been interpreted, are such that while the particular Dasein drifts along towards an ever-increasing groundlessness as it floats, the uncanniness of this floating remains hidden from it under their protecting shelter. (1962, p.214)

For Heidegger, anxiety has the role of shaking us out of the disposition to misinterpret ourselves and lose ourselves in idle talk. When an existential orientation falters, we can no longer take it for granted. It becomes phenomenologically conspicuous in its erosion.

Conviction and doubt

Phenomenological critique can also be employed to dismiss certain cases of so-called *sceptical doubt*. Take the classic case of Cartesian doubt. Can one really doubt the existence of the world or of one's body? One can think of one's body as an object, or of the world as a collection of objects, and then think 'it is not the case that object p exists'. But can one genuinely conceive of one's disembodied existence, as a Cartesian mental substance or a brain in a vat, when all of one's experience is structured by a tacit background of feeling? And can the reality of the world be doubted, when the sense of 'reality' does not consist in an object being presented to consciousness but in a presupposed possibility space that enables things to be experienced as 'real'? Can one, in a detached, indifferent manner, doubt the sense of reality itself or of one's bodily being in the world? I suggest not. One can doubt the existence of an object but experience of body and world does not just consist in experiencing objects; it is a framework through which objects are experienced and thought of as real or unreal. So doubting the existence of 'world as object' or 'body as object' does not add up to genuine doubt concerning their existence.

Returning to the three kinds of doubt mentioned earlier in this chapter, the world's existence cannot really be doubted unless the sense of reality is shaken in some way, perhaps weakened, changed, or consistently susceptible to changes. If one asserts that the world does not exist without even making explicit the practical, felt affirmation of the world's being that underlies experience and thought, let alone contemplating its absence, then one does not really doubt. One has instead mischaracterized what it is to believe in the world's existence and then doubted the reliability of this mischaracterized conviction. The feeling of reality and belonging has not wavered at all during this process.

We cannot doubt, in a purely propositional sense, the existence of the world, because the conviction that the world exists does not have a propositional form. The relevant doubt must involve a changed existential orientation, which is quite different in nature from a within-world doubt concerning the potential non-existence of some entity. In the latter, one has a sense of what it is to be the case and doubts that p is the case. However, what is lost in the former is a sense of what it is to be the case; the 'doubt' is an erosion of the feeling of reality. So the sentence 'I am not sure that the world exists', when used to express an erosion of felt reality, does not express the same content as that utterance when it is made by a sceptic who is obliviously at home in the world. Regardless of whether or not the sceptic sincerely affirms her claim, she cannot really think what she thinks that she thinks without undergoing an existential upheaval. And, if she did undergo such an upheaval, she could not think it either, because the modalities of conviction would have shifted and she would not 'believe' anything in quite the same way.[8]

This kind of criticism is not restricted to doubts; it applies equally to claims that are assented to or even proclaimed to be indubitable. To take a familiar example, Descartes 'believes' that he cannot doubt his existence and yet the certainty he achieves is only an intellectual, propositional certainty. It would

---

[8] I have offered a phenomenological argument to the effect that doubts of this kind are unthinkable. However, other non-phenomenological arguments could lead us to much the same conclusion. See, for example, Wittgenstein's (1975, p.22) claim that certain propositions 'stand fast' in a given context, in such a way as to render incoherent the question of whether or not they are *known* to be true. However, it should be emphasized that a sense of the world's existence is not in any sense 'propositional'.

be of little comfort to a psychiatric patient whose existential orientation no longer incorporated a sense of her existence. This is something that Jaspers (1962, p.94) recognizes:

> Descartes' 'cogito ergo sum' holds even for the person in a state of derealisation who says paradoxically: 'I am not but have to go on being nothing for ever'. Descartes' phrase therefore cannot convince us by logic alone; in addition it requires the primary awareness of Being and the awareness of one's existence in particular.[9]

However much such a patient repeats 'cogito ergo sum', she cannot recover something that is altogether removed from the space of possibilities. It becomes an empty assertion, a proposition that is assented to without any possibility of genuine conviction.

Wisdom (1964, p.170) makes some complementary points concerning the nature of philosophical doubt and conviction:

> …no philosopher becomes really a Sceptic; because if a man really feels what the Sceptic says he feels then he is said to have 'a sense of unreality' and is removed to a home. In fact the sceptical philosopher never succeeds in killing his primitive creduli-ties which, as Hume says, reassert themselves the moment he takes up the affairs of life and ceases to murmur the incantations which generate his philosophic doubt.

Like James, Wisdom distinguishes genuine doubt and conviction from the hollow affirmation and denial of propositions. Philosophical doubts, he says, are often not real doubts. He suggests that the philosopher's 'doubts' are more akin to those of the neurotic than the psychotic. The neurotic engages in a kind of dithering, a reluctance to end the uncertainty and get on with things:

> …we have all read of the man who cannot be sure that he has turned off the tap or the light. He must go again to make sure, and then perhaps he must go again because though he knows the light's turned off he yet cannot *feel* sure. He is obsessed by a chronic doubt. (Wisdom, 1964, p.172)

The neurotic does not really 'believe' that the tap or the lights have been left on. Unlike the psychotic, he is well-grounded enough to know that he really has turned them off. Nevertheless, he goes back to check all the same, due to a persistent feeling of uncertainty. But the option of going back is not open to a philosopher who doubts, in a similar way, that the world exists. So there is no comparable checking ritual that can be employed to placate the feeling of doubt. Unlike the neurotic who does at least act upon his feelings, the philoso-pher's activities all presuppose his practical groundedness in the world,

---

9 The 'cogito' is also discussed by Young and Leafhead (1996), who contrast Cartesian cer-tainty regarding one's own existence with the utterances of patients suffering from the Cotard delusion.

the only exception being some of his utterances. There is no more to his doubts than his saying that he doubts:

> The neurotic, we might say, doesn't believe what he says. Still he does go back at the risk of losing his train to make sure that the lights are off. The philosopher doesn't. His acts and feelings are even less in accordance with his words than are the acts and feelings of the neurotic. He, even more than the neurotic and much more than the psychotic, doesn't believe what he says, doesn't doubt when he says he's not sure. (Wisdom, 1964, p.174)

However, the sceptical philosopher is not insincere in what she says. As Wisdom notes, although she does not really doubt, she is not a liar either. She is in a kind of conceptual muddle, partly symptomatic of being comfortably at home in the world and oblivious to the contingency of an existential orientation that even her 'doubts' take for granted. Wisdom adds that:

> There is a big difference between the philosopher and both the psychotic and the obsessional neurotic. It lies in the flow of justificatory talk, of rationalization, which the philosopher produces when asked why he takes the extraordinary line he does. (1964, p.174)

The philosopher's rationalizations, he says, 'impress' us, although not quite enough to be duped by them. Those of the psychotic and neurotic do not, even though they do sometimes offer something in the way of reasons to support their claims. But the difference runs deeper than that, I think. The sceptic is quite unlike the psychotic in her existential orientation. The former utters what she does because she is well grounded and the latter because she is not. And, unlike the feelings of the neurotic, which at least have practical consequences, the philosopher's feelings of doubt concern only what is said.

In addition, it is debatable whether the feelings of doubt that the philosopher has are of the same *kind* as those experienced by the neurotic. Affirmation of the proposition 'there is doubt as to whether the world exists' could well be accompanied by a range of different feelings, perhaps wonder, awe, horror, a reassuring sense of conviction, a slight worry, a feeling that there is something that needs to be resolved or a feeling of curiosity. Of course, another possibility, which may apply to some cases, is that the philosopher is inauthentic in her utterances, as opposed to being authentic but confused. There may be no motivating feeling at all, other than perhaps a playful sense of satisfaction associated with putting the word 'not' in front of a sentence. To further complicate things, an explicit position that is detached from an existential orientation in this way might still be partly constituted by that existential orientation, given that certain ways of finding oneself in a world incorporate a comfortable obliviousness to the fact that one does occupy a contingent existential orientation.

A question I have not yet addressed is that of whether there is a right kind of existential feeling, a set of dispositions that is best equipped to facilitate fruitful enquiry. Some philosophers endorse the broadly Aristotelian view that having the right emotional dispositions is central to successful thought and activity, and that it is possible to culture these dispositions. For example:

> If we do not have the right emotional dispositions, prudential and moral, that properly attune us to the world, then, I will argue, our emotions can distort perception and reason so that the world seems to us other than it really is: as I will put it, the emotions *skew* the *epistemic landscape*. (Goldie, 2004, p.92)

> ...a large part of education is evoking, shaping, developing relevant care and concern, and [...] an important feature of good intellectual work is continuing to have and exercise relevant care and concern. (Stocker, 2004, pp.135–48)

When it comes to intellectual activity, some existential feelings are clearly preferable to others. It goes without saying that the feeling typical of full-blown schizophrenia is sub-optimal for philosophical enquiry and for enquiry more generally. The same no doubt applies to a range of other existential feelings too. Nevertheless, there will not be a single, optimal kind of existential feeling. As pointed out by Hookway (2002), a diverse range of dispositions on the part of individuals can add up to a better outcome collectively than a single set of 'optimal' dispositions shared by everyone. However, there is a further case to be made in favour of a diversity of existential feelings in philosophical and, more specifically, phenomenological enquiry, the diversity in question being both intra-personal and inter-personal.

The structure of existential feeling is revealed through changes in existential feeling. We can scrutinize descriptions of extreme changes that occur in psychiatric illnesses but we can also reflect upon the lesser fluctuations in existential feeling that we ourselves undergo. Changes in existential feeling thus facilitate phenomenological enquiry, in addition to being part of its subject matter. Phenomenological study does not require a single, complete *epoché* or a moment of anxiety that eradicates the natural attitude in one blow, allowing us to catch sight of what we usually inhabit. The 'natural attitude' is changeable and takes on a plethora of different forms. It is this changeability that reveals its structure to us. When we reflect upon changes, we come to recognize that there is a question to be addressed regarding the nature of our sense of reality, a question that cannot be asked if reality is taken as given. This recognition, this refusal to take the sense of reality for granted, is adopted as a methodological principal. It need not take the form of a consistent and total suspension of an ordinarily taken-for-granted reality. The relevant enquiry can be pursued gradually, revealing, interpreting and re-interpreting the structure of experience a bit at a time. What is required for this is not an existential feeling that is unchanging and closed off to alternative possibilities but one that is susceptible to shifts and involves a sense of openness to different modes of belonging to the world. The relevant shifts are not under direct volitional control in the way that moving one's arm is but, as with feelings more generally, one can do various things to elicit them and become progressively skilled at attending to and interpreting them.

A stance of openness, involving some degree of changeability, can be contrasted both with existential chaos and with inflexibility. Existential chaos is not conducive to any enquiry. Inflexibility, however, is characteristic of doctrines such as scientific naturalism, which incorporate the suffocating certainty that some contingent set of epistemic practices will ultimately be able to encompass absolutely everything. A sense of the world as something that cannot be wholly captured by any contingent stance that we might adopt is integral to a sense of reality. Thus an existential orientation that involves some humility, some sense of its own incompleteness and fragility, of how the space of possibilities might open up, fall away or change, does not add up to a diminished sense of reality but, rather, a heightened one. In contrast to this, an unchangeable way of being in the world, although maybe comforting, is a rigidly constrained and inflexible possibility space, a comparatively diminished world.

Hence some of the points I make about the role of existential feelings in my own method do not apply exclusively to a particular kind of phenomenological enquiry. Existential feelings play a role in philosophy more generally, in making explicit what one previously took for granted, in contemplating alternatives, in understanding positions that differ from one's own and in thinking through problems. Rational philosophical thought includes a lot more than the exchange of arguments. The practical skills of suspending implicit stances, making them explicit and moving between them are important aspects of critical enquiry. In addition, an understanding of existential feeling also casts light on the ways in which people can fail to 'connect' in philosophical debates. It also makes explicit certain confusions that occur when philosophers discuss the world, our relationship to it and the nature of experience. Of course, phenomenological enquiry alone will not always be able to arbitrate between rival positions and, needless to say, there is enormous scope for debate within phenomenology itself. Nevertheless, it is at least clear that existential feelings can be part of a critical enquiry, rather than sources of inflexible, dogmatic positions that are immune from critique and that can, at best, be confessed.

Chapter 10

Pathologies of existential feeling

I have discussed the role of existential feelings in everyday life, psychiatric illness and philosophical enquiry. The contrast between everyday feelings and those that feature in illness indicates that some existential feelings are pathological and others not. There is also the issue of whether some of the feelings that motivate philosophical thought are pathological. In this final chapter, I address the question of what it is that distinguishes pathological from non-pathological existential feelings. To do so, I focus on the topic of religious experience. Religious experience has often been compared to psychotic experience and thus serves as a suitable case study through which to explore some of the philosophical problems involved in determining whether or not an existential orientation is pathological. Again, I refer to what William James has to say on the matter. Drawing on his work, I suggest that existential feelings are central to religious experience but that the relevant feelings are not themselves intrinsically religious. Then I consider whether some or all of these feelings are pathological, drawing a distinction between biological, epistemic, pragmatic and existential pathologies in the process. (Hence I use the word 'pathological' in a broad way, to refer to something going *wrong* in the context of a human life, rather than to something going wrong in a specifically *biological* way.) I go on to offer an account of what it is for a predicament to be *existentially pathological* and argue that a complete or partial loss of openness to interpersonal possibilities is central to all such cases. I bring the book to a close by returning to those attitudes in philosophy, science and everyday life that involve a surreptitious denial of our existential predicament. I suggest that they are not existentially pathological but that they do amount to a kind of intellectual pathology, an extreme but unacknowledged form of scepticism that is sometimes accompanied by existential unsettledness.

The nature of religious experience

Many of those experiences that are referred to as *religious* incorporate changed existential feeling and I will turn to these experiences in order to address the question of what it is that makes an existential feeling pathological. Before doing so, it is important to make clear what a religious experience actually is.

There is, of course, more to being religious than having religious experiences. Much of the structure of religion cannot be understood in terms of the experiences of religious individuals, given that religion is also a cultural–historical framework into which those individuals are born or introduced and then shaped. A religion is not just a matter of what an individual experiences; it is a shared way of life, through which one's own and others' words, deeds and experiences are interpreted (see, for example, Phillips, 1986). To further complicate matters, religions differ in all manner of ways, as do the contents of religious experiences.

It is therefore difficult to pin down what religious experiences consist of and to determine whether the different experiences have anything interesting in common. One option is to claim that a religious experience is an experience of God. This view is popular in so-called 'neurotheology', a fairly new field of study that explores the neural correlates of religious experiences and religious dispositions. For instance, Persinger (2002), in his work on the neurobiology of religious experience, frequently refers to 'the God experience', suggesting that a distinctive kind of experience has been identified, the neural correlates of which can be investigated.[1] However, this is rather simplistic and many philosophers, theologians and others offer more sophisticated, nuanced accounts, which distinguish different kinds of religious experience, some of which do not include anything resembling the God of monotheism. For example, Franks Davis (1989, chapter 2) offers the following taxonomy:

1 Interpretive experiences: experiences such as fortuitous co-incidences, which are interpreted in religious terms.

2 Quasi-sensory experiences: these include visions, voices, dreams and tactile sensations.

3 Revelatory experiences: sudden moments of insight that seem to come from elsewhere.

4 Regenerative experiences: profound feelings of strength, comfort or joy.

5 Numinous experiences: feelings of insignificance before the majesty of God.

6 Mystical experiences: the experience of encountering ultimate reality, often associated with feelings of oneness, serenity and a loss of the sense of space and time.

The specific contents of these experiences are both diverse and culturally influenced. Hence it is highly doubtful that all religious experiences share a common content. In addition, it is debatable as to whether some of the contents

---

[1] See Ratcliffe (2006) for a critique of 'neurotheology'.

reported by people are intrinsic to the relevant experience. They might instead consist of interpretations of the experience that accord with the pre-existent religious beliefs of the person having the experience or at least with beliefs that she has been exposed to by her culture. Furthermore, the line between those contents that are intrinsic to the experience and those that are not may be a difficult one to draw.

An alternative approach is to consider whether these experiences have a common structure, rather than a common content. This is the approach I adopt here. To say that something is a 'God experience' is no more informative than saying that something is a 'car experience' or a *Star Wars* film experience'. That experiences have a common content does not imply that they have anything else of interest in common. Two people's '*Star Wars* film experiences' could well be very different in nature. In Chapters 5, 6 and 7, I made the same point with respect to the contents of delusions. What instances of a delusion such as the Capgras or Cotard delusion have in common with each other is not, first and foremost, an experiential or propositional content but an existential feeling. The content is an expression of that feeling. Although the contents of some other delusions (including many of those found in schizophrenia) do not express existential feelings so directly, these too are symptomatic of kinds of existential change.

However, it is possible that religious experiences do not share a common structure any more than they share a common content. James (1902) offers an account which concedes that both content and structure are heterogeneous but maintains at the same time that religious experiences all share a common 'nucleus'. The experiential contents that people report are, according to James, symptomatic of historically and culturally diverse interpretive tendencies. They arise due to the imposition of what he calls 'over-beliefs', narratives that people spin around an underlying experience. Even 'God', for example, is not intrinsic to the experience. It is one over-belief amongst others, in terms of which a core experience might be interpreted and communicated to others. The experience itself is neither intrinsically monotheistic nor polytheistic; it does not match up with any specific religious doctrine (1902, pp.507–14). If doctrinal contents consist of over-beliefs, the diverse contents of religious experiences need not imply that the underlying experiences have nothing in common. However, it does suggest that the term 'religious' is misleading when employed to characterize the core experience; experiences are *interpreted* in terms of religious doctrines rather than being *intrinsically* religious.

James claims that the relevant experiences are not only made to fit in with pre-existent religious narratives but also motivate the construction of such narratives. In fact, they are the source from which all explicit religious belief originates. The true believer, for James, is not one who performs in accordance with a pre-established doctrine but one who undergoes an existential transformation, who feels the truth of her convictions and communicates them in the form of a religious narrative. Those who just follow a doctrine do not *live* the religious life in the same way. So religion, for James, originates in pre-articulate feelings:

> I do believe that feeling is the deeper source of religion, and that philosophic and theological formulas are secondary products, like translations of a text into another tongue. (1902, p.431)[2]

The kind of conviction that arises in religious experience is not at all like assuming or inferring that a specific experiential content is veridical. The feeling embodies a different kind and degree of conviction, which runs much deeper than any propositional attitude:

> Individuality is founded in feeling; and the recesses of feeling, the darker, blinder strata of character, are the only places in the world in which we catch real fact in the making, and directly perceive how events happen, and how work is actually done. Compared with this world of living individualized feelings, the world of generalized objects which the intellect contemplates is without solidity or life. (James, 1902, pp.501–2)

Religious belief originates in these 'living individualized feelings'. Hence the difference between a resolute atheist and someone who authentically asserts the existence of a monotheistic deity does not consist solely, or even primarily, of their holding different propositional attitudes. A belief in God is symptomatic of a felt way of belonging to the world. It is not like believing that the Eiffel Tower is in Paris. For many believers, it is a very different *kind* of commitment. It is imbued with feeling rather than being a proposition that one can indifferently assert from a standpoint of neutral detachment. The feeling is integral to religious experience and commitment, rather than just accompanying it.

Philosophical discussion of religious belief is littered with attempts to prove the existence of God or at least provide good grounds for religious belief, on the basis of reason and evidence. There are also many kinds of argument that

---

2 The view that feeling is central to religious experience is corroborated by recent neurobiological studies that measure emotional changes which happen when people have such experiences. In reflecting upon one such study, Ramachandran comments, 'I find it ironic that this sense of enlightenment, this absolute conviction that Truth is revealed at last, should derive from limbic structures concerned with emotions rather than from the thinking, rational parts of the brain that take so much pride in their ability to discern truth and falsehood' (Ramachandran and Blakeslee, 1998, p.179). However, it does not seem remarkable at all once it is appreciated that all experiences and thoughts presuppose backgrounds of existential feeling.

seek to show that religious belief is unwarranted. For example, there are arguments starting from the well-known *problem of evil*, which conclude that the world contains too much evil for it to be the product of an all good, all knowing, all loving God.[3] Although such arguments and counter-arguments are technically sophisticated, they fail to connect with the realities of religious belief, in so far as religious utterances are symptomatic of existential feelings. Belief in God is not, in some cases at least, a matter of assenting to a proposition on the basis of reason or evidence; it is something that originates in feeling. And the same can be said for other *spiritual* and *mystical* convictions that do not incorporate a monotheistic God.

Are all 'religious' experiences united by a common existential feeling? I think this is unlikely, as does James. In addition to admitting that the feelings in question are not themselves intrinsically religious, he acknowledges that they are not all of the same kind. There 'seems to be no one elementary religious emotion, but only a common storehouse of emotions upon which religious objects may draw' (1902, p.28). That different kinds of feeling are involved is also apparent from his account of religious temperaments, where he contrasts the religion of the 'healthy minded' person with that of the 'sick soul'. These broad categories group together a range of different kinds of feeling, some of which are interpreted by some people in religious terms. The experience of the sick soul can be strikingly similar to an existential predicament reported in schizophrenia: 'a thick veil alters the tone and look of everything' and 'I weep false tears. I have unreal hands: the things I see are not real things' (James, 1902, p.152). However, it does not always take quite this form. Another quotation he offers suggests a kind of anxious depression, involving an all-enveloping, nameless threat and the loss of everyday significance, rather than a world that is impenetrable and artificial: 'the world now looks remote, strange, sinister, uncanny. Its color is gone, its breath is cold, there is no speculation in the eyes it glares with' (1902, p.151).

A sick soul is sometimes rescued by religious conversion. This, for James, is a shift in existential orientation; a 'transfiguration of the face of nature' (1902, p.151). Again, he does not claim that the feelings implicated in the change are the same in every case. Nevertheless, he does propose that all such existential changes have something in common. In the shift from an everyday or a sick orientation, there is also the recognition that the mundane world is incomplete, that reality is not exhausted by it contents. This recognition includes the sense of there being a higher order to which one harmoniously belongs, a higher power from which one is inextricable. Through it, the torment of the

---

[3] See Mackie (1982) for one of many good discussions of such arguments.

sick soul is relieved. This shift from a feeling of uneasiness to a sense of its solution is, according to James, the common 'nucleus' of religious experience (1902, pp.507–8).

The experience James describes might be thought of in terms of a specific experiential content that is revealed, an object of experience that is outside of mundane reality. However, his descriptions suggest that it is an existential change, rather than the appearance of some new experiential content. This change can, I think, be interpreted in terms of existential feeling. A world that is drained of life, painfully mundane or otherwise limited in its possibilities can be shaken up so as to reveal a different and perhaps wider space of possibility, something *more*, something *greater*. In the process, the contingency of one's earlier orientation is also revealed. Several different kinds of existential change all embody this common element, the appreciation that things are not exhausted by the space of possibilities in which one previously resided.

Such shifts need not involve a revelation of order, harmony and communion with being. The revelation in question could be the feeling that a previously dependable, everyday world is contingent and fragile. The changed space of possibilities might take the form of an all-enveloping threat or a sinister presence that infiltrates everything, leaving nowhere to hide. Rather than escaping from a world of painful uncertainty and doubt or from a suffocating prison bereft of all meaning, one might fall from the safe, familiar, warming, reassuringly limited world into a realm of disempowerment, lack of control, limitless threat or terrifying uncertainty. In neither the positive nor the negative existential transformations are the relevant feelings intrinsically *religious*. The common revelation is the contingency of what one took for granted and a sense of there being something more, which can be felt as reassuring or threatening in a number of different ways. Thus, although James states that 'God is the natural appellation, for us Christians at least, for the supreme reality' (1902, p.516), interpreting these experiences in terms of existential feeling suggests that their common content may be even further removed from anything specifically theistic or religious than even James suggests.

James's account explicitly focuses on those unusual individuals for whom religion is an 'acute fever', rather than a 'dull habit' (1902, p.6). But I have emphasized throughout this book that changes in existential feeling are not rare occurrences. The *natural attitude* is interpersonally variable and, in addition, we all experience a variety of subtle changes in how we find ourselves in the world. Granted, some changes are much more extreme than others but there is no strict contrast to be drawn between those who undergo the relevant existential changes and those who remain firmly anchored in the mundane world. Even if we use the terms 'mystical' or 'spiritual', rather than 'religious', it is misleading to contrast spiritual or mystical experiences with mundane experiences and to regard the former as exceptional events. There is more continuity than that.

The distinction made by James between core experiences and over-beliefs is also problematic. According to James, the over-beliefs are imposed *upon* the core experience. He thus fails to acknowledge that contingent conceptual systems shape the ways in which we *experience* things, rather than just being laid *on top of* pre-given experiences. For example, consider a sign that says 'no smoking'. It is well nigh impossible to look at this sign without comprehending its meaning, a grasp of which is inseparable from *experience* of the sign. In order to experience it *as* a 'no smoking' sign, one must know how to read a particular language and also be a competent participant in a culture that recognises the practices of smoking and of prohibiting certain things in certain places. Generalizing from any number of such examples, it is arguable that the notion of a core religious experience, untainted by culture, is untenable. As Taylor puts it:

> The ideas, the understanding with which we live our lives, shape directly what we could call religious experiences; and these languages, these vocabularies, are never those simply of an individual. (2002, p.28)

The *over-beliefs* are not optional add-ons to an experience comprised of pre-conceptual feeling. Rather, contingent conceptualizations participate in the experience; we cannot prize the experience apart from its religious content.

However, in all fairness to James, it is not clear that he does regard the over-beliefs as distinct from the experience. The conceptualizations could be construed as part of an experience that also incorporates a non-conceptual existential feeling. He emphasizes the importance of the latter over the former, rather than making a firm distinction between an experience and all historically and culturally contingent conceptualizations. The plausible assumption that religious experiences involve existential feeling is compatible with the view that these experiences are not solely a matter of existential feeling.

Even so, the implication remains that 'religious experience' is not itself an informative experiential category. Types of contingent content do not serve to distinguish experiential kinds. Furthermore, the existential shifts involved in these experiences are not themselves intrinsically religious, the same existential shift being compatible with a range of religious and non-religious experiential contents. Hence existential feelings are to be distinguished from specifically religious experiential contents and from doctrinal commitments. This distinction will be important in addressing the issue of whether and why these and other existential feelings should be regarded as *pathological*.

Medical and existential perspectives

Some existential changes, such as those involved in severe schizophrenia, are clearly pathological rather than just unusual. However, the matter is far less clear in the case of religious experiences, where there is considerable disagreement. What one person takes to be the veridical disclosure of a higher being another takes to be a delusional state, perhaps something to be interpreted in medical terms. When we consider what James calls 'religious geniuses', there is a fine line between religious experience and pathology:

> They have known no measure, been liable to obsessions and fixed ideas; and frequently they have fallen into trances, heard voices, seen visions, and presented all sorts of peculiarities which are ordinarily classed as pathological. Often, moreover, these pathological features in their career have helped to give them their religious authority and influence. (James, 1902, p.7)

However, James is scornful of attempts to cast the predicament of such people in exclusively medical terms:

> Medical materialism finishes up Saint Paul by calling his vision on the road to Damascus a discharging lesion of the occipital cortex, he being an epileptic. It snuffs out Saint Teresa as a hysteric, Saint Francis of Assisi as a hereditary degenerate. (1902, p.13)

He admits that their experience and conduct is, in some way, pathological, but claims that it can at the same time have genuine spiritual significance. So the question of whether something is to be understood medically or existentially does not require an either/or answer. The possibility of a medical interpretation does not imply that an experience has no value or that it is wholly misleading with respect to the contents of reality.[4]

James observes that the manner in which bodily feelings contribute to religious experience and belief is by no means exceptional. They contribute to our lives more generally and any aspect of human experience, thought or activity could equally be interpreted in medical terms:

> Scientific theories are organically conditioned just as much as religious emotions are; and if we only knew the facts intimately enough, we should doubtless see 'the liver' determining the dicta of the sturdy atheist as decisively as it does those of the Methodist under conviction anxious about his soul. (1902, p.14)

Hence the fact that we can understand something in terms of changes in body and brain does not exclude other interpretations.

---

4 Jaspers (1962, p.108) similarly claims that 'religious experience remains what it is, whether it occurs in saint or psychotic or whether the person in whom it occurs is both at once'.

It might be objected that not all experience, thought and activity are on a par here. When a way of experiencing, thinking or acting arises due to illness or disease, we are indeed warranted in claiming it to be of no existential significance. In such cases, it occurs due to processes in brain and/or body going *wrong* and it is therefore unlikely to disclose the world in an informative way. However, the distinction between pathological and non-pathological existential feelings cannot be drawn in this way. As discussed in Chapter 4, changed existential feelings are not restricted to psychiatric illness and occur in many other illnesses that are referred to as 'bodily' or 'somatic' rather than 'psychological' (although I also questioned the legitimacy of such distinctions). In many 'somatic' cases, although an existential feeling arises due to something that has gone wrong with the body, the feeling itself need not be considered pathological. When suffering from influenza, one might feel detached from everything or that the world is no longer quite as it was. But feeling that way when one has influenza is not itself what is wrong. One does not treat the feeling of estrangement but treats other symptoms of illness to which a feeling of estrangement might be a *natural* or even *appropriate* rather than pathological response.

Furthermore, existential feelings that arise due to illness are not always *misleading* and might well offer genuine insight. For example, a feeling of detachment and estrangement can be partly constitutive of the recognition that one is ill. And, as van den Berg (1966) points out, some sense of vulnerability and fragility is part of an existentially healthy predicament and this is something that experience of illness can foster. However, pathological and non-pathological existential feelings cannot be distinguished on the basis that only the latter offer us genuine insight. By analogy, people can learn many things from severe illness and acknowledging this certainly does not imply that what gives them insight is non-pathological. Likewise, even if some existential feelings involved in illness are pathological and others not, it might well be possible to gain genuine understanding from both. Hence some other criterion is required in order to determine whether or not an existential feeling is pathological.

In response to the distinction I have drawn between existential feelings and the illnesses in which they sometimes arise, it could be argued that diagnoses of mental disorders, in contrast to diagnoses of somatic disorders, do not allow us to make a distinction between the underlying pathology and the existential feelings that are symptomatic of it. Types of 'bodily' pathology are usually identified by injuries, the presence of other bodily changes, toxins in the body or the intrusion of alien organisms. Characteristic feelings of discomfort and the like, some of which may be existential feelings under a partial description, are *effects* of the condition rather than *parts* of it. However, the presence of a so-called 'mental disorder', as classified by systems such as the DSM, is not inferred from a cluster of symptoms but identified by the presence of those symptoms. In addition, many of the symptoms of disorders such as schizophrenia are either identical with existential changes or arise in the context of existential changes. Hence, unlike influenza, these disorders are not separable from existential feelings.

By suggesting that schizophrenia and at least some other psychiatric conditions are identified by changes in existential feeling and inseparable from them, I mean that the symptom-based classifications that are used to diagnose them *refer* to changed existential feeling, rather than that they actually *describe* the relevant existential changes. The feelings in question are only partially described, in ways that are often misleading.[5] Changes in the sense of reality cannot be understood if one takes the sense of reality for granted when interpreting them. Even so, it is possible to refer to a changed existential feeling without fully understanding what it is that one is referring to. For example, an existential change could be referred to as a 'lack of affective response'.

If existential changes are constitutive of certain *disorders*, then surely these feelings are pathological regardless of how they are referred to. However, it could be maintained that they are pathological when interpreted in one way but not when interpreted in another. For example, it might be that the phenomenological stance required to interpret feelings as *existential* feelings is purely descriptive and so does not incorporate normative judgements to the effect that an existential orientation is or is not pathological. Furthermore, existential feelings are ways of finding oneself in a world and, when we are interpreting them as such, there is no further standpoint we can retreat to in order to determine whether or not they are pathological. When viewing them as pathological, we switch from treating them as ways of being in the world to something that we encounter within the world, in the context of another existential predicament that we ourselves take for granted. So we cannot treat something as pathological and at the same time as an existential feeling. Whatever it is for something to be 'pathological', the term does not apply to existential orientations understood as existential orientations.

However, even if this is so (and I will suggest otherwise), it does not rule out the possibility of criteria for determining whether or not an existential feeling

---

5 For a recent statement of the view that a medical point of view is limited when it comes to interpreting psychiatric illness, see Martin's (1999) discussion of depression, which advocates an intertwining of both 'therapeutic' and 'moral' perspectives. See also Hansen (2004) for a discussion of existential, medical and other approaches to the understanding of depression. See Matthews (2007) for a critique of either/or approaches to illness and existential orientation, which draws on Merleau-Ponty's distinction between the lived body and the medicalized body.

is pathological, given that the relevant criteria could refer to existential feelings whilst not engaging with them *as* existential predicaments. Certain existential feelings, as described in other ways, are partly or even wholly constitutive of mental *disorders*. So there is the question of what it is that makes these feelings pathological. I will consider three different answers, rejecting two but cautiously endorsing the third. Then I will go on to propose a criterion for identifying an existential feeling as *existentially* pathological.

Medical, epistemic and pragmatic pathologies

Could there be objective medical grounds for determining whether or not an existential feeling is pathological? By 'medical', I mean *biological* criteria for distinguishing health from disease. There is considerable disagreement over which are the right biological criteria with which to do so.[6] A popular approach is to maintain that pathologies are biological *malfunctions*. That is, parts of the body fail to do what they are biologically adapted to do. However, a simple malfunction criterion would accommodate too much. Our bodies do many things that they are not evolutionarily adapted to do, such as sitting on a chair for hours on end writing a book.

Even if an account could be elaborated and modified in such a way as to rule out certain things that we would not wish to regard as pathological, there are other objections to the practice of identifying pathologies in terms of biological malfunction. For example, Amundson (2000) criticizes the distinction that is often presupposed between a species-typical *normal* or *proper* function and a range of pathological deviations from it. Evolution, he says, gives us diversity rather than a single, species-typical way of doing things. Within a species, there are many ways in which organisms and their parts manage to perform tasks, and they can employ quite different strategies that are equally efficient. Amundson distinguishes between *level* and *mode* of performance, the former being a measure of how successful something is at achieving a given end and the latter being the *way* in which it achieves that end. Biological success, he says, is about level rather than mode; but, regardless of this, medical approaches tend to emphasize proper mode of function over level. People who deviate from it are treated with a view to restoring normal mode as far as is possible, even though level of performance can actually be impaired by the process. According to Amundson, this practice is a reflection of social attitudes that favour cosmetic adjustments and has no genuine medical rationale— some of the pathologies which are identified in terms of deviant mode of function are not pathological at all.

---

[6] See Cooper (2005) for a discussion of different criteria that are employed to identify 'disease'.

Thus, even if pathologies of existential feeling could, in principle, be identified according to biological criteria, there would still be difficult issues to address concerning both the relevant criteria and which so-called pathologies really were pathological. So I do not wish to imply that we currently have at our disposal wholly reliable medical criteria in place for distinguishing disease from health, which might or might not be applicable to existential feeling. What I do want to suggest though is that, even if some such criteria were universally accepted, they *still* could not be employed to identify pathologies of existential feeling.

As already noted, current methods for diagnosing conditions such as schizophrenia do not rely upon the identification of distinctive biological impairments that are common to all cases of schizophrenia and occur only in cases of schizophrenia. Observed psychological and behavioural changes are central to the diagnosis. One option is to maintain that to have these symptoms *is* to have schizophrenia, regardless of how the symptoms might have originated, a view that Radden (2003, p.41) calls 'ontological descriptivism'. If ontological descriptivism is accepted, existential feelings cannot be pathological in virtue of their being identified with something that has gone *biologically* wrong because the criteria for being a mental disorder are independent of anything we might discover about biological functions and malfunctions.

Of course, it could conceivably turn out that all instances of these symptoms have a common, underlying, biological cause. Hence, rather than identifying schizophrenia with the observed symptoms, it might then be identified with that cause. Let us suppose that a distinctive pattern of biological changes were discovered and that the condition were then identified with this. Would the relevant existential changes be properly regarded as medically pathological? The answer is again that they would not. They would be symptoms of a biological malfunction and, as already discussed, symptoms of a malfunction need not themselves be malfunctions. The biological changes involved could relate to the psychological symptoms in any number of complicated ways.

I should add that this conclusion does not rely upon a distinction between the realms of the 'psychological' and the 'biological'. The point is that a symptom is distinct from what causes it, regardless of whether or not the former is described in biological and the latter in psychological terms. The pathological status of the cause does not imply that the effect is also pathological.

Furthermore, even if a strong case could be made for describing a given symptom as *biologically* pathological, it need not add up to something *psychologically* pathological and vice versa. The criteria are different. Many psychologically painful and debilitating conditions that we might want to treat could turn out to be biologically normal and many psychological conditions that are not a cause for psychiatric concern could turn out to be pathological according to biological criteria. Psychiatric criteria address psychological rather than biological concerns and so they are unlikely to map onto biological criteria when it comes to the identification of pathology. In the case of existential feelings, it is the existential predicament rather than any biological abnormality that is troubling, painful or debilitating and it is this predicament that diagnostic criteria, such as loss of observable affect, refer to.

An alternative approach is to appeal to epistemological criteria. Existential predicaments are constitutive of some delusions and cultivate the formation of others. Delusions are clearly pathological in an *epistemic* sense. They are not just false beliefs but false beliefs that stem from consistently faulty epistemic practices, practices that have gone *wrong*. Even if we cannot come up with criteria for something's being *existentially* pathological, we can identify epistemic pathologies and, in so far as these are associated with distinctive existential changes, we can regard those changes as pathological on epistemic grounds.

Of course, there are problems involved in identifying something as epistemically pathological. Epistemic practices in the general population are varied and it is not always clear which are reliable and which are not. The matter is complicated by the possibility that, as suggested by James, there are cases where one must commit oneself in a certain way before a truth can be revealed. A belief might look epistemically pathological to someone because she has not committed herself in the right way. Even so, certain delusional claims are so far-fetched that there is no ambiguity; they are clearly false. And the person who holds them clearly has a deficient epistemic strategy.

As I argued in Part II, it is misleading to treat delusions simply as false beliefs. At least some delusions arise due to changed existential orientations and thus changed modes of conviction. The deluded person does not take things to be the case in the way that she once did and so she does not claim to 'know' in the way she once did either. But let us assume, just for the sake of argument, that delusions can be treated as relevantly like knowledge claims or statements of belief. Can they be used to identify pathological existential feelings? The first problem is that not all existential changes that we might regard as pathological do result in delusions. Indeed, most do not. When it comes to identifying more subtle epistemic failings, matters are complicated by the fact that many conflicting criteria could be invoked to distinguish effective from ineffective epistemic strategies. Religious experiences are particularly problematic, given that there is debate over whether experiences of communion with God and the like are veridical or delusional, and over whether or not religious belief should be regarded as an epistemic pathology. Furthermore, the relationship between a specific religious content and an existential feeling is contingent, thus weakening the link between epistemic pathology and existential feeling.

Even if such problems are set aside, it would seem that something can be epistemically pathological without implying that the associated existential feelings are themselves in any way pathological. It is often simply assumed that delusions and the like are pathological. For example, Currie and Jureidini (2001, p.159) state that 'delusions, we all agree, are pathological'. However, the sense in which they are supposed to be pathological is not clear. Evolutionary and various other approaches can be employed to plausibly argue that some kinds of delusion are advantageous to those who have them. As suggested by James's account of the religious genius, a delusional temperament might at the same time render a person influential or even inspiring, serving to that person's advantage in both personal and biological terms (a 'biological' advantage being an enhanced chance of survival and reproduction). Furthermore, epistemic pathologies, if construed as systematic tendencies to form certain kinds of false belief, are certainly not restricted to anomalous and extreme existential orientations. It is arguable that the majority of the population hold on to convictions that are scarcely more plausible or better grounded than many delusions:

> Delusions are seen as abnormal, but who decides this? Abnormal compared to whom? Abnormal in what sense? Opinion surveys regularly demonstrate that large sections of the population believe in UFOs, ghosts, telepathy, and so on. (Harper, 2004, p.56)

In addition, as argued in the last chapter, commonplace existential orientations dispose their occupants to misinterpret how they find themselves in the world. Hence existential feelings cannot be reliably identified as pathological on the basis that they are associated with epistemic pathologies. Indeed, the more comfortable, unremarkable existential predicaments are themselves dispositions to misconstrue the structure of world-experience.

There is a need to distinguish between what is not intellectually respectable and what impairs the ability to deal with everyday practical situations. People cling to countless dubious beliefs, yet go about their business quite happily and do not suffer from anomalous existential feeling. An emphasis on daily life suggests a more pragmatic, person-centred approach, and I think some such approach, although resisting rigid formulation, can offer more plausible criteria for distinguishing between healthy and unhealthy existential predicaments. For example, Jackson and Fulford (1997) propose that a psychological change be regarded as pathological when it prevents a person from doing what she ordinarily does, and also that value judgements are required on the part of both clinician and patient. They argue that both sets of judgements should play an interdependent role in determining whether something is pathological.

The clinician should take account of the patient's values and, in the process, critically reflect upon the way in which her own values shape her judgements. Pathology is not a matter of medical facts alone but of whether the trait is valued positively or negatively, whether or not it is best construed as the loss of something important.

This kind of approach can be applied to many of the existential feelings found in psychiatric illness, which involve impoverished experience, thought or activity. There may be a loss of the sense of others, a feeling of disconnectedness from the world, a feeling of being imprisoned in a limited world, a loss of feeling, a feeling of the loss of feeling, a draining away of significance, a breakdown of coherence and so on. Most of the existential predicaments that are the concern of psychiatry can be described in terms of some kind of loss, which the patient is often aware of. Experience might be structured by an incapacitating 'pain', which takes the form of loneliness, anxiety or objectless terror. Of course, the boundaries are blurred. For example, intense grief includes a painful sense of absence, a loss of the significance of things and much else besides. But most instances of grief would be regarded as non-pathological by clinician and patient alike. Many other kinds of existential feeling that involve some form of pain, loss or incapacity need not be treated as pathological. For example, it is arguable that some such feelings constitute the recognition that a radical change in routine is required. As noted by Jackson and Fulford (2002, p.388), an anomalous or even psychotic experience might sometimes be best construed as an adaptive response to an 'existential crisis', a painful re-orientation but one that has beneficial long-term repercussions and so ultimately warrants a positive evaluation.

When it comes to religious experiences, the judgement is especially difficult to make. Jackson and Fulford (1997, 2002) focus specifically on this issue and propose that non-pathological 'spiritual' experiences differ from pathological experiences in that the former are valued positively and enable, rather than disable. Even when they involve psychotic elements, which fall under the category of what I have called 'epistemic pathology', they can still be of positive value to a person and enhance a life. They are to be interpreted in terms of that person's values, rather than just the values of the clinician.[7] But the pathological/non-pathological distinction remains a difficult one to draw here. James (1902) makes clear that the 'religious genius' is not always enabled by

---

[7] See Fulford (2004) for a more general discussion of 'values-based medicine', defined as 'the theory and practice of effective health-care decision making for situations in which legitimately different (and hence potentially conflicting) value perspectives are in play' (p.205).

her experiences. The experience that drives her and might enable her in some ways can also disable her in lots of others.[8] Indeed, the predicament of many sick souls seems indistinguishable from that of many psychiatric patients and the conversion experience is not always so much a return to health as a descent into religious fervour, eccentric claims and bizarre behaviour. The person who *lives* the religious life can be tortured, troubled, in a near constant state of existential torment. She herself might or might not value all this positively. And she might value certain aspects of it but wish away others that are inextricable from them.

There will be many cases where evaluations diverge significantly. What for almost everyone else looks like a stripped down, diminished, unstructured and painful life may be filled with significance for the person who lives it, incorporating a resolute pursuit from which he will not be swayed by anyone. In such cases, there might well be a growing isolation and disconnectedness from others, a diminished space of possibilities. It is this isolation from others, this retreat from a shared world, which often prompts them to regard the person as ill, even if that person seems quite happy. And it is this, I will now suggest, that serves to identify an existential feeling as *existentially* pathological.

Existential pathology

As acknowledged by Jackson and Fulford (1997, 2002), certain 'spiritual' experiences have much in common with others that are judged to be 'psychotic'. In some cases, the difference between the two may come down to how they are evaluated in the context of a person's life, rather than to a clear difference in their form or content. Of course, we should be wary of imposing exclusively psychiatric interpretations upon experiences that are understood by a patient and perhaps also by many others in religious terms. Labelling them as '*psychotic* but perhaps not unhealthy' is to neglect a different framework of interpretation that can also be brought to bear on them, so as to give them a different significance (Marzanski and Bratton, 2002). However, the account of existential feeling I have offered in earlier chapters is founded upon neither a psychiatric nor a religious perspective. Hence my account can acknowledge that feelings treated by psychiatrists as pathologies are much like feelings that some people regard as profound spiritual revelations, without advocating the supremacy of either interpretive framework over the other.

---

[8] See also Marzanski and Bratton (2002) for the view that spiritual experience need not be benign or enhancing.

It does indeed appear that some of the existential feelings reported in these different contexts are very similar. For example, Brett observes that both psychotic and spiritual or mystical experiences can involve:

> ...radical change of belief, time distortion, perception of and communication with supernatural entities, perception of meaning in events and purpose in life, social withdrawal, and so on. [...] the content of both kinds of experience can bear striking similarities, religious themes being common in psychotic delusions, and the epistemological revelations of spiritual experiences often contrasting sharply with the everyday view of reality. (2002, p.321)

In addition to noting the frequent similarity in experiential *contents*, she also acknowledges similarities in existential orientation, in suggesting that the 'mystical' states central to some Eastern traditions are indistinguishable from the 'delusional mood' typical of early psychosis (2002, p.322).

When making such comparisons, it is important not to draw too clear a distinction between an 'everyday view of reality' and the existential predicaments involved in both psychosis and mystical experience. References to an 'everyday view' are ambiguous. I pointed out in Chapter 9 that how people conceptualize the world is often at odds with how they find themselves in it. Thus, if the everyday view is a *conception* of our relationship with the world, then it is at odds with most spiritual/religious, psychotic *and* everyday experiences. So the issue to address is that of how the everyday way in which we actually *do* find ourselves in the world differs from psychotic and mystical existential orientations.

The everyday feeling of being is not the mundane, dull thud of a wholly disenchanted, mechanistic world. The reality that we inhabit is not simply a realm of objects that are arranged in spatiotemporal patterns, bereft of all significance and consisting only of actualities. The world is a space of meaningful possibilities and it is imbued with a practical significance that intensifies and fades. And, as I have emphasized throughout, the way in which we find ourselves in the world is inter- and intra-personally variable. Compare, for example the background of familiarity that one takes for granted in a safe and well-known place with the pervasive sense of dislocation, uncertainty and conspicuousness associated with starting a new job in a new city. We can feel at one with the world in many different ways—at one with nature, at home with others, like a smooth-running component harmoniously integrated into a bigger machine, at peace with things or part of things. We can feel detached from it in all sorts of ways too, which take on a range of different overall feeling tones, from indifference to loneliness to terror. Given this variety, the difference between everyday experiences and anomalous experiences in religious and psychiatric contexts is not quite as extreme as it is often assumed to be.

Brett points out that the question of whether or not an experience is pathological is complicated by the fact that judgements are made against the backdrop of culturally variable assumptions about the nature of reality. For example, in some Eastern religions:

> ...the epistemologies of the systems examined validate the experience of psychosis, in a sense, in that the material world, and the embodied, thought-composed, independently existent, and discrete self are held to be delusions of the ordinary mind, obscuring a more unified fundamental reality that transcends the relative phenomenal world perceived via the categories of understanding. (2002, p.334)

I think this is right. I have claimed that certain popular conceptions of how we relate to the world contribute to the persistent misinterpretation of world-experience. This also applies to the more specific case of 'spiritual' experiences. It is very likely that not all cultures share the same misleading interpretive assumptions. It might well turn out that some experiences labelled as pathological can be reinterpreted through a different set of assumptions in such a way as to legitimate them. Hence, in some cases at least, assignment of pathological status may reflect tacit cultural prejudice.

This concern should not however be overstated. That an experience has a religious content does not in itself preclude the possibility of its being pathological. Likewise, the categories 'spiritual/mystical' and 'pathological' are not mutually exclusive; a contrast could surely be drawn between pathological and non-pathological mystical/spiritual experiences. And there will indeed be borderline cases where differing background assumptions contribute to conflicting judgements on the matter. Nevertheless, there is a substantial difference between many of the existential feelings typical of religious, spiritual or mystical experience and other feelings that are generally regarded as pathological. Brett (2002, pp.335–6) suggests that what is pathological about some ways of experiencing the world is not their content but the inability to escape from them:

> It consists of an inability to return to the ontological framework of consensus reality; in psychological isolation, and inability to accommodate to the subjectivity of others; in a focus of interest in the mental realm and loss of practical concerns that leads to paucity of action and neglect of self-care.

So the two kinds of experience could be identical in both structure and content, the relevant difference being an ability to escape from one but not the other.

However, a sense of an existential orientation as contingent and changeable is *part of* that orientation, rather than something separate from it. Given this, there is a substantial difference between fixed and changeable orientations. As proposed in Part II, some existential feelings are more open than others.

They comprise a sense that 'how the world is revealed to me now does not exhaust the way that it is' and that 'the way in which I belong to the world is fragile'. Once it is acknowledged that experience is not just a matter of perceived actualities but also of possibilities, the difference between healthy mystical experiences and pathological experiences looks to be quite pronounced. One experience is open to possibilities in a way that the other is not. One incorporates the possibility of escape, a sense of its own contingency, and the other does not. An important difference between healthy spiritual experiences and pathological experiences is that the former 'are not an engulfing totality' (McGhee, 2002, p.345).

This contrast, I suggest, is the key to an understanding of what makes something *existentially* pathological. The phenomenologist is not obliged to make a normative judgement as to the pathological or non-pathological status of the existential orientations that she explores. Even so, such a distinction can be drawn. An existential change is never simply a *loss*; all existential feelings can be described in terms of loss, addition and change. But what distinguishes a predicament as *existentially* pathological is a particular kind of *loss*, a loss of the sense of other people or a loss of possibilities involving access to other people. The sense of reality is changeable and there is no single, healthy, normal mode of belonging. A sense of other people varies too. Experience as a whole might be shaped by a feeling of ease with respect to other people or perhaps by the feeling that others in general are a threat. However, what characterizes all everyday experience is a sense of others as *people*, and an ability to relate to and commune with them in personal ways. Most of the possibilities that structure our experience implicate other people. A sense of reality is partly constituted by an appreciation of accessibility to others, of the possibilities not being exclusively mine. The world I find myself in is a world where I have my point of view *amongst* others. It is not exhausted by the within-world perspectives that I identify as belonging to me and to nobody else; it is disclosed as a space of possibilities that are not just mine. There are possibilities that appear as being 'for us', possibilities that are there 'for me but not for others' and possibilities that belong 'to others but not to me'. Without these other-involving possibilities, a distinction between experiences that are *mine* and the shared world in which I have them would no longer be part of my experience.

All the pathological experiences I have discussed in this book involve either a changed sense of other people or a felt loss of access to other people. Plath's bell jar is not so much a suffocating isolation from a reality independent of her as it is from other people; it is a failure to be affected by them. The inflexibility of the existential feeling she describes is at the same time a painful inability to be moved by others or by the social world that moves them. I also argued that the Capgras delusion and schizophrenia involve a diminished or absent sense of others as people. People appear as robots, puppets, mannequins, mechanisms. In some cases, the loss is felt; the absence of others or their inaccessibility shapes experience as a whole in a way that is often deeply unpleasant. However, once the schizophrenic person has fallen into a delusional realm of her own, perhaps others are no longer missed. At this point, it is not only a sense of others as people that is absent from experience but also the sense of something being absent.

Granted, the existential changes found in these and other conditions involve more than just other people. They are also changes in the experience of self and of the impersonal world. But it is the loss of others that condemns the person to a diminished existential realm. A sense of other people *is* an openness to alternative possibilities, the feeling that what is given to one now is not all that there is. With their loss or inaccessibility, an experiential world becomes a place that offers no possibility of escape. There is no chance of help, no way out, no alternative to where one is. It is difficult to describe such experiences without referring to loss, impoverishment, inaccessibility, diminishment and the like. For example, here is how Tracy Thompson describes the lack of interpersonal connectedness so central to her own depressive illness and to the illnesses of other psychiatric patients whom she encountered during a stay in hospital:

> I wanted a connection I couldn't have; I did not understand or value the ones I did have. It was a story I saw again and again in the ward. 'Only connect!' E. M. Forster had written, but we hadn't, or couldn't, or never had. There was the doctor, lost in his personal torment, or Heather, grasping for superficial symbols of connectedness, or Luisa, looking for it through sex. It seemed to me the basic definition of any mental illness, this persistent, painful inability to simply *be* with someone else. It might be lifelong, or it might descend like a sudden catastrophe, this blankness between ourselves and the rest of the world. The blankness might not even be obvious to others. But on our side of that severed connection, it was hell, a life lived behind glass. The only difference between mild depression and severe schizophrenia was the amount of sound and air that seeped in. (1995, pp.199–200)

The wrongness of it all often features as a conspicuous part of the relevant experience. The existential orientation embodies a sense of itself as lacking, an exception to this being when the loss is so extreme that even the sense of loss disappears. As van den Berg (1972) stresses, 'loneliness is the nucleus of psychiatry' (p.105). Jaspers (1962) likewise emphasizes the centrality of changed interpersonal experience in psychiatric illness. There is, he says, either a '*failure of empathy*', where an appreciation of others as people is diminished or absent, or there is an '*unpleasantly forceful empathy*', where intersubjectivity breaks down due to a sense of others as threatening (pp.63–4). He also observes that people with schizophrenia 'feel they have lost contact with things. They feel distant and lonely' (p.117). Regardless of whether a pathological existential feeling amounts to an excess of possibilities, a lack of possibilities, the diminishment or enhancement of certain kinds of possibility or a chaotic possibility space, it will always include an impaired sense of the personal or a feeling of isolation from people.

The poverty of the mechanistic world

The healthiness of an existential feeling can be largely independent of whether and to what extent it is understood by oneself and others. However, it is likely that a shared understanding of existential feelings will be of value in a clinical context. When a patient is already painfully isolated from other people, the inability to communicate her predicament, coupled with the clinician's inability to understand it, could well exacerbate it. An existential understanding can also inform a more pragmatic value judgement as to whether and how a condition is pathological.[9] In other contexts too, it is arguable that the extent to which we understand how we find ourselves in the world has at least some effect upon the structure of our existential orientation. I argued in Chapter 9 that obliviousness to the sense of reality can be symptomatic of being cosily embedded in the world. Nevertheless, the predominance of conceptions of the world that do not acknowledge the manner in which we belong to it can, I think, be existentially unsettling for some people, resulting in the subtle but all-pervasive feeling that something is missing or not quite right.

Doctrines that go by names such as 'scientific naturalism' tend to assume that being in a world is a matter of being physically situated in a realm of objects. The reality of this world, it is maintained, can be wholly captured by the deliverances of empirical science. It is a world of matter, to be understood in mechanistic terms and manipulated accordingly, people themselves being increasingly included in this mechanistic scheme of things. The fact that we belong to the world in a way that is presupposed by any such conception is not merely something that goes unacknowledged. It is *denied*, by the insistence that a particular set of current epistemic practices, which concerns itself only with the actual, is able in principle to tell us *everything* there is to know about the world. The outcome of this insistence is a form of what I earlier referred to

---

[9] Jackson and Fulford (2002, p.390) suggest that the integration of phenomenological understanding into clinical practice may help to rectify 'an institutionalized dumbing down of clinicians' sensitivity to the person and to their unique experiences as individual human beings'.

as 'epistemic pathology', where the world we live in is ignored altogether and replaced by an abstract, meaningless realm. In this place, subjects somehow hook up with objects by having 'intentional states', states that do not fit in with the scientific view of things themselves and so need to be 'naturalized'.

Sass (1992, 1999) discusses at length the parallels between experiential changes that occur in schizophrenia and ways of thinking that are prevalent in the modern world:

> ...in the realms both of madness and of modernism, we find, tightly intertwined, a solipsism that would elevate the mind and derealize the world along with a self-objec-tification that would rob the subject of its transcendental role as a centre of power and knowledge. (1999, pp.333–4)

The comparison applies more specifically to the kind of mechanistic thinking that is so common in philosophy and many other disciplines. For example, Stanghellini (2004, 2007) observes that schizophrenic people often experience, think and speak about themselves in a mechanistic way:

> ...he describes himself [...] as a mechanical scanner [....] He conceives of himself, and especially of his brain, as a computational device. [...] the living body becomes a functioning body, a thing-like mechanism. (2007, pp.131–3)

This is not unlike the way in which many philosophers talk about human beings and claim to conceive of themselves. Now an intellectual pathology is distinct from an existential pathology. However, the mechanistic view of things is not only endorsed by a few obliviously well-grounded philosophers. Mechanistic thinking is widespread, as is the view that how we find ourselves in the world can be wholly accommodated by empirical science. In some people, this might well contribute to existential feelings of unsettledness, to the sense that something is missing or that one is somehow lost and does not belong. The phenomenologist Gabriel Marcel observes that the modern age is typified by an explicit absence of ontological worries, due largely to the establishment of a mechanistic materialism that many people take to be ontologically complete. He suggests though that these worries remain in the background, taking the form of pre-articulate feelings. The individual increasingly comes to think of himself and others in a mechanistic way, 'as an agglomeration of functions' (1948, p.1). However, the fact that this view does not accommodate his being but denies it altogether continues to haunt him:

> ...besides the sadness felt by the onlooker, there is the dull, intolerable unease of the actor himself who is reduced to living as though he were in fact submerged by his functions. This uneasiness is enough to show that there is in all this some appalling mistake, some ghastly misinterpretation, implanted in defenceless minds by an increasingly inhuman social order and an equally inhuman philosophy. (1948, p.3)

Marcel claims that the mechanistic world does not acknowledge its own groundedness in a presupposed reality that it can never accommodate. Knowledge of the mechanistic world is, he says, 'contingent on a participation in being for which no epistemology can account because it continually pre-supposes it' (1948, p.8). Or, to put it in my terms, an account of what reality consists of will never accommodate the presupposed sense of reality and belonging.[10]

The conceptions of how we find ourselves in the world that are assumed by many philosophical and scientific discussions of experience and thought are not just incomplete. In fact, they amount to an extreme but unacknowledged form of scepticism. What they leave out of the world is precisely what binds us to it. The background of belonging that *is* our 'belief' in the world's existence is something they do not even consider. Experiences of things are instead con-strued as taking place in some phenomenological nowhere, devoid of all sense of belonging and reality. To endorse any account of how the *internal* mental realms of worldless subjects manage to connect up with *external* objects is not to reject scepticism. It is the ultimate expression of scepticism. Rather than being a mere *doubt* in the reality of some object or objects of experience and thought (typically, a very big object called the world or lots of little objects called people), it is a *denial* of the sense of reality itself. It is the affirmation of a view that resolutely refuses to recognize the ground beneath its feet. In the face of this, the sceptic who doubts the existence of the world is right to doubt. If that were what our relationship with the world consisted of, it would indeed be unclear how we could ever connect up to it in experience and thought.

---

[10] Heidegger makes a somewhat similar claim in his essay 'The question concerning tech-nology' (1978b), where he complains that a mechanistic, functionalized world, where everything is disclosed as an object of use, serves to obscure an appreciation of how we belong to the world. Although the technological view of things is limited, he claims that it is also well-nigh impossible to escape from, a framework through which we think rather than an explicitly formulated view that can be held up for critical scrutiny and modified or rejected. Heidegger offers a complementary critique of mechanistic, scientistic think-ing in his *Zollikon Seminars*, warning of the increasing tendency to model our understanding of human beings upon the physical sciences, the 'unavoidable result' being the 'technical construction of the human being as machine' (2001, p.135). More recently, David Cooper (2002) has drawn on Heidegger's view to offer a critique of doctrines like scientific naturalism, which assume their own ability to encompass absolutely everything. They are, he says, guilty of 'hubris'. He also makes the point that if these doctrines were actually lived they would be existentially unbearable. As an alternative to such approaches, Cooper recommends that we attune ourselves to mystery, by cultivating a sense of some-thing indescribable to which we are ultimately answerable; 'there is a way the world independently is, but this way is not discursable'. He calls this a 'doctrine of *mystery*' (p.279).

Thankfully though, the mechanistic world is not actually lived in by its proponents. If it were, their experience would involve a derealization so crippling as to prohibit them from assenting to any doctrine.

None of this is to dismiss, criticize or downplay empirical science. Amongst many other things, science can tell us a great deal about feelings, including existential feelings. The point is simply that the perspective of empirical science, which accepts the world as given and enquires as to its nature, is not adequate to the task of understanding absolutely everything. And existential feeling is a case in point. Scientific study of existential feeling will be informative but unavoidably incomplete, given that these feelings constitute a sense of reality that scientific practices and theories take for granted. The additional perspective offered by phenomenology can contribute something important to psychiatric understanding that no biological or other empirical scientific perspective can wholly encompass. Binswanger (1975) makes a case along such lines in relation to a specifically Heideggerian phenomenology:

> Martin Heidegger's analytic of existence is doubly significant for psychiatry. It affords empirical psychopathological research a new methodological and material basis that goes beyond its previous framework, and its treatment of the existential concept of science places *psychiatry in general* in a position to account for the actuality, possibility, and limits of its own scientific world design or, as we may also call it, transcendental horizon of understanding. (1975, p.206)[11]

However, it is possible for psychiatry to engage with phenomenological thought without adopting the thinking of any particular phenomenologist. We can seek to understand anomalous forms of experience by means of phenomenology and we can *do* phenomenology in the process. In addition to applying the insights of phenomenologists, we can make phenomenological discoveries. The emphasis in this book has been upon a dialogue between the fields of phenomenology and psychiatry. But phenomenological understanding can be employed *within* psychiatry too, in understanding and interacting with patients. It is my hope that the account of existential feeling offered here can be put into practice in such a way.

---

[11] Although Heidegger approved of the idea of a psychiatry grounded in his philosophy, he disapproved of the specific way in which Binswanger interpreted and appropriated his ideas. See Askay (2001) for a discussion.

References

American Psychiatric Association. (2004). *Diagnostic and Statistical Manual of Mental Disorders* (Fourth Edition, Text Revision). Washington, DC: American Psychiatric Association.

Amundson, R. (2000). Against Normal Function. *Studies in History and Philosophy of Biological and Biomedical Sciences* **31**: 33–53.

Askay, R. (2001). Heidegger's Philosophy and its Implications for Psychology, Freud, and Existential Psychoanalysis. In: Heidegger's *Zollikon Seminars: Protocols—Conversations—Letters* (ed. Boss, M.; Trans. Mayr, F and Askay, R.). Evanston: Northwestern University Press: 301–315.

Atwood, M. (1994). *The Robber Bride*. London: Virago.

Austin, J. L. (1962). *Sense and Sensibilia*. Oxford: Clarendon Press.

Baker, L. R. (2001). Are Beliefs Brain States? In: Meijers, A. (ed.) *Explaining Beliefs: Lynne Rudder Baker and her Critics*. Stanford: CSLI Publications: 17–38.

Baker, D., Hunter, E., Lawrence, E. and David, A. (2007). *Overcoming Depersonalization and Feelings of Unreality: A Self-Help Guide using Cognitive Behavioral Techniques*. London: Robinson.

Bayne, T. and Pacherie, E. (2004). Bottom-up or Top-down? Campbell's Rationalist Account of Monothematic Delusions. *Philosophy, Psychiatry & Psychology* **11**: 1–11.

Bayne, T. and Pacherie, E. (2005). Defence of the Doxastic Conception of Delusions. *Mind & Language* **20**: 163–188.

Bentall, R. (2003). *Madness Explained: Psychosis and Human Nature*. London: Penguin.

Ben-Ze'ev, A. (2004). Emotion as a Subtle Mental Mode. In: Solomon, R. C. (ed.) *Thinking about Feeling: Contemporary Philosophers on Emotions*. Oxford: Oxford University Press: 250–268.

Bermúdez, J. L. (2001). Normativity and Rationality in Delusional Psychiatric Disorders. *Mind & Language* **16**: 457–493.

Berrios, G. and Luque, R. (1995). Cotard's Delusion or Syndrome? A Conceptual History. *Comprehensive Psychiatry* **36**: 218–223.

Binswanger, L. (1975). *Being-in-the-world: Selected Papers of Ludwig Binswanger*. (Trans. Needleman, J.). London: Souvenir Books.

Blankenburg, W. (2001). First Steps Toward a Psychopathology of 'Common Sense'. (Trans. Mishara, A. L.). *Philosophy, Psychiatry & Psychology* **8**: 303–315.

Bleuler, E. (1950). *Dementia Praecox or the Group of Schizophrenias* (Trans. Zinkin, J.). New York: International Universities Press.

Bortolotti, L. (2005). Delusions and the Background of Rationality. *Mind & Language* **20**: 189–208.

Brett, C. (2002). Psychotic and Mystical States of Being: Connections and Distinctions. *Philosophy, Psychiatry & Psychology* **9**: 321–341.

Brewer, B. (2002). Emotion and Other Minds. In: Goldie, P. (ed.) *Understanding Emotions: Mind and Morals*, Aldershot: Ashgate: 23–36.

Broome, M. R. (2004). The Rationality of Psychosis and Understanding the Deluded. *Philosophy, Psychiatry & Psychology* 11: 35–41.

Broome, M. R., Woolley, J. B., Tabraham, P., Johns, L. C., Bramon, E., Murray, G. K., Pariante, C., McGuire, P. K. and Murray, R. M. (2005). What Causes the Onset of Psychosis? *Schizophrenia Research* 79: 23–34.

Campbell, S. (1997). *Interpreting the Personal: Expression and the Formation of Feelings*. Ithaca: Cornell University Press.

Campbell, J. (1999). Schizophrenia, the Space of Reasons, and Thinking as a Motor Process. *The Monist* 82: 609–625.

Campbell, J. (2001). Rationality, Meaning, and the Analysis of Delusion. *Philosophy, Psychiatry and Psychology* 8: 89–100.

Carnap, R. (1959). The Elimination of Metaphysics through Logical Analysis of Language. In: Ayer, A. J. (ed.) *Logical Positivism*. New York: The Free Press: 60–81.

Cataldi, S. L. (1993). *Emotion, Depth and Flesh: A Study of Sensitive Space*. Albany: State University of New York Press.

Cole, J. (1995). *Pride and a Daily Marathon*. Cambridge MA: MIT Press.

Cole, J. (1998). *About Face*. Cambridge MA: MIT Press.

Cooper, D. E. (2002). *The Measure of Things: Humanism, Humility and Mystery*. Oxford: Clarendon Press.

Cooper, W. (2002). *The Unity of William James's Thought*. Nashville: Vanderbilt University Press.

Cooper, R. (2005). *Classifying Madness: A Philosophical Examination of the Diagnostic and Statistical Manual of Mental Disorders*. Dordrecht: Springer.

Crane, T. and Mellor, D. H. (1990). There is no Question of Physicalism. *Mind* 99: 185–206.

Currie, G. and Jureidini, J. (2001). Delusion, Rationality, Empathy: Commentary on Davies *et al. Philosophy, Psychiatry & Psychology* 8: 159–162.

Cutting, J. (1991). Delusional Misidentification and the Role of the Right Hemisphere in the Appreciation of Identity. *British Journal of Psychiatry* 159 (Supp. 14): 70–75.

Damasio, A. (1995). *Descartes' Error: Emotion, Reason and the Human Brain*. London: Picador.

Damasio, A. (1996). The Somatic Marker Hypothesis and the Possible Functions of the Prefrontal Cortex. *Philosophical Transactions of the Royal Society of London, Series B (Biological Sciences)* 351: 1413–1420.

Damasio, A. (2000). *The Feeling of What Happens: Body, Emotion and the Making of Consciousness*. London: Vintage.

Damasio, A. (2003). *Looking for Spinoza: Joy, Sorrow and the Feeling Brain*. London: Heinemann.

Damasio, A. (2004). Emotions and Feelings: A Neurobiological Perspective. In: Manstead, S. R., Frijda, N. and Fischer, A. (ed.) *Feelings and Emotions: The Amsterdam Symposium*. Cambridge: Cambridge University Press: 49–57.

David, A. (1999). On the Impossibility of Defining Delusions. *Philosophy, Psychiatry & Psychology* 6: 17–20.

Davidson, D. (2001). *Subjective, Intersubjective, Objective*. Oxford: Oxford University Press.

Davies, M. and Coltheart, M. (2000). Introduction: Pathologies of Belief. In: Coltheart, M. and Davies, M. (ed.) *Pathologies of Belief*. Oxford: Blackwell: 1–46.

Davies, M., Coltheart, M., Langdon, R. and Breen, N. (2001). Monothematic Delusions: Towards a Two-Factor Account. *Philosophy, Psychiatry and Psychology* **8**: 133–158.

Dennett, D. C. (1987. *The Intentional Stance*. Cambridge MA: MIT Press.

Depraz, N. (2003). Putting the Epoché into Practice: Schizophrenic Experience as Illustrating the Phenomenological Exploration of Consciousness. In: Fulford, K. W. M., Morris, K., Sadler, J. and Stanghellini, G. (ed.) *Nature and Narrative: An Introduction to the New Philosophy of Psychiatry*. Oxford: Oxford University Press: 187–198.

De Sousa, R. (1980). The Rationality of Emotions. In: Rorty, A. (ed.) *Explaining Emotions*, Berkeley: University of California Press: 127–152.

De Sousa, R. (1990). *The Rationality of Emotion*. Cambridge MA: MIT Press.

De Sousa, R. (2004). Emotions: What I know, what I'd like to think I know, and what I'd like to think. In: Solomon, R.C. (ed.) *Thinking about Feeling: Contemporary Philosophers on Emotions*. Oxford: Oxford University Press: 61–75.

Downing, G. (2000). Emotion Theory Reconsidered. In: Wrathall, M. and Malpas, J. (ed.) *Heidegger, Coping, and Cognitive Science: Essays in Honor of Hubert L. Dreyfus Volume 2*, Cambridge Mass: MIT Press: 245–270.

Dreyfus, H.L. (1991). *Being-in-the-world: A Commentary on Heidegger's Being and Time, Division I*. Cambridge MA: MIT Press.

Drummond, J. J. (2004). 'Cognitive Impenetrability' and the Complex Intentionality of the Emotions. In: Zahavi, D. (ed.) *Hidden Resources: Classical Perspectives on Subjectivity*. Exeter: Imprint Academic: 109–126.

Eilan, N. (2001). Meaning, Truth, and the Self: Commentary on Campbell, and Parnas and Sass. *Philosophy, Psychiatry & Psychology* **8**: 121–132.

Ellis, H. D. and Lewis, M. B. (2001). Capgras Delusion: A Window on Face Recognition. *Trends in Cognitive Sciences* **5**: 149–156.

Ellis, H. D. and Young, A. W. (1990). Accounting for Delusional Misidentifications. *British Journal of Psychiatry* **157**: 239–248.

Ellis, H. D., Young, A. W., Quayle, A. H. and de Pauw, K. W. (1997). Reduced Autonomic Responses to Faces in Capgras Delusion. *Proceedings of the Royal Society of London* **B264**: 1085–1092.

Faulks, S. (1990). *The Girl at the Lion d'Or*. London: Vintage.

Fine, C., Craigie, J. and Gold, I. (2005). Damned if you do, Damned if you don't: The Impasse in Cognitive Accounts of the Capgras Delusion. *Philosophy, Psychiatry & Psychology* **12**: 143–151.

Franks Davis, C. (1989). *The Evidential Force of Religious Experience*. Oxford: Oxford University Press.

Freud, S. (2003). *The Uncanny*. London: Penguin.

Frewen, P. A., Lanius, R. A., Dozois, D. J. A., Neufeld, R. W., Pain, C., Hopper, J. W., Densmore, M. and Stevens, T. K. forthcoming. Clinical and Neural Correlates of Alexithymia. *Journal of Abnormal Psychology* **117**: 171–181.

Frith, C. (1992). *The Cognitive Neuropsychology of Schizophrenia*. Hove: Psychology Press.

Fuchs, T. (2005). Corporealized and Disembodied Minds: A Phenomenological View of the Body in Melancholia and Schizophrenia. *Philosophy, Psychiatry & Psychology* **12**: 95–107.

Fulford, K. W. M. (1994). Value, Illness and Failure of Action. In: Graham, G. and Stephens, G. L. (ed.) *Philosophical Psychopathology*. Cambridge MA: MIT Press: 205–233.

Fulford, K. L. M. (2004). Facts / Values: Ten Principles of Values-based Medicine. In: Radden, J. (ed.) *The Philosophy of Psychiatry: A Companion*. Oxford: Oxford University Press: 205–234.

Gallagher, S. (2001). The Practice of Mind: Theory, Simulation, or Interaction? *Journal of Consciousness Studies* **8** (5–7): 83–107.

Gallagher, S. (2005). *How the Body shapes the Mind*. Oxford: Oxford University Press.

Gallagher, S. (2007). Logical and Phenomenological Arguments against Simulation Theory. In: Hutto, D. D. and Ratcliffe, M. (ed.) *Folk Psychology Re-assessed*. Dordrecht: Springer: 63–78.

Gerrans, P. (1999). Delusional Misidentification and Subpersonal Disintegration. *The Monist* **82**: 590–608.

Gerrans, P. (2000). Refining the Explanation of Cotard's Delusion. In: Coltheart, M. and Davies, M. (ed.) *Pathologies of Belief*. Oxford: Blackwell: 111–122.

Gerrans, P. (2002). A One-Stage Explanation of the Cotard Delusion. *Philosophy, Psychiatry & Psychology* **9**: 47–53.

Ghaemi, S. N. (2004). The Perils of Belief: Delusions Reexamined. *Philosophy, Psychiatry & Psychology* **11**: 49–54.

Gibson. J. J. (1979). *The Ecological Approach to Visual Perception*. Hillsdale, New Jersey: Lawrence Erlbaum Associates.

Glas, G. (2003). Anxiety—Animal Reactions and the Embodiment of Meaning. In: Fulford, K. W. M.., Morris, K., Sadler, J., and Stanghellini, G. (ed.) *Nature and Narrative: An Introduction to the New Philosophy of Psychiatry*. Oxford: Oxford University Press: 231–249.

Goldie, P. (2000). *The Emotions: A Philosophical Exploration*. Oxford: Clarendon Press.

Goldie, P. (2002). Emotions, Feelings and Intentionality. *Phenomenology and the Cognitive Sciences* **1**: 235–254.

Goldie, P. (2004). Emotion, Feeling, and Knowledge of the World. In: Solomon, R. C. (ed.) *Thinking about Feeling: Contemporary Philosophers on Emotions*. Oxford: Oxford University Press: 91–106.

Goldie, P. and Spicer, F. (2002). Introduction. In: Goldie, P. (ed.) *Understanding Emotions: Mind and Morals*, Aldershot: Ashgate: 1–22.

Goodman, N. (1978). *Ways of Worldmaking*. Indianapolis: Hackett.

Goodman, N. (1984). *Of Mind and Other Matters*. Cambridge Mass: MIT Press.

Gordon, R. M. (1987). *The Structure of Emotions: Investigations in Cognitive Philosophy*. Cambridge: Cambridge University Press.

Gray, R. (2005). On the Concept of a Sense. *Synthese* **147**: 461–475.

Greenfield, S. (2000). *The Private Life of the Brain*. London: Penguin Books.

Greenspan, P. (2004). Emotions, Rationality, and Mind / Body. In: Solomon, R. C. (ed.) *Thinking about Feeling: Contemporary Philosophers on Emotions*. Oxford: Oxford University Press: 125–134.

Griffiths, P. (1997). *What Emotions Really Are: The Problem of Psychological Categories.* Chicago: Chicago University Press.

Hamilton, A. J. (2007). Against the Belief Model of Delusion. In: Chung, M. C., Fulford, K. W. M. and Graham, G. (ed.) *Reconceiving Schizophrenia.* Oxford: Oxford University Press: 217–234.

Hansen, J. (2004). Affectivity: Depression and Mania. In: Radden, J. (ed.) *The Philosophy of Psychiatry: A Companion.* Oxford: Oxford University Press: 36–53.

Harper, D. J. (2004). Delusions and Discourse: Moving Beyond the Constraints of the Modernist Paradigm. *Philosophy, Psychiatry & Psychology* 11: 55–64.

Harr, M. (1992). Attunement and Thinking. In: Dreyfus, H.L. and Hall, H. (ed.) *Heidegger: A Critical Reader.* Oxford: Blackwell: 159–172.

Heal, J. (1995). Replication and Functionalism. In: Davies, M. and Stone, T. (ed.) *Folk Psychology.* Oxford: Blackwell: 45–59.

Heidegger, M. (1962). *Being and Time* (Trans. Macquarrie, J. and Robinson, E.). Oxford: Blackwell.

Heidegger, M. (1978a). What is Metaphysics? (Trans. Krell, D. F.). In: Heidegger, M. *Basic Writings* (ed. D. F. Krell). London: Routledge: 93–110.

Heidegger, M. (1978b). The Question Concerning Technology. (Trans. Lovitt, W.). In: Heidegger, M. *Basic Writings* (D. F. Krell, ed.). London: Routledge: 311–341.

Heidegger, M. (1982). *Basic Problems of Phenomenology* (Trans. Hofstadter, A.). Bloomington: Indiana University Press.

Heidegger, M. (1983). *The Fundamental Concepts of Metaphysics.* Bloomington: Indiana University Press.

Heidegger, M. (1996). *Being and Time* (Trans. Stambaugh, J.). New York: State University of New York Press.

Heidegger, M. (2001). *Zollikon Seminars: Protocols—Conversations—Letters* (ed. Boss, M.; Trans. Mayr, F. and Askay, R.). Evanston: Northwestern University Press.

Hobson, R. P. (2002). *The Cradle of Thought.* London: Macmillan.

Hohwy, J. and Rosenberg, R. (2005). Unusual Experiences, Reality Testing and Delusions of Alien Control. *Mind & Language* 20: 141–162.

Hookway, C. (2002). Emotions and Epistemic Evaluations. In: Carruthers, P, Stich, S. and Siegal, M. (ed.) *The Cognitive Basis of Science.* Cambridge: Cambridge University Press: 251–262.

Hookway, C. (2003). Affective States and Epistemic Immediacy. *Metaphilosophy* 34: 78–96.

Hull, J. (1990). *Touching the Rock: An Experience of Blindness.* New York: Pantheon Books.

Husserl, E. (1960). *Cartesian Meditations: An Introduction to Phenomenology* (Trans. Cairns, D.). The Hague: Martinus Nijhoff.

Husserl, E. (1970). The Vienna Lecture. In: *The Crisis of European Sciences and Transcendental Phenomenology.* (Trans. Carr, D.) Evanston: Northwestern University Press: 269–299.

Husserl, E. (1989). *Ideas Pertaining to a Pure Phenomenology and to a Phenomenological Philosophy*, Second Book (Trans. Rojcewicz, R. and Schuwer, A.). Dordrecht: Kluwer.

Husserl, E. (2001). *Analyses concerning Passive and Active Synthesis: Lectures on Transcendental Logic* (Trans. Steinbock, A. J.). Dordrecht: Kluwer.

Hutto, D. D. and Ratcliffe, M. (ed.) (2007). *Folk Psychology Re-assessed.* Dordrecht: Springer.

Ihde, D. (1983). *Sense and Significance*. Atlantic Highlands, NJ: Humanities Press.

Jackson, M. C. and Fulford, K. W. M. (1997). Spiritual Experience and Psychopathology. *Philosophy, Psychiatry & Psychology* 4: 42–65.

Jackson, M. C. and Fulford, K. W. M. (2002). Psychosis Good and Bad: Values-Based Practice and the Distinction between Pathological and Nonpathological Forms of Psychotic Experience. *Philosophy, Psychiatry & Psychology* 9: 387–394.

James, W. (1879). The Sentiment of Rationality. *Mind* 4: 317–346.

James, W. (1884). What is an Emotion? *Mind* 9: 188–205.

James, W. (1890). *The Principles of Psychology*, Volume II. New York: Holt.

James, W. (1894). The Physical Basis of Emotion. *Psychological Review* 1: 516–529.

James, W. (1897). *The Will to Believe and Other Essays in Popular Philosophy*. New York: Longmans, Green and Co.

James, W. (1902). *The Varieties of Religious Experience*. New York: Longmans, Green and Co.

James, W. (1905). The Place of Affectional Facts in a World of Pure Experience. *The Journal of Philosophy, Psychology and Scientific Methods,* Volume II/**11**: 281–287.

James, W. (1912). *Essays in Radical Empiricism*. New York: Longmans, Green and Co.

James, W. (1970). *The Meaning of Truth*. Ann Arbor Paperbacks: University of Michigan Press.

James, W. (1981). *Pragmatism*. Indianapolis: Hackett.

Jaspers, K. (1962). *General Psychopathology*. Manchester: Manchester University Press.

Johnson-Laird, P. and Oatley, K. (1992). Basic Emotions, Rationality and Folk Theory. *Cognition and Emotion* 6: 201–223.

Jonas, H. (1954). The Nobility of Sight. *Philosophy and Phenomenological Research* **14**: 507–519.

Keller, E. F. and Grontowski, C. R. (1996). The Mind's Eye. In: Keller, E. F. and Longino, H. E. (ed.) *Feminism and Science*. Oxford: Oxford University Press.

Kelly, S. D. (2002). Merleau-Ponty on the Body. *Ratio* XV: 376–391.

Kraepelin, E. (1919). *Dementia Praecox and Paraphrenia* (Trans. Barclay, R. M.). Edinburgh: E. & S. Livingstone.

Kraus, A. (2007). Schizophrenic Delusion and Hallucination as the Expression and Consequence of an Alteration of the Existential A Prioris. In: Chung, M. C., Fulford, K. W. M. and Graham, G. (ed.) *Reconceiving Schizophrenia*. Oxford: Oxford University Press: 97–111.

Ladyman, J. (2000). What's Really Wrong with Constructive Empiricism? Van Fraassen and the Metaphysics of Modality. *British Journal for the Philosophy of Science* **51**: 837–856.

Laing, R. D. (1960). *The Divided Self: A Study of Sanity and Madness*. London: Tavistock Publications.

Leder, D. (1990). *The Absent Body*. Chicago: University of Chicago Press.

Leder, D. (2005). Moving beyond 'Mind' and 'Body'. *Philosophy, Psychiatry & Psychology* **12**: 109–113.

Lewontin, R. C. (1978). Adaptation. *Scientific American* 239:156–169.

Lewontin, R. C. (1982). Organism and Environment. In: Plotkin, H. (ed.) *Learning, Development and Culture: Essays in Evolutionary Epistemology*. Chichester: John Wiley and Sons: 151–170.

Lyons, W. (1980). *Emotion*. Cambridge: Cambridge University Press.

Lysaker, P. H., Johannesen, J. K. and Lysaker, J. T. (2005). Schizophrenia and the Experience of Intersubjectivity as Threat. *Phenomenology and the Cognitive Sciences* **4**: 335–352.

Mackie, J.L. (1982). *The Miracle of Theism: Arguments for and against the Existence of God.* Oxford: Oxford University Press.

Maher, B. (1999). Anomalous Experience in Everyday Life: Its Significance for Psychopathology. *Monist* **82**: 547–570.

Malloy, P., Cimino, C. and Westlake, R. (1992). Differential Diagnosis of Primary and Secondary Capgras Delusions. *Neuropsychiatry, Neuropsychology, and Behavioral Neurology* **5**: 83–96.

Marcel, G. (1948). *The Philosophy of Existence* (Trans. Harari, M.). London: The Harvill Press.

Marr, D. (1982). *Vision.* New York: W. H. Freeman.

Martin, M. (1992). Sight and Touch. In: Crane, T. (ed.) *The Contents of Experience.* Cambridge: Cambridge University Press: 196–215.

Martin. M. (1993). Sense Modalities and Spatial Properties. In: Eilan, N., McCarthy, R. and Brewer, B. (ed.) *Spatial Representation: Problems in Philosophy and Psychology.* Oxford: Blackwell: 206–218.

Martin, M. (1995). Bodily Awareness: A Sense of Ownership. In: Bermúdez, J. L., Marcel, A. and Eilan, N. (ed.) *The Body and the Self.* Cambridge MA: MIT Press: 267–289.

Martin, M. W. (1999). Depression, Illness, Insight and Identity. *Philosophy, Psychiatry & Psychology* **6**: 271–286.

Marzanski, M. and Bratton, M. (2002). Psychpathological Symptoms and Religious Experience: A Critique of Jackson and Fulford. *Philosophy, Psychiatry & Psychology* **9**: 359–371.

Matthews, E. (2007). Suspicions of Schizophrenia. In: Chung, M. C., Fulford, K. W. M. and Graham, G. (ed.) *Reconceiving Schizophrenia.* Oxford: Oxford University Press: 307–327.

McGhee, M. (2002). Mysticism and Psychosis: Descriptions and Distinctions. *Philosophy, Psychiatry & Psychology* **9**: 343–347.

Medford, N., Sierra, M., Baker, D. and David, A. S. (2005). Understanding and Treating Depersonalisation Disorder. *Advances in Psychiatric Treatment* **11**: 92–100.

Merleau-Ponty, M. (1962). *Phenomenology of Perception* (Trans. Smith, C.). London: Routledge.

Merleau-Ponty, M. (1964a). *Sense and Non-sense* (Trans. Dreyfus, H. L. and Dreyfus, P. A.). Evanston: Northwestern University Press.

Merleau-Ponty, M. (1964b). *Signs* (Trans. McCleary, R. C.). Evanston: Northwestern University Press.

Merleau-Ponty, M. (1964c). *The Primacy of Perception* (ed. Edie, J. M.). Evanston: Northwestern University Press.

Merleau-Ponty, M. (1968). *The Visible and the Invisible* (Trans. Lingis, A.). Evanston: Northwestern University Press.

Millikan, R. (1984). *Language, Thought and Other Biological Categories.* Cambridge MA: MIT Press.

Minkowski, E. and Targowla, R. (2001). A Contribution to the Study of Autism: The Interrogative Attitude (Trans. Ziadeh, S.). *Philosophy, Psychiatry & Psychology* **8**: 271–278.

Montagu, A. (1986. *Touching: The Human Significance of the Skin* (Third Edition). New York: Harper and Row.

Morris, C. (2002). This is not Here. *Philosophy, Psychiatry & Psychology* **9**: 281–283.

Myers, G. E. (1986). *William James: His Life and Thought*, New Haven: Yale University Press.

Nagel, T. (1986). *The View from Nowhere*. Oxford: Oxford University Press.

Nagel, T. (1995). *Other Minds: Critical Essays 1969–1994*. Oxford: Oxford University Press.

Noé, A. (2004). *Action in Perception*. Cambridge MA: MIT Press.

Nussbaum, M. (2001). *Upheavals of Thought: The Intelligence of Emotions*. Cambridge: Cambridge University Press.

Nussbaum, M. (2004). Emotions as Judgments of Value and Importance. In: Solomon, R. C. *Thinking about Feeling: Contemporary Philosophers on Emotions*. Oxford: Oxford University Press:183–199.

O'Regan, J. K. and Noé, A. (2001). A Sensorimotor Account of Vision and Visual Consciousness. *Behavioral and Brain Sciences* **24**: 939–1031.

O'Shaughnessy, B. (1989). The Sense of Touch. *Australasian Journal of Philosophy* **67**: 37–58.

O'Shaughnessy, B. (1995). Proprioception and the Body Image. In: Bermúdez, J. L., Marcel, A. and Eilan, N. (ed.) *The Body and the Self*. Cambridge MA: MIT Press: 175–203.

O'Shaughnessy, B. (2000). *Consciousness and the World*. Oxford: Clarendon Press.

Papineau, D. (1987). *Reality and Representation*. Oxford: Blackwell.

Parnas, J. and Sass, L. A. (2001). Self, Solipsism and Schizophrenic Delusions. *Philosophy, Psychiatry & Psychology* **8**: 101–120.

Persinger, M. (2002). The Temporal Lobe: The Biological Basis of the God Experience. In: Joseph, R. (ed.) *Neurotheology: Brain, Science, Spirituality, Religious Experience*. San Jose, California: University Press: 273–278.

Phillips, D. Z. (1986). *Belief, Change and Forms of Life*. London: MacMillan.

Phillips, M. L., Medford, N., Senior, C., Bullmore, E. T., Suckling, J., Brammer, M. J., Andrew, C., Sierra, M., Williams, S. C. R. and David, A. S. (2001). Depersonalization Disorder: Thinking without Feeling. *Psychiatry Research: Neuroimaging Section* **108**: 145–160.

Plath, S. (1966). *The Bell Jar*. London: Faber & Faber.

Poland, J. (2007). How to Move beyond the Concept of Schizophrenia. In: Chung, M. C., Fulford, K. W. M. and Graham, G. (ed.) *Reconceiving Schizophrenia*. Oxford: Oxford University Press: 167–191.

Polt, R. (1999). *Heidegger: An Introduction*. London: UCL Press.

Prinz, J. (2004). *Gut Reactions: A Perceptual Theory of Emotion*. Oxford: Oxford University Press.

Radden, J. (2003). Is this Dame Melancholy? Equating Today's Depression and Past Melancholia. *Philosophy, Psychiatry & Psychology* **10**: 37–52.

Radovic, F. and Radovic, S. (2002). Feelings of Unreality: A Conceptual and Phenomenological Analysis of the Language of Depersonalization. *Philosophy, Psychiatry and Psychology* **9**: 271–279.

Ramachandran, V.S. and Blakeslee, S. (1998). *Phantoms in the Brain*. London: Fourth Estate.

Ratcliffe, M. (2002). Heidegger's Attunement and the Neuropsychology of Emotion. *Phenomenology and the Cognitive Sciences* **1**: 287–312.

Ratcliffe, M. (2004). Interpreting Delusions. *Phenomenology and the Cognitive Sciences* **3**: 25–48.

Ratcliffe, M. (2005a). William James on Emotion and Intentionality. *International Journal of Philosophical Studies* **13**: 179–202.

Ratcliffe, M. (2005b). The Feeling of Being. *Journal of Consciousness Studies* **12** (8–10): 43–60.

Ratcliffe, M. (2006). Neurotheology: A Science of What? In: McNamara, P. (ed.) *Where God and Science Meet, Volume 2, The Neurology of Religious Experience*. Westport, Connecticut: Praeger: 81–104.

Ratcliffe, M. (2007). *Rethinking Commonsense Psychology: A Critique of Folk Psychology, Theory of Mind and Simulation*. Basingstoke: Palgrave Macmillan.

Ratcliffe, M. (2008a). Touch and Situatedness. *International Journal of Philosophical Studies* **16** (in press).

Ratcliffe, M. (2008b). The Phenomenological Role of Affect in the Capgras Delusion. *Continental Philosophy Review* **41** (in press).

Ratcliffe, M. (2008c). Stance, Feeling and Phenomenology. *Synthese* (in press).

Ratcliffe, M. (forthcoming). Existential Feeling and Psychopathology. *Philosophy, Psychiatry & Psychology*.

Rea, M. (2002). *World without Design: The Ontological Consequences of Naturalism*. Oxford: Clarendon Press.

Roberts, R. (1988). What an Emotion is: A Sketch. *Philosophical Review* **97**: 183–209.

Rorty, A. (1980). Introduction. In: Rorty, A. (ed.) *Explaining Emotions*: Los Angeles: University of California Press: 1–8

Rowbottom, D. (2005). The Empirical Stance vs. The Critical Attitude. *South African Journal of Philosophy* **24**: 200–223.

Sacks, O. (1987). Nothingness. In: Gregory, R. L. (ed.) *The Oxford Companion to the Mind*. Oxford: Oxford University Press: 564–565.

Sartre, J. P. (1963). *Nausea* (Trans. Baldick, R.). London: Penguin.

Sartre, J. P. (1989). *Being and Nothingness* (Trans. Barnes, H. E.). London: Routledge.

Sartre, J.P. (1994). *Sketch for a Theory of the Emotions* (Trans. Mairet, P.). London: Routledge

Sass, L. A. (1992). *Madness and Modernism: Insanity in the Light of Modern Art, Literature and Thought*. New York: Basic Books.

Sass, L. A. (1994). *The Paradoxes of Delusion: Wittgenstein, Schreber, and the Schizophrenic Mind*. Ithaca: Cornell University Press.

Sass, L. A. (1999). Schizophrenia, Self-consciousness and the Modern Mind. In: Gallagher, S. and Shear, J. (ed.) *Models of the Self*. Exeter: Imprint Academic: 319–341.

Sass, L. A. (2003). 'Negative Symptoms', Schizophrenia, and the Self. *International Journal of Psychology and Psychological Therapy* **3**: 153–180.

Sass, L. A. (2004a). Some Reflections on the (Analytic) Philosophical Approach to Delusion. *Philosophy, Psychiatry & Psychology* **11**: 71–80.

Sass, L. A. (2004b). Affectivity in Schizophrenia: A Phenomenological View. In: Zahavi, D. (ed.) *Hidden Resources: Classical Perspectives on Subjectivity*. Exeter: Imprint Academic: 127–147.

Sass, L. A. (2007). Contradictions of Emotion in Schizophrenia. *Cognition & Emotion* **21**: 351–390.

Sass, L. A. and Parnas, J. (2007). Explaining Schizophrenia. The Relevance of Phenomenology. In: Chung, M. C., Fulford, K. W. M. and Graham, G. (ed.) *Reconceiving Schizophrenia*. Oxford: Oxford University Press: 63–95.

Schachter, S. and Singer, J. (1962). Cognitive, Social and Physiological Determinants of Emotional State. *Psychological Review* **63**: 379–399.

Scheler, M. (1992). *On Feeling, Knowing and Valuing*. (Bershady, H. J., ed.). Chicago: University of Chicago Press.

Schreber, D. P. (2000). *Memoirs of my Nervous Illness*. New York: New York Review of Books.

Schutz, A. (1967). *The Phenomenology of the Social World* (Trans. Walsh, G. and Lehnert, F.). Evanston: Northwestern University Press.

Scott, M. (2001). Tactual Perception. *Australasian Journal of Philosophy* **79**: 149–160.

Searle, J. R. (2000). The Limits of Phenomenology. In: Wrathall, M. and Malpas, J. (ed.) *Heidegger, Coping and Cognitive Science. Essays in Honor of Hubert L. Dreyfus. Volume 2*. Cambridge MA: MIT Press: 71–92.

Sechehaye, M. (1970). *Autobiography of a Schizophrenic Girl*. New York: Signet.

Sheets-Johnstone, M. forthcoming. Schizophrenia and the Comet's Tail of Nature: A Case Study in Phenomenology and Human Psycho-Pathology. *Philoctetes*.

Sizer, L. (2006). What Feelings can't do. *Mind & Language* **20**: 108–135.

Solomon, R. C. (1980). Emotions and Choice. In: Rorty, A. (ed.) *Explaining Emotions*, Berkeley: University of California Press: 251–281.

Solomon, R. C. (1993). *The Passions: Emotions and the Meaning of Life* (revised edition). Cambridge: Hackett.

Solomon, R. C. (2003). *Not Passion's Slave: Emotions and Choice*. Oxford: Oxford University Press.

Solomon, R.C. (2004*a*). Emotions, Thoughts, and Feelings: Emotions as Engagements with the World. In: Solomon, R. C. (ed.) *Thinking about Feeling: Contemporary Philosophers on Emotions*. Oxford: Oxford University Press: 76–88.

Solomon, R. C. (2004*b*). On the Passivity of the Passions. In: Manstead, S. R., Frijda, N. and Fischer, A. (ed.) *Feelings and Emotions: The Amsterdam Symposium*. Cambridge: Cambridge University Press: 11–29.

Solomon, R. C. (ed.) (2004). *Thinking about Feeling: Contemporary Philosophers on Emotions*. Oxford: Oxford University Press.

Stanghellini, G. (2001). Psychopathology of Common Sense. *Philosophy, Psychiatry & Psychology* **8**: 201–218.

Stanghellini, G. (2004). *Disembodied Spirits and Deanimated Bodies: The Psychopathology of Common Sense*. Oxford: Oxford University Press.

Stanghellini, G. (2007). Schizophrenia and the Sixth Sense. In: Chung, M. C., Fulford, K. W. M. and Graham, G. (ed.) *Reconceiving Schizophrenia*. Oxford: Oxford University Press: 129–149.

Stawarska, B. (2006). Mutual Gaze and Social Cognition. *Phenomenology and the Cognitive Sciences* **5**: 17–30.

Stephens, G. L. and Graham, G. (2000). *When Self-consciousness Breaks: Alien Voices and Inserted Thoughts*. Cambridge MA.: MIT Press.

Stern, D. (1993). The Role of Feelings for an Interpersonal Self. In: Neisser, E. (ed.) *The Perceived Self: Ecological and Interpersonal Sources of Self-Knowledge*. Cambridge: Cambridge University Press: 205–215.

Stocker, M. (2004). Some Considerations about Intellectual Desire and Emotions. In: Solomon, R. C. (ed.) *Thinking about Feeling: Contemporary Philosophers on Emotions.* Oxford: Oxford University Press: 135–148.

Stocker, M. and Hegeman, E. (1996). *Valuing Emotions.* Cambridge: Cambridge University Press.

Stone, T. and Young, A. W. (1997). Delusions and Brain Injury: The Philosophy and Psychology of Belief. *Mind & Language* **12**: 327–364.

Strasser, S. (1977). *Phenomenology of Feeling: An Essay on the Phenomena of the Heart.* Pittsburgh: Duquesne University Press.

Styron, W. (2001). *Darkness Visible.* London: Vintage.

Taylor, C. (2002). *Varieties of Religion Today: William James Revisited.* Cambridge MA: Harvard University Press.

Teller, P. (2004). What is a Stance? *Philosophical Studies* **121**: 159–170.

Thompson. T. (1995). *The Beast: A Reckoning with Depression.* New York: Putnam.

Tolstoy, L. (1996). *A Confession.* New York: W.W. Norton.

Tolstoy, L. (1960). *The Death of Ivan Ilych.* New York: Signet.

Vallelonga, D. S. (1992). A Phenomenological Response to James's View of Emotion. In: Donnelly, M. E. (ed.) *Reinterpreting the Legacy of William James*, Washington D.C.: American Psychological Association: 231–241.

Van den Berg, J. H. (1952). The Human Body and the Significance of Human Movement: A Phenomenological Study. *Philosophy and Phenomenological Research* **13**: 159–183.

Van den Berg, J. H. (1966). *The Psychology of the Sickbed.* Pittsburgh: Duquesne University Press.

Van den Berg, J. H. (1972). *A Different Existence: Principles of Phenomenological Psychopathology.* Pittsburgh: Duquesne University Press.

Van Fraassen, B. (1994). Against Transcendental Empiricism. In: Stapleton, T. J. (ed.) *The Question of Hermeneutics.* Amsterdam: Kluwer: 309–335.

Van Fraassen, B. (2002). *The Empirical Stance.* New Haven: Yale University Press.

Varela, F. J., Thompson, E. and Rosch, E. (1991). *The Embodied Mind: Cognitive Science and Human Experience.* Cambridge MA: MIT Press.

Viney, W. (1992). A Study of Emotion in the Context of Radical Empiricism. In: Donnelly, M. E. (ed.) *Reinterpreting the Legacy of William James*, Washington D.C.: American Psychological Association: 243–50.

Weinstein, E. A. (1996). Reduplicative Misidentification Syndromes. In: Halligan, P. W. and Marshall, J. C. (ed.) *Method in Madness: Case Studies in Cognitive Neuropsychiatry.* Hove: Psychology Press.

Wiggins, O. P. and Schwartz, M. A. (2007). Schizophrenia: A Phenomenological-Anthropological Approach. In: Chung, M. C., Fulford, K. W. M. and Graham, G. (ed.) *Reconceiving Schizophrenia.* Oxford: Oxford University Press: 113–127.

Wisdom, J. (1964). *Philosophy and Psychoanalysis.* Oxford: Blackwell.

Wittgenstein, L. (1975). *On Certainty* (Trans. Paul, D. and Anscombe, G. E. M.). Oxford: Blackwell.

Wolpert, L. (1999). *Malignant Sadness: The Anatomy of Depression.* London: Faber & Faber.

Wright, S, Young, A. W. and Hellawell, D. (1993). Sequential Cotard and Capgras Delusions. *British Journal of Clinical Psychology* **30**: 345–249.

Young, A. W. (2000). Wondrous Strange: The Neuropsychology of Abnormal Beliefs. In: Coltheart, M. and Davies, M. (ed.) *Pathologies of Belief*. Oxford: Blackwell: 47–73.

Young, A. W. and Leafhead, K. (1996). Betwixt Life and Death: Case Studies of the Cotard Delusion. In: Halligan, P. and Marshall, J. (ed.) *Method in Madness: Case Studies in Cognitive Neuropsychiatry*. Hove: Psychology Press: 147–171.

Young, A. W. and de Pauw, K. W. (2002). One Stage is not Enough. *Philosophy, Psychiatry & Psychology* 9: 55–59.

Young, I. M. (2005). *On Female Body Experience: 'Throwing Like a Girl' and Other Essays*. Oxford: Oxford University Press.

Index

Printed in the United States
By Bookmasters